Clinical Pharmacology
for Dental Professionals

Sebastian G. Ciancio, D.D.S.

Professor and Chairman
Department of Periodontics-Endodontics
Clinical Professor of Pharmacology
State University of New York at Buffalo
Diplomate, American Board of Periodontology

Priscilla C. Bourgault, B.S., Ph.D.

Assistant Professor of Pharmacology
Department of Physiology-Pharmacology
Loyola University

McGraw-Hill Book Company

New York St. Louis San Francisco Auckland Bogotá Düsseldorf
Johannesburg London Madrid Mexico Montreal New Delhi
Panama Paris São Paulo Singapore Sydney Tokyo Toronto

This book was set in Times Roman by Bi-Comp, Incorporated.
The editors were Laura A. Dysart, Stuart D. Boynton, and Henry C. De Leo;
the cover was designed by Robin Hessel;
the production supervisor was Jeanne Selzam.
The drawings were done by ECL Art Associates, Inc.
Kingsport Press, Inc., was printer and binder.

CLINICAL PHARMACOLOGY FOR DENTAL PROFESSIONALS

1 2 3 4 5 6 7 8 9 0   KPKP   7 8 3 2 1 0 9

Library of Congress Cataloging in Publication Data

Ciancio, Sebastian G
    Clinical pharmacology for dental professionals.

    Bibliography: p.
    Includes index.
    1. Dental pharmacology.   2. Materia medica, Dental.   3. Dental auxiliary personnel.   I. Bourgault, Priscilla C., joint author.   II. Title. [DNLM: 1. Dental auxiliaries.   2. Pharmacology.   QV50 C566c]
RK701.C57   615'.1'0246176   79-10416
ISBN 0-07-010953-2

To my wife for her love and understanding.
To my children for trying to understand.
To my parents for their ideals and sacrifices.

Sebastian G. Ciancio

To my friends and "second family" at Village-on-the-Lake and to Rae for their friendship, understanding, and lack of demands.
To Don Doemling, the Department Chairman for his patience.
To Lou Blanchet, my fellow pharmacologist, and the members of the Department of Anatomy for their encouragement and moral support.

Priscilla C. Bourgault

Contents

3

DRUGS THAT MAY ALTER DAILY PRACTICE   147

4

EMERGENCY DRUGS AND ADVERSE EFFECTS   183

5

APPLIED PHARMACOLOGY   221

6

APPENDIX   241

7

GLOSSARY

Preface

Dental auxiliary personnel are essential to the delivery of complete dental care. This book is directed toward providing clinical pharmacologic knowledge to dental professionals so that they can feel competent in their interactions with patients receiving medications from a dentist or physician.

The book is written in a manner meaningful to all members of the dental team relative to their role in the overall management of the dental patient. The underlying theme throughout is the application of basic principles of pharmacology to chairside dental care. Most chapters begin with a clinical situation applicable to that chapter so that the reader is oriented to its contents and their clinical value. Answers to these cases are given at the end of each chapter so that the reader's interest will be such that he will read the chapter and then obtain the answer. The questions at the end of each chapter summarize the most important points in that section. Also, reading references are included for those who would like to delve further into specific topics.

The reader will find general comments regarding drugs not usually prescribed by dentists and will find detailed comments regarding drugs usually prescribed by dentists. Also, when both a generic name and trade name of a drug are used, common trade names will be placed in parentheses. The various principles discussed throughout the book are summarized in the section entitled Case Reports and the reader will find this section especially valuable to the daily practice of dentistry.

Although this text is designed to teach clinical pharmacology to dental professionals, the practicing dentist will find it to be an excellent review of pharmacology for himself. We feel that this book will be as valuable to the reader as the instruments used daily and that the reader will include it as part of all chairside armamentarium.

We would like to acknowledge, with appreciation, the editorial comments of Ms. Elizabeth Rose, Mrs. Angela Ritz, Ms. Suzanne Chudy, Edward Montgomery, William Feagans, Hans Mühlemann, Ms. V. Mehrlust, and the staff of the University of Zurich Dental School. We would also like to acknowledge the organizational efforts of Ms. Nancy Borsuk. Drawings in this text were skillfully prepared by Ms. Lynn Pelonero, and technical assistance was appreciated from Ms. Bobbi Schaff. A special acknowledgement is given to Russell Nisengard, for his editorial review.

Sebastian G. Ciancio
Priscilla C. Bourgault

Clinical Pharmacology
for Dental Professionals

Part One

The Basic Principles of Pharmacology

Drug Transport

Ms. Smith, the aspirins that I took after surgery the last time I came upset my stomach. This time, Dr. Jones gave me a prescription for enteric-coated aspirin. He said that this type would be easy on my stomach. Can you explain what the difference is? I thought all aspirins were the same.

INTRODUCTION

The science of pharmacology deals with the way chemical substances interact with living systems. The living body and all the substances that it produces or ingests are constructed of molecules. The interaction of these molecular substances provides the basis for all the processes of life.

Various chemical agents that are introduced into the body can mimic natural substances, block the action of natural substances, or alter in other ways the functions of the body. Frequently, but not in all instances, chemicals are able to do this because of structural similarities to the natural substances of the body. It is important to realize that chemicals never impart a new function to cells, but simply increase or decrease the activity that cells normally possess. Chemicals are called drugs when they are administered for the purpose of producing a desirable change. A drug may therefore be defined as a chemical substance used in the diagnosis, prevention, modification, and cure of disease, as well as the prevention of conception, the elimination of pain, and the alteration of mood and behavior.

DEFINITIONS

The broad field of *pharmacology* is divided into several subdivisions and related disciplines. Many aspects of these areas are of limited interest at the present time to members of the health team. *Parmacognosy* deals with the knowledge of the natural sources of drugs. At one time this knowledge was important to clinicians who had to prepare crude drugs from plants. Presently most drugs are highly purified or completely synthesized so that knowledge of the sources is not as important for proper therapy. However, knowledge of new sources of drugs continues to grow. At the present time pharmaceutical manufacturers are systematically investigating the animal and plant life of the sea, where they are finding previously unknown compounds from these natural sources.

The field of *pharmacy* deals with the knowledge of the compounding and dispensing of drugs. At one time clinicians did a great deal of their own preparation and dispensing. Most of this work eventually was done by a specialist, the pharmacist. Pharmacy has evolved so that at the present time most of the compounding of drugs is done by the pharmaceutical manufacturer. Pharmacists are now essentially dispensers of drugs, using their skills to assure maximum effectiveness and safety in the distribution and use of medication. They maintain a drug history, and may make judgments as to appropriateness of medications. They are specialists on dosage forms, storage needs, and the stability characteristics of drugs. The pharmacist is frequently the only source of information for the over-the-counter (nonprescription) drugs.

Toxicology is the field of study which deals with the adverse effects of drugs, as well as industrial poisons, environmental contaminants, pesticides, and household chemicals. The toxicologist is concerned with the chemical detection of hazardous compounds, the levels which produce toxicity, public health measures to control toxic substances, and the selection of antidotes. The toxicologist also has to understand the pharmacological principles involved in the intake, accumulation, and removal of toxic substances from the body, as well as the ability of these substances to damage genes or the unborn child, and to cause cancer.

Pharmacokinetics involves the study of all factors which affect the concentration of a drug at the specific area in the body which produces a response. This includes the manner in which a drug is administered, absorbed, distributed, stored, transformed, and excreted.

The biological effect of a drug and the mechanism by which this effect is produced is termed *pharmacodynamics*. Drug effects can be achieved by:

1 Enhancing or blocking the action of ingested compounds or compounds made by the body that produce a biochemical or physiological response (for example, acetylcholine released by the motor nerve stimulates muscle contraction; this action is blocked by neuromuscular blocking drugs).
2 Directly stimulating or depressing cellular function (for example, the central nervous system stimulants and depressants).
3 Exerting mechanical, chemical, and purely physical actions (antacids, for example, decrease the acidity of the stomach).
4 Replacing natural body chemicals such as hormones (for example, insulin in diabetics).
5 Destroying parasites which produce diseases (for example, antibiotics used for the treatment of bacterial infections).

Pharmacotherapeutics is the proper sphere of clinicians since it deals with the way drugs prevent or cure diseases. This science is based upon understanding disease processes and their alterations by drugs. Knowledge of certain aspects of toxicology, pharmacodynamics, and pharmacokinetics is necessary for a proper understanding of pharmacotherapeutics.

TRANSPORT OF DRUGS ACROSS CELL MEMBRANES

A drug may be administered by various routes. Once it reaches the circulation it can be distributed to many areas of the body. When a responsive cell is reached, a drug activity is initiated. The action of the drug is ended by biotransformation and excretion. Biotransformation is the process by which the body changes the molecular structure of drugs. Frequently, but not always, this process converts active drugs to inactive forms. Both unchanged drugs and metabolites (converted forms) may be excreted from the body, primarily by the kidney. All these processes are influenced by the ease or difficulty of the movement of drugs across cell membranes. Drugs move across membranes by passive diffusion or specialized transport.

Passive Diffusion

Everyone is familiar with the process of diffusion. The sugar allowed to dissolve and spread through a cup of tea is an example. So is the dispersal of an odor through the still air of a room. In both cases the principle is movement of a dissolved substance from a region where it is in greater concentration to a region where it is in lesser concentration. Under ideal conditions the substance eventually becomes evenly distributed through the medium in which it is dissolved.

In the body we are concerned with diffusion through cell membranes. The cell membrane is the outer layer of any cell which separates the contents of the cell from its environment.

Many cells are joined to others at the surface of their outer membranes. The cells may be arranged in hollow tubes, as in the walls of the gastrointestinal tract or in blood vessels. They may be clustered as tissues, such as muscle, bone, or nerves, or in combinations of tissues as organs. From wherever drugs enter the body, several such cell membrane barriers will be crossed as the molecules spread through the body. Because the cell membrane may speed, retard, or even deny passage to molecules, it is worth reviewing its structure.

The cell membrane is composed primarily of phospholipids and proteins (Fig. 1-1). The phospholipids are arranged so that the polar (charged) ends of the molecules form the two outer layers of the membrane while the lipid (fat) portion forms the two inner layers of the membrane. Here and there large protein molecules extend through the membrane from outside the cell. Some are attached to the polar group on the cell surface.

Molecules that do not have ionic charges pass through cell membranes because they are soluble in the lipid layer of the membrane. No barrier exists for these lipid-soluble drugs, and they are able to penetrate all cells of the body. Because of this, they are able to exert their pharmacological actions within cells or on the

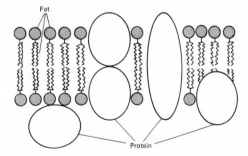

Figure 1-1 Membrane structure. The charged hydrophilic (water-loving) ends of the phospholipid molecules are represented by small circles while the lipophilic (fat-loving) ends are represented by wavy lines. (*From L. Langley, I. Telford, and J. Christensen, Dynamic Anatomy and Physiology, 5th ed., McGraw-Hill, 1980. Used by permission.*)

inner surface of cellular membranes. How fast these drugs move across membranes is dependent on the degree of lipid solubility. Drugs which are very lipid soluble penetrate rapidly, while poorly lipid-soluble drugs penetrate slowly. (Lipid solubility is not an absolute term. Nonionic drugs are soluble in both fat and water. It is the ratio of these two solubilities that determines the speed of movement across membranes. Some degree of water solubility is necessary to enable these drugs to pass through the charged outer layer of the cell membrane.)

Drugs that possess ionic charges (ions) are water soluble but not fat soluble. Therefore, they cannot diffuse through the lipid layers of the membranes. Ions can only pass through pores in membranes. It is postulated that the large proteins extending through the cell membrane serve as watery channels for these compounds. Ions move through pores according to size. However, these pores are so small that only small molecules like water and urea can get through. Most drugs with ionic charges are too large to diffuse across these pores. Therefore they can only produce their effects by acting on cell surfaces. However, some of these drugs can be taken across cell membranes into the interior of cells by specialized transport systems, to be described later.

Ionic drugs can reach cell surfaces because they are able to move in and out of the circulation by means of capillaries. Capillaries are fine blood vessels whose tube structure is made up of a single layer of cells. Drugs distributed through the bloodstream must in most cases enter and leave capillaries before reaching responsive cells in tissues. Ionic drugs that cannot penetrate through the small pores of capillary cell membranes can follow a different route across capillary boundaries. Spaces larger than membrane pores exist between the cells of the capillary. Furthermore, these spaces vary considerably in size, depending on the area of the body in which the capillaries

are located. In other words, water-soluble drugs possessing ionic charges pass through capillary walls by moving between the cells of which the walls are composed. In this manner they are able to pass out of the circulation into the extracellular fluid which bathes the outer surface of cells where they can exert their pharmacological action. (Lipid-soluble drugs pass through the capillary membrane itself.) How fast these ionic drugs move through capillaries is dependent on the size of the drug molecule (in the same manner that ions move across pores). The small molecules move rapidly, while the larger ones take more time. Some very large molecules are not able to cross many of the body's capillaries.

Many drugs have the ability to attach themselves to molecules of protein in the cell or plasma. When this "binding" occurs, the portion that is bound is not available to move across cell membranes. The consequences of protein binding are described later in the chapter.

Effect of pH and pK_a on Transport   Drugs that are weak acids or weak bases do not fall into the simple categories described above but exist in either of two forms: an ionized (charged), water-soluble form or a nonionized (uncharged), lipid-soluble form. The degree of ionization depends upon the pH of the body fluid as well as the readiness of the drug to give up or accept hydrogen ions. To describe this there is a measure of dissociation, abbreviated as pK_a. In order to understand the influence of pH and pK_a on transport of weak acids and bases it is important to understand thoroughly the meaning of these two terms.

A measure of the acidity of a solution is pH. Acidity is defined as the concentration of hydrogen ions (H^+) in a solution. The pH number has an inverse relationship to the H^+ concentration. A solution which has a high concentration of H^+ will nevertheless have a low pH, while one that has a low concentration of H^+

will have a high pH. By convention a solution is said to be acidic when it has a pH lower than 7, the pH of water, and basic when the pH is greater than 7. However, these terms can also be used in a relative manner. For instance, one can say that a solution with a pH of 6 is more basic than one with a pH of 5 and more acidic than one with a pH of 7.

Figure 1-2 illustrates the usual pH of various body fluids. A wide range of pH values compatible with life can exist in the fluids of the gastrointestinal and urinary tracts because these fluids do not come in direct contact with internal body tissues. For instance, urine has a usual pH of 6, but the value can range between 4 and 8, depending on how much acid is excreted. Intracellular (pH 6 to 7) and extracellular (pH 7.0 to 7.8) fluids that come in contact with the internal environment have a narrower range that is compatible with life.

While the pH is a characteristic of the solution or body fluid, the pK_a is a characteristic of the solute, that is, the drug molecule. The pK_a tells one how easily a compound will release or pick up hydrogen ions when placed in a solution. A weak acid releases hydrogen ions, and the remaining dissociated molecules become charged. On the other hand, most drugs that are weak bases pick up hydrogen ions and so become charged. This is because the uncharged nitrogen (N)-containing molecule is capable of picking up a hydrogen ion and retaining its charge. As has been said, a charged molecule is insoluble in lipid. For weak acids we have

$$R\text{—}O\text{—}H \rightleftharpoons R\text{—}O^- + H^+$$

Undissociated   Dissociated
nonionized   ionized

And for weak bases we have

$$R\text{—}\overset{\displaystyle H}{\underset{}{N}}\text{—}H + H^+ \rightleftharpoons R\text{—}\overset{\displaystyle H^+}{\underset{\displaystyle H}{N}}\text{—}H$$

Dissociated   Undissociated
nonionized   ionized

Each drug has its own pK_a; this is a value that does not change. The ability of a drug to combine with hydrogen is also influenced by the pH of the solution in which it is dissolved. Large numbers of H^+ in a solution make it more difficult for an acid to release hydrogen and easier for a base to combine with hydrogen. In order to be able to compare various compounds and to be consistent, the pK_a of a drug is defined as the number which is equivalent to the pH value of a solution in which 50 percent is nonionized. In other words, a drug like salicylic acid which is 50 percent ionized in a solution having a pH of 3 will have a pK_a of 3. The change in ionization which occurs with different pH values is illustrated in Table 1-1 (top two are acids; bottom two are bases).

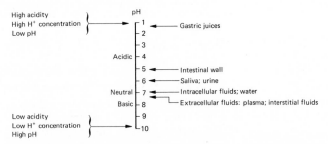

Figure 1-2 The pH values of various body fluids are indicated on a scale of 1 to 10. Each pH decrease of 1 represents a tenfold increase in H^+ concentration.

Table 1-1 Effect of pH on Ionization of Weak Acids and Bases*

Salicylic acid, pK_a = 3		
pH	Ionized, %	Nonionized, %
1	00.99	99.01
2	9.09	90.91
3	50.00	50.00
4	90.91	9.09
5	99.01	0.99
6	99.90	0.10

Phenobarbital, pK_a = 7.3		
3.3	<0.10	>99.90
4.3	0.10	99.90
5.3	0.99	99.01
6.3	9.09	90.00
7.3	50.00	50.00
8.3	90.91	9.09

Codeine, pK_a = 7.9		
3.9	>99.90	<0.10
4.9	99.90	0.10
5.9	99.01	0.99
6.9	90.91	9.09
7.9	50.00	50.00
8.9	9.09	90.91

Quinine, pK_a = 8.4		
4.4	>99.90	<0.10
5.4	99.90	0.10
6.4	99.01	0.99
7.4	90.91	9.09
8.4	50.00	50.00
9.4	9.09	90.91

* Italics indicate 50 percent ionization at the pH that is equivalent to the pK_a. Weak acids become less ionized and bases become more ionized with decreasing pH. Note the degree of ionization that occurs near the pH values of body fluids as illustrated in Fig. 1-2.

Passage of a Weak Acid between the Stomach and the Circulation The influence of pH on the movement of weak acids and bases is well shown by the diffusion of these substances across the membranes between the stomach and circulation. The difference in pH of these two body compartments is great, and the degree of ionization will be very different in the stomach (pH = 1.4) when compared with the plasma (pH = 7.4).

In the strong acidic content of the stomach a weak acid exists mostly in the nonionized undissociated form. This occurs because the presence of many hydrogen ions (H^+) increases the possibility that a molecule of the drug will combine with hydrogen. This undissociated molecule is no longer charged. Since it is now lipid soluble, it is capable of passing across the gastric membrane into the plasma. In the plasma, where the pH is 7.4, there are fewer hydrogen ions present so the molecule easily releases the hydrogen ion. Once this occurs the drug becomes negatively charged (ionized) and does not diffuse back across the membrane, which it otherwise might do as the concentration of these molecules increases in plasma.

Passage of a Weak Base between the Stomach and the Circulation The opposite occurs when a weak base is in the gastric juices. Again, because many hydrogen ions are present in the stomach, the molecules combine with the hydrogen ions with ease. Now, however, these combined molecules are charged and cannot penetrate the gastric membrane. Very few molecules remain in the nonionized state that are capable of diffusing into the plasma. As a result, little or no absorption takes place in the stomach. If a weak base is already present in the circulation because of parenteral administration, it will diffuse into the stomach where it will become ionized, and thus little back diffusion can occur. Knowledge of this concept is utilized to identify narcotics (weak bases) when death occurs due to overdosage. Even when taken intravenously these drugs can be identified in the gastric juices.

Examples of Passage of a Weak Acid and a Weak Base between the Stomach and the Circulation In the first example in Fig. 1-3, a weak acid (HA), pK_a = 3, is present mostly in the nonionized form at the low pH of the gastric juices. The nonionized molecules pass rapidly across the gastric membrane into the plasma, where most of the molecules become ionized

Plasma   Gastric   Stomach
pH 7.4   membrane   pH 1.4

$$H^+ + A^- \rightleftharpoons HA \qquad \rightleftharpoons \qquad HA \rightleftharpoons H^+ + A^-$$

$$\begin{bmatrix} 2.5 \\ \text{million} \end{bmatrix} \quad [10.0] \qquad\qquad [10.0] \qquad\qquad [1.0]$$

$$HB^+ \rightleftharpoons H^+ + B \qquad \rightleftharpoons \qquad B \rightleftharpoons H^+ + HB^+$$

$$[1.0] \qquad\qquad [10.0] \qquad\qquad [10.0] \qquad \begin{bmatrix} 2.5 \\ \text{million} \end{bmatrix}$$

Figure 1-3 Examples of passage of (top) a weak acid and (bottom) a weak base between the stomach and the circulation.

because of the high pH. Only a few nonionized molecules are capable of back diffusion. In the second example, the exact opposite occurs with a base (B) that has the same pK_a (3). Most of the drug is ionized in the stomach. The small number of nonionized molecules that pass into the plasma will remain mostly in the nonionized form and be capable of back diffusion. Numbers represent the proportion of ionized and nonionized molecules in each compartment at equilibrium. Note that the same number of nonionized molecules is present on both sides of the membrane for the acid and the base.

If the pK_a of a weak acid is 3, most of the drug in the stomach will be nonionized while most of the drug in the circulation will be ionized (Table 1-1). However, if the pK_a of a weak acid is 7.3, it would be mostly nonionized in the gastric juices but only 50 percent ionized in the plasma (Table 1-1). The nonionized 50 percent in the plasma would be lipid soluble and thus available for back diffusion and for passage across other body membranes. Diffusion back into the stomach is limited only by action of the circulation in carrying the drug to other parts of the body. If this drug is administered so that it is first present in the circulation, rather than in the alimentary canal, some of it will diffuse into the stomach.

Passage between the Intestines and Plasma of Weak Acids and Bases Most drugs with a pK_a in the range of 3 to 7.8 are well absorbed in the intestines. The absorbing surface in the gut has a pH of 5.3. This allows a sufficient portion of most weak acids and bases to be present in the nonionized state and therefore well absorbed. Absorption in the intestines is facilitated because there is an extensive absorption surface when compared to the stomach.

Changes in Body pH Because weak acids and bases can be ionized, changing the pH of body tissues will influence drug movement. For example, raising the pH of the stomach by ingesting sodium bicarbonate (base) will delay absorption of certain weak acids and improve absorption of weak bases. The treatment of phenobarbital poisoning includes intravenous administration of bicarbonate. The extracellular and urinary fluids become more basic, and an increasing amount of the drug is converted to its ionic form. This form cannot be reabsorbed by the kidney tubules and is eliminated in the urine. Since less drug is now present in the body, the toxicity is decreased. Local anesthetics which are weak bases are less effective when injected into inflamed tissue because inflammation causes a drop in pH and more of the anesthetic remains in an ionic form so that it penetrates poorly to its site of action.

Lipid Solubility of the Nonionized Form In addition to the factors influencing ionization, the nonionized form of various drugs differ in their lipid solubility. For instance, the weak acids secobarbital and phenobarbital have similar pK_a values, but secobarbital is absorbed much more rapidly because its nonionized form is much more lipid soluble than the nonionized form of phenobarbital.

Specialized Transport

Some water-soluble drugs barred by their size from passing across membranes through pores can do so with special help, the specialized transport processes. These processes, active transport, facilitated diffusion, and pinocytosis, are the same as those used by the cells to transport selectively essential substances that are vital to cell survival and which cannot be transported by passive diffusion.

Active Transport   In this process a carrier molecule within the membrane combines with a drug molecule and transports it across the cell membrane where the drug molecule is released. Proteins in the membrane which traverse the lipid core are believed to be the carrier molecules. Molecules can be transported in either direction from the outside to the inside of a cell, or from the inside to the outside. In the active transport process energy is required because the molecules are moved against a concentration gradient, that is, from an area of low concentration to one of high concentration. Carrier proteins are very specific and transport only those agents that are closely related structurally to natural chemicals of the body. For example, penicillin, an organic acid, is transported from the circulation through the tubular cells of the kidney into the tubular urine by an active process that is used to remove certain naturally occurring organic acids, like uric acid, from the body. Unlike passive diffusion, the number of molecules that can pass by active transport through the membrane is limited by the number of carrier molecules available. Active transport processes are available for the movement of certain ions, sugars, amino acids, and vitamins.

Facilitated Diffusion   This process is similar to active transport except that movement pro-

ceeds along a concentration gradient. A solute moves from a highly concentrated to a less concentrated area in the same manner as passive diffusion. Energy is not necessary to maintain this process. Some water-soluble drugs may be transported in this manner.

Pinocytosis   The transfer process called *pinocytosis* involves the engulfing of fluids or macromolecules by the cell membrane, which forms a vesicle around the content. The vesicle is then pinched off and released on the other side of the membrane. Botulinus toxin and certain proteins may be absorbed by this process.

ABSORPTION

Absorption refers to the movement of drugs from the area of administration to the blood stream. The ease or difficulty of absorption will affect the onset, intensity, and duration of drug activity. Factors which influence absorption include the routes of administration, the blood flow to the area where the drug is administered, and the physical state of the drugs, as well as the factors affecting drug transport across cell membranes, discussed above.

Routes of Administration

Enteral   The term *enteral* refers to absorption through the gastrointestinal tract and includes the oral, sublingual, and rectal routes. The easiest way to administer a drug is *orally* (po), so it is the route which is most commonly used. It is safer, more convenient, and more economical than other routes. There are, however, certain disadvantages associated with ingesting drugs. A drug may irritate the gastric mucosa and cause nausea and vomiting or irritate the intestinal mucosa and colon and cause diarrhea. The presence of food will make it more difficult for a drug to reach the absorption surfaces of the gastrointestinal tract. A drug may combine with substances in the food or cause a delay in gastric emptying. Drugs may be inactivated by digestive juices and enzymes and may be altered by variations in pH. Absorption through the gastrointestinal tract is usually slower than absorption by the intramuscular (IM), subcutaneous (SC), or intravenous (IV) routes.

When drugs are absorbed from the stomach and intestines, they first pass by means of the portal circulation into the liver which is the body's most important site for drug inactivation. Certain drugs like nitroglycerin are inactivated so rapidly here that not enough active drug remains to produce an effect. When other routes of administration are used, the drugs are delivered to the liver at a slower rate, inactivation is slower, and the drug is more effective.

Absorption also may occur through the mucous membranes of the oral cavity. This route is infrequently used since it is difficult to hold a drug in the mouth for a sufficient length of time. However, if it is held here, absorption will occur according to the same principles that govern drug movement across other membranes. Good absorption can be expected because of the thin epithelium, high vascularity, and slightly acidic pH of the saliva (pH of approximately 6). Many weak acids and bases are sufficiently nonionized at this pH to be well absorbed, and changes in salivary pH will affect their rate of absorption. A drug may be administered in this manner if it is readily soluble in saliva and rapidly absorbed. This route is convenient for the administration of nitroglycerin since absorption takes place within a few minutes and drugs absorbed from this area do not pass through the portal circulation into the liver immediately. Nitroglycerin is administered *sublingually*, that is, it is placed underneath the tongue. Absorption is facilitated by the rich blood supply to this area.

Drugs may be administered rectally, but absorption is better in the upper part of the gastrointestinal tract; also, the rectal mucosa is easily irritated. This route is sometimes useful in children when vomiting occurs or when a patient is unconscious.

Parenteral These routes include all types of drug administration outside the gastrointestinal tract. The most used are the IV, IM, and SC routes. When compared to the oral route these methods of administration will give a more uniform rapid response. However, administration is more difficult since it usually has to be performed by a second person, and strict aseptic technique must be observed. An intravascular injection may occur when not intended, and pain may accompany the injection.

Drugs administered IV, that is, directly into a vein, will act rapidly because the absorption process is bypassed and the drug is immediately available for distribution to its site of activity. The IV route is useful for administration of drugs that are poorly absorbed by other routes.

The IV route is important for administering drugs which cause local tissue damage because they become rapidly diluted by the blood when given slowly and also because the blood vessel walls are generally less sensitive to irritating substances. A drug administered IV tends to produce more undesirable reactions than other routes because it arrives at its site of action rapidly and at a higher concentration. Rapid injections of any substance can lead to a fall in blood pressure, cardiac irregularities, and respiratory disturbances. It is essential to administer slowly drugs that are given IV.

Continuous infusion is important for the administration of large amounts of fluids and for the administration of drugs with small margins of safety, especially if they are rapidly excreted or metabolized. The plasma level can easily be controlled by either increasing or decreasing the infusion rate.

If particles precipitate in an IV solution, venous thrombosis can result. Thrombosis can also result from damage to veins caused by prolonged infusions.

A drug injected IM will usually have a slower onset than one given IV and a faster onset than one given SC. Absorption is affected by ionization and lipid solubility. A drug which is insoluble at body pH will be absorbed very slowly. Irritating drugs cause less pain and tissue damage by this route than by the subcutaneous route. Decrease in blood flow through muscle will slow absorption, while increases will speed absorption. Absorption will be delayed by cooling the area or by application of a tourniquet. Exercise, on the other hand, will increase blood flow through muscles and improve absorption.

SC injections are affected by the same factors as IM injections. However, generally there is less blood flow through subcutaneous sites, and consequently absorption is slower. Absorption will be delayed and drug response at the site of injection will be prolonged by simultaneous administration of a vasoconstrictor like epinephrine. The action of local anesthetics is improved in this manner. On the other hand, drugs with vasodilator activity will be absorbed very rapidly. Drugs with irritating properties will cause pain and damage to subcutaneous tissues, producing necrosis and sloughing at the site of injection.

Other less common methods of injection include intrathecal, intraarterial, and intraperitoneal. Intrathecal involves injection into the spinal subarachnoid space. This method is used for spinal anesthesia and to treat infections of the central nervous system. The intraarterial method is used occasionally to produce a localized effect and should be given with great care by an expert. Cancer drugs are sometimes given in this manner in order to treat a localized tumor. Injection into the peritoneal cavity is used mostly in laboratory animals.

Inhalation   Volatile anesthetics are administered by inhalation. These drugs are lipid soluble and easily cross the mucous membranes of the lung. This surface area is large, and absorption is very rapid. Drugs may also be given by inhalation of aerosols (an aerosol contains small droplets of a drug in solution suspended in air). Drugs are administered in this manner for treatment of asthma and other types of lung disease. It is difficult to control the dose, and undesirable systemic effects may occur. Occasionally, aerosols may be taken for their systemic effects.

Other Mucous Membranes   Drugs are administered topically to the mucous membranes of the vagina, urethra, bladder, eye, nose, and throat in order to produce a local effect. Undesirable systemic responses may occur because drugs are readily absorbed from these sites.

Skin   Water-soluble drugs do not penetrate the horny outer layer of the epidermis, while lipid-soluble drugs pass more slowly through this thick membrane than through other body membranes. Lipid-soluble drugs may be applied in ointments for their topical effects, but water-soluble drugs must be given by other routes in order to treat the deeper layers of the skin. Many industrial compounds like carbon tetrachloride and some insecticides are highly lipid soluble and may cause poisoning and death when absorbed through the skin.

Physical State of Drugs

The term *bioavailability* is used to describe the amount and rate of entrance of drugs into the circulation and tissues. It has become increasingly apparent that pharmaceutical preparations containing equal amounts of the same drug may have different rates of absorption. Many factors may be responsible for this difference. Since a solid form of a drug will disintegrate and go into solution from its outer surface to its inner core, small particles with a proportionally larger surface area will be absorbed at a faster rate than large particles. Inert substances in a tablet or the thickness of a capsule wall may affect the rate of disintegration. Differences in bioavailability can be found in different lots of a drug produced by the same manufacturer as well as in lots of the same drug produced by various manufacturers. Serious results can occur if the condition being treated is serious and the blood level is critical for safety and effectiveness.

Various formulations are used in order to change the absorption of drugs. Some compounds are coated with fatty substances (enteric coating) that will not disintegrate in the stomach but will do so in the intestines. This is useful in preventing destruction of certain drugs or in preventing nausea and vomiting that is caused by the irritation of the gastric mucosa.

More complicated coatings are incorporated into sustained release medication. Drugs incorporated into the outer and inner layers are released at different times. An immediate effect can be produced, as well as a prolonged action, and the frequency of administration is decreased. Greater variability in absorption occurs with sustained release preparations than with the standard forms. Since larger amounts are administered at one time, faulty, rapid dissolution may release toxic amounts. If release from any of the layers is delayed, therapeutic levels may be inadequate.

Absorption from SC and IM injection sites may be prolonged by administering suspensions of poorly soluble forms of drugs. Even and sustained blood levels of insulin and penicillin can be achieved in this manner.

Drugs dissolved in oil instead of water will also be absorbed slowly from intramuscular sites. Very slow, even absorption over a period of weeks or months will occur when drugs are incorporated into flat disks and inserted underneath the skin. Various hormones are administered in this manner.

DISTRIBUTION

Once drugs have been absorbed, they move from the bloodstream to other parts of the body, including the site where a response takes place.

Drugs must first move across capillaries in order to reach the various compartments of the body. Passage is affected by ionization, size, and lipid solubility, as previously described. In addition, the characteristics of capillaries, the blood flow through each organ, and storage will alter the rate and amount of drug delivered at different sites. Most water-soluble and all lipid-soluble molecules will pass through the capillary walls into the interstitial fluid where they reach other cell surfaces. Only the lipid-soluble molecules will penetrate the membranes of these cells. Drug activity will differ depending on this distribution. The water-soluble drugs can only interact with responsive sites if these are present at cell surfaces, while the lipid-soluble drugs can interact with responsive sites within as well as on the exterior of cells.

How fast molecules move from the circulation to a particular site or organ is influenced by the blood flow to that area. An organ which is well supplied with blood vessels will receive molecules at a faster rate than a poorly perfused one. The brain, cardiac muscle, kidney, and liver have rich blood supplies, while fat and bone are poorly perfused. All other tissues are moderately perfused. For example, if other factors are equal, solutes in the circulation will reach the brain much faster than they can be deposited in muscle or fatty tissue. Although drugs are initially distributed unequally to various organs, they will with time tend to become equally distributed in all body compartments that they can penetrate. Complete diffusion rarely occurs since drugs are biotransformed and excreted at the same time that they are distributed.

Storage Due to Plasma Protein and Tissue Binding

Distribution of some drugs may be further altered because drugs combine with proteins in the circulation and with protein and other elements of cells after distribution. The drug which is bound to protein is not available to reach a site of action or produce a pharmacological effect. Binding varies in importance depending on the strength and reversibility of the bond which in turn affects the amount of drug bound. For instance, approximately 97 percent of the anticoagulant drug Warfarin is bound, while only 3 percent is available to produce an effect.

In the circulation, drugs are bound principally to albumin, an important plasma protein. The amount that is bound is in equilibrium with the amount that is free. If the bond is weak, a larger proportion of the drug will be free. When the drug leaves the circulation, some of the bound drug is released to replace it and equilibrium is maintained. When the dose is increased, an increasing number of binding sites become occupied and a larger fraction of the total molecules remains free. When all sites are bound, any additional drug administered will remain free.

Binding by plasma proteins delays the rate at which a drug is released at its site of action. The result is a pharmacological response of long duration.

Drugs that bind to plasma proteins also bind to cellular proteins, as well as to other cellular elements such as nucleoproteins and phospholipids. This binding can contribute substantially to the total storage of the drug.

Other drugs may compete for these various binding sites and displace the drug that was initially administered. More of the drug is now free than was anticipated. This could lead to a toxic response because only the free drug can initiate an action. This displacement from inactive binding sites of one drug by another is the basis of many drug interactions.

Storage in Fat

Lipid-soluble drugs will accumulate in fat. However, since the blood flow to this tissue is poor, storage as well as return to the circulation is slow. The stored drug is usually released too slowly to contribute to the maintenance of a sustained drug response.

Other Storage Sites

Many drugs will accumulate in various cells of the body because of either binding or active transport. This process can provide a substantial reservoir if enough of the drug accumulates and the binding is reversible. For example, the antimalarial drug quinacrine when administered chronically becomes several thousand times more concentrated in the liver than in the plasma. Release of quinacrine from the liver provides a sustained drug response.

Other drugs like tetracycline and heavy metals will accumulate in bone and teeth. In this situation, tetracycline can be removed from the circulation and will form an inactive complex with calcium. However, this complex does not serve as a reservoir since it is essentially irreversible. Lead is also deposited in bone, but storage here can be affected by the ingestion of calcium and vitamin D. Calcium mobilizes lead from bone while vitamin D increases storage.

Liver and Kidney

The biotransformation of drugs takes place primarily in the liver, and the excretion of water-soluble compounds occurs in the kidney. Water-soluble and lipid-soluble drugs pass very rapidly from the circulation to the liver and kidney. This is due to good blood flow and rapid movement through capillaries. The small blood vessels of the liver, called sinusoids, which serve the same purpose as capillaries in other organs, have an incomplete endothelial wall so that even very large molecules can pass rapidly through these openings. The kidney capillaries contain larger spaces than other capillaries, which also facilitates movement of solutes into the kidney tubules. This movement is further aided by the capillary pressure which is greater here than in other capillary beds.

The Blood-Brain Barrier

Lipid-soluble drugs penetrate the brain with the same ease that they pass into other tissues of the body. In addition, good blood flow is responsible for rapid distribution of these drugs to this area. (Approximately 17 percent of the blood that passes through the heart is circulated to the brain.)

Water-soluble drugs, except for very small molecules and those few drugs that move across by specialized transport, are effectively prevented from leaving the blood vessels of the brain. This is because tight junctions exist between the endothelial cells of these capillaries. There is virtually no space between the cells for molecules to pass. In addition, unlike other capillaries, the endothelial cells of capillaries within the central nervous system do not engage in pinocytosis. Because of this blood-brain barrier, water-soluble molecules which can pass into the interstitial fluid across other capillaries in the body cannot reach the interstitial fluid bathing the brain, and are therefore prevented from having any contact with neurons of the central nervous system.

The Placenta

Solutes moving from the maternal circulation to the fetus must pass through maternal capillaries. Before solutes can reach fetal capillaries they must pass through a layer of epithelial cells of the chorion, a membrane surrounding the fetus. This is a situation similar to that of the blood-brain barrier, except that this barrier is more freely permeable to water-soluble molecules than the barrier of the central nervous system. This tissue layer also becomes progressively thinner from early pregnancy to term. There is indication that it is much easier for solutes to cross this membrane in late pregnancy. The placental barrier is of limited effectiveness, and there is no guarantee that any drug in the maternal blood will not reach the fetus.

Equilibration between maternal and fetal blood of highly lipid-soluble molecules is relatively slow. This is due to a limited blood flow. A drug administered just before delivery may not reach significant levels in the fetus. However, if delivery is delayed the fetus may be affected. The placenta contains numerous drug-metabolizing enzymes which may inactivate many drugs that would otherwise reach the fetus.

Drugs which bind to plasma proteins will also bind to the proteins of the fetal circulation, further limiting the amount of free drug available to other fetal tissues. Return of drugs from fetal to maternal circulation is also slow because of limited blood flow. Drugs that cross the placenta can cause deformities of the fetus, especially when taken by the mother during the first trimester of pregnancy. These drugs include certain sulfonamides, some anticancer drugs, and the products of nuclear fission such as radioactive calcium and strontium. Many other drugs may increase the risk of malformation. Knowledge in this area is limited, so it is advisable for pregnant women to refrain from taking all drugs including alcohol, aspirin, or nicotine unless the need is great.

ANSWER TO CHAPTER CASE

The enteric-coated aspirin is covered by a fatty substance that does not disintegrate in the stomach but passes unchanged into the small intestines. In this manner the drug does not come in contact with the gastric mucosa, therefore avoiding the nausea, vomiting, and gastric discomfort that may be produced by the irritating properties of this drug.

QUESTIONS

1 What are the factors which influence the movement of drugs across cell membranes?
2 What are the advantages and disadvantages of various routes of administration?

3 How does inflammation at a site of injection affect local anesthetic activity?

4 How is distribution affected by the size, lipid and water solubility, and tissue binding of drugs, as well as blood flow to various organs?

5 What is the blood-brain barrier, and what types of drugs are prevented from entering the brain?

6 What are the dangers of administering drugs to pregnant women?

READING REFERENCES

Goldstein, A., L. Aronow, and S. M. Kalman, *Principles of Drug Action: The Basis of Pharmacology,* Wiley, New York, 1974, pp. 129–154, 227–289.

Goodman, L. S., and A. Gilman, *The Pharmacological Basis of Therapeutics,* Macmillan, New York, 1975, pp. 1–46.

Goth, A., *Medical Pharmacology,* Mosby, St. Louis, 1976, pp. 24–51.

LaDu, B. N., H. G. Mandel, and E. L. Way, *Fundamentals of Drug Metabolism and Drug Disposition,* Williams and Wilkins, Baltimore, 1971.

Levine, R., *Pharmacology, Drug Actions and Reactions,* Little, Brown, Boston, 1973, pp. 113–194.

Melmon, K. L., and H. F. Morelli, *Clinical Pharmacology: Basic Principles in Therapeutics,* Macmillan, New York, 1972.

Modell, W., O. Schild, and A. Wilson, *Applied Pharmacology,* Saunders, Philadelphia, 1976, pp. 1–94.

Smith, M. C., and D. A. Knapp, *Pharmacy Drugs and Medical Care,* Williams and Wilkins, Baltimore, 1976.

Drug Activity and Termination

Mr. Smith, the last time that I had a tooth extracted, Dr. Jones told me to take a couple of aspirins for pain, but she also gave me a prescription for a more effective drug in case I might need it. It seems to me that instead of that I could have taken four aspirins. Why wouldn't that produce the same results?

DRUG ACTIVITY

Drug activity is produced when a drug interacts with a responsive site. This can be specialized areas of cells called *receptors* or reactive sites or *enzymes*. Drugs can also interact in a *nonspecific manner* by producing changes in cells by their presence. The *mechanical* presence of certain drugs can protect sensitive tissue or destroy undesirable growths such as warts. Drugs may also bring about their responses by interacting with body chemicals in the way antacids neutralize stomach acidity.

Action of Drugs on Receptors

Receptors are specialized molecules on the surface or within cells that have the ability to combine with complementary parts of drugs. When an active drug combines with a sufficient number of receptors, a change occurs at the site of action which initiates some form of activity. For instance, acetylcholine (ACh) combines with receptors present on the surface of skeletal muscle fibers at the junction of muscles and nerves (Fig. 2-1). Activation of these receptors produces a change in the mus-

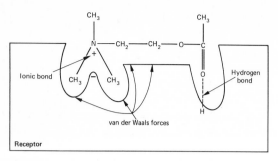

Figure 2-1 Acetylcholine is shown combined with an active receptor at a cell surface. The nitrogen (N⁺) containing a positive charge is attracted to a negative charge on the cell surface (ionized bond). The methyl (CH₃) groups fit in three-dimensional pockets, and the oxygen is held in another pocket by a hydrogen (H) bond. van der Waals forces help the formation of a tight fit.

cle cell membrane, which initiates conduction of a muscle impulse, which in turn produces muscle contraction. In a similar manner, epinephrine combines with receptors in cardiac muscle, resulting in an increase in cardiac rate and force of contraction.

The entity formed when a drug combines with receptors is called the *drug-receptor complex*. This complex is like a key in a lock. A drug, like a key, has to have an exact three-dimensional part which fits into a complementary receptor, the lock. Opening the lock can be compared to initiating drug activity. A key that fits into a lock but cannot turn the latch will prevent another key from opening the lock as long as it remains there. In the same manner a drug can occupy an active receptor without producing an effect but will prevent another drug from actively interacting with the receptor. This is called *pharmacological antagonism*. A key which cannot enter a lock because it has a different shape is like a drug which will bypass many receptors it does not fit.

Besides the three-dimensional fit of drugs and receptors (steric fit) chemical forces are needed to attract a drug to a receptor and to help maintain contact until an effect takes place. These forces include covalent bonds, ionic bonds, hydrogen bonds, and van der Waals forces. (See Glossary for definitions.)

With a *covalent bond* two atoms share an electron. A stable complex between drug and receptor molecules results. Because of this, these drugs have a long duration of action. Covalent binding is rare. For most drugs the ionic bond is the important force which first attracts a drug to a receptor. An *ionic bond* is the attractive force that exists between atoms carrying opposite charges. Figure 2-1 demonstrates the positively charged nitrogen of ACh interacting with a negatively charged atom on the receptor. This ionic force may be sufficiently strong to pull a drug molecule to a receptor but may not be strong enough to hold it there. This is where *hydrogen bonds* may come into play.

Hydrogen bonds can form whenever a molecule contains a hydrogen bound to oxygen, nitrogen, or fluorine. The hydrogen in this combination has a strong positive attracting force, while the oxygen, nitrogen, or fluorine to which it is attached has a strong negative force. The hydrogen of these molecules will be attracted to the oxygen, nitrogen, or fluorine of similar molecules. For example, in Fig. 2-1 the oxygen of ACh forms a bond with a hydrogen on the receptor. Hydrogen bonds are weaker than true ionic bonds and alone are not strong enough to attract a drug to a receptor. They will, however, reinforce the drug-receptor interaction brought about by ionic binding.

Once the drug and receptor are very close together, van der Waals forces contribute to the formation of a tight fit. These very weak attractive forces that exist between neutral atoms are very important in tightening the drug-receptor fit which initiates drug action.

It is apparent, then, that the ability of a drug to combine with a specific receptor and produce a drug action is dependent on the three-dimensional structures and the various attractive forces of both the drug and receptor. Any alteration in these structures or bonds can interfere with drug activity.

When a drug-receptor complex produces a

pharmacological effect, the receptors involved are called *primary* or *active receptors*. Receptors that cannot initiate a pharmacological response, such as those on plasma proteins, are known as *silent* or *secondary receptors*. Frequently silent receptors are more numerous than active receptors and will store an important fraction of the total drug administered (see Chap. 1, Storage).

Affinity and Intrinsic Activity

The degree of attraction between a drug and receptor is called *affinity*. The greater the affinity of a drug, the more drug-receptor complexes are formed. When the drug-receptor complex initiates an action, the drug is said to have *intrinsic activity*. Drugs that possess both affinity and intrinsic activity are called *agonists*. Acetylcholine interacting with its receptor as demonstrated in Fig. 2-1 is such an agonist. When the ACh receptors of the heart are activated, cardiac slowing results, while activation of ACh receptors on skeletal muscle produces muscle contraction. If the affinity of a drug is weaker than the affinity of another drug, larger amounts of the first will be needed to produce the same effect. Ephedrine activates adrenergic receptors of the heart and produces cardiac stimulation in milligram doses, while epinephrine produces this same effect in microgram doses, which are much smaller (a milligram is a thousand times greater than a microgram).

If a drug has affinity but no intrinsic activity, it is a pharmacological *antagonist*. As mentioned earlier, the antagonist produces its effect by preventing another drug or chemical produced by the body from occupying its receptor site. For instance, the drug atropine combines with the ACh receptors of the heart and prevents ACh released by the vagus nerve from slowing the heart (the vagus nerve is part of the parasympathetic division of the autonomic nervous system which controls the function of internal organs). As a consequence of this block, the heart rate increases.

Some drugs have both agonist and antagonist properties. Initially, they exhibit both affinity and intrinsic activity, but later they lose their intrinsic activity and are only capable of blocking. Succinylcholine initially activates ACh receptors on skeletal muscle and produces muscle contraction. This is quickly followed by muscle relaxation. Drugs that have this mixed effect are called *partial agonists* or *partial antagonists*. The degree of affinity of a drug is one factor which influences the potency of a drug while the intrinsic activity may well influence effectiveness of drugs, but this is less well defined. (Potency and efficacy are discussed below.)

Action of Drugs on Enzymes

A similar situation exists when drugs interact with enzymes. The reactive area on the enzyme is like a receptor and requires similar, complementary, three-dimensional fit and attractive forces in order to combine with a drug. The formation of a drug-enzyme complex usually results in interference in normal enzyme activity. For instance, ACh produced by the body is rapidly metabolized by the enzyme cholinesterase. Neostigmine, an inhibitor of cholinesterase, combines with the enzyme and prevents it from metabolizing ACh. Acetylcholine accumulates and produces more intense actions.

Nonspecific Activity

Although the majority of drugs produce a response by combining with receptors in a very specific manner, some drugs produce effects in a nonspecific way. General anesthetics and sedative-hypnotic drugs produce their effects, drowsiness and anesthesia, by occupying the membranes of the neurons of the central nervous system. These compounds vary considerably in chemical and three-dimensional structure and therefore could not be expected to combine with receptors that possess a discrete three-dimensional shape like a lock even though some nonspecific binding does take place. Potency and effectiveness of these compounds appear to be related to the total concentration achieved at the site of action. Differences are to a great extent related to characteristics like lipid solubility, which affects absorption, distribution, and termination, rather than to affinity and intrinsic activity, which characterize drugs that interact with specific receptors.

MECHANICAL AND CHEMICAL ACTIVITY

Some drugs act locally by mechanical or chemical means. These agents generally have a simple mode of action; they frequently are sold in over-the-counter preparations and are vigorously promoted by manufacturers. Some of these drugs, especially laxatives and antacids, are used extensively by the public when they are not needed. Examples of drugs that act by mechanical means include demulcents, emollients, adsorbents, and laxatives.

Demulcents like glycerin and gum arabic, when applied locally, form a protective coating over abraded skin or mucous membranes which prevent air and irritating substances from making contact. They may be administered in the form of ointments, throat lozenges, or as demulcent drinks to sooth the gastrointestinal tract.

Emollients composed of fats and oils include substances like cocoa butter, lanolin, petrolatum, and beeswax. They are used to protect and soften the skin and as vehicles for more active drugs. Softening of the skin occurs because these substances produce an oily film which prevents the evaporation of water from the deeper layers of the skin.

Adsorbents like kaolin, pectin, and activated charcoal help remove noxious gases, bacteria, and toxins from the gastrointestinal tract. The adsorbents combine with these substances in a mechanical way like a sponge picks up water. The adsorbed substances are no longer active, they cannot be absorbed, and they will be removed along with the adsorbents by defeca-

tion. Unfortunately, adsorbents will also combine with many drugs and essential nutrients, which reduces the bioavailability of these compounds.

Several types of *laxatives* produce evacuation of feces by mechanical means. Bulk laxatives like bran and methylcellulose swell in water to form a viscous solution which softens and increases the bulk of the feces. Saline laxatives like magnesium sulfate (Epsom salt) and magnesium hydroxide (milk of magnesia) are poorly absorbed and retain water by osmotic forces. In both of these instances the increased bulk promotes gastrointestinal motility and defecation. On the other hand, emollient laxatives like mineral oil promote defecation by producing a mild softening of feces.

Examples of drugs which act by chemical means include antacids, astringents, and antiseptics.

Antacids act by decreasing the acidity of stomach juices. These drugs are basic in nature and produce their effects by combining with hydrogen ions. Some typical antacids include magnesium hydroxide, calcium carbonate, and sodium bicarbonate. The first two compounds produce an antacid effect that is confined to the gastrointestinal tract, while the third compound can also neutralize the acidity of the extracellular fluids. Disturbance in acid-base balance may result due to this systemic effect. Changes in pH produced by these drugs will also affect the absorption of acids and bases.

Astringents produce their effects by precipitating proteins. This action is limited to the surface of cells and is transient. When proteins of capillaries and tissues as well as blood are precipitated, fluid exchange is inhibited, blood clots, and tissue contraction occurs. Because of these characteristics, astringents are useful in dentistry to prevent oozing of blood from tissues and capillary bleeding, to reduce inflammation of mucous membranes, and to produce contraction of gingival tissues for taking impressions. Aluminum chloride is a commonly used astringent in dentistry.

Antiseptics are drugs that are applied to tissues in order to inhibit growth or kill bacteria. Many act by denaturing proteins and can be harmful to the host as well as to the bacteria. They are useful mainly for cleansing the skin of patients and surgeons before an operation. Generally they should not be used to treat fresh or infected wounds since simple cleansing with a sodium chloride solution is better. They are beneficial for the treatment of localized infections that are resistant to systemic treatment.

There are many other compounds that act by mechanical or chemical means, but the examples presented here should be sufficient to differentiate these locally acting compounds from drugs that interact with receptors of body cells and enzymes.

DOSAGE, POTENCY, AND EFFICACY

Before discussing potency and efficacy it is necessary to understand the meaning of drug dosage. A drug dose refers to the amount of drug that will produce a particular biological response. Dosage affects the length of time before a response takes place (latency), the maximum effect reached, and the time at which a peak effect will occur, as well as the duration of a drug effect. For instance, when a large dose is compared to a small dose of a drug, the drug given in large amounts will reach its site of action sooner, its greatest effect will occur sooner, its maximum effect will be greater (unless the maximum possible effect was reached at a lower dose), and the amount of drug at the site of action will remain for a longer period producing a more sustained effect than when a small dose is given. Since the ability to produce an effect is dependent on the concentration of the drug as well as the length of time that the drug remains in contact at the active site, all factors that affect absorption, distribution, metabolism, excretion, and drug activity

will influence the required dosage necessary to produce an effect. When the dosage required is small, a drug is said to be *potent*. For instance, morphine is more potent than codeine because it takes only 10 mg of morphine to alleviate pain while it takes 120 mg of codeine to produce a similar effect. Potency, by itself, is rarely important since drugs of different potencies can produce the same response if given in sufficient quantity. The term *efficacy* is only related to the ability of a drug to produce a maximum response. A drug is said to be more effective if the maximum response that it can produce is greater than the maximum response produced by another drug. Efficacy is important since some poorly effective drugs cannot produce a response that is adequate for many conditions. For instance, severe dental pain may not be relieved by taking 2 tablets of aspirin every 3 to 4 h. This is usually the limit of effectiveness of aspirin, and increasing the dose will not bring further relief. It is necessary to give a more effective drug like codeine.

Dose-response curves are commonly used to examine and illustrate characteristics of potency and efficacy of drugs. A dose-response curve is the curve produced when increasing doses of a drug are plotted against the degree of response produced in an individual or a population. The dose is increased until the maximum response is achieved. Usually an S-shaped curve is produced.

Figure 2-2 illustrates the type of information that can be obtained from examining dose-response curves. The positioning of a curve on the left side of the graph indicates greater potency for the drug represented than positioning on the right side. The top of each curve which flattens out tells the maximum response which can be achieved by a particular drug. One can see that drug A is more potent than all the other drugs, drug B is less potent than drug A but equally effective, drug C is less potent and less effective than drug B, drugs C and D are equally effective, but the difference in the shapes of the curves makes it difficult to eval-

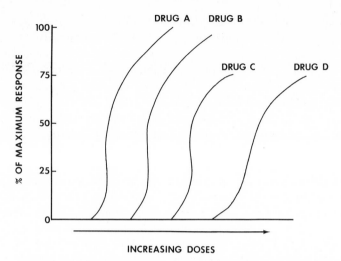

Figure 2-2 Drug A is the most potent and drug D the least potent of the four drugs. Drug A has the same efficacy as drug B. Drugs A and B are more effective than drugs C and D. Drugs C and D are equally effective. Drug D is less potent than drug C, but the difference in potency varies with the dose.

uate potency. The flat curve for drug D indicates that the drug dose must be doubled many times before the maximum effect is reached. On the other hand, the steep curve for drug C indicates that doubling of doses only a few times will be required before obtaining the maximum response. Since the difference in potency of these two drugs increases with increasing doses, potency has to be compared at each dose level. It is easier to overmedicate or undermedicate with drug C because of the narrow dose range. One can see from the dose-response curves that the effects of a range of doses must be studied in order to acquire reliable knowledge about the potency and efficacy of drugs.

FACTORS AFFECTING DRUG ACTIVITY

Many factors come into play that can alter a desired drug response. Beneficial effects may be enhanced or undesirable side effects may be antagonized by other drugs. The activity of some drugs may be increased or decreased after repeated administration, depending on their inherent properties. Individual differences, genetic abnormalities, weight, age, diseases, and psychological factors will modify drug activity.

Pharmacological Antagonism

Pharmacological antagonism, as previously mentioned, involves the occupation of a receptor site by a drug which cannot produce a response. By remaining on the receptor, this drug prevents other drugs or natural chemicals found in the body from activating the receptor. Therefore the latter compounds will not be able to produce their usual effects. For example, tubocurarine blocks receptors on skeletal muscles. This prevents ACh released by the nerve from occupying receptors and initiating muscular contraction.

Physiological Antagonism

Two drugs acting at different sites may produce opposite effects on the same system. For example, diuretics lower blood pressure because they produce a loss of fluid from the circulation, while sympathomimetic amines, such as those used in the treatment of asthma, may raise the blood pressure because they cause constriction of blood vessels.

Another example involves the antagonism between histamine and epinephrine. Both drugs produce opposing effects by acting on their respective receptors. Histamine produces dilation, while epinephrine produces constriction. The net result will depend on which effect dominates. Epinephrine will not only counteract the vasodilator action of histamine but will also produce additional vasoconstriction. One can see that in both of these examples of physiological antagonism the site of action of each drug is independent of the other, even though the responses have an opposite effect on one function.

Chemical Antagonism

The effects of a drug can also be antagonized without body tissue becoming involved. Chemical antagonism occurs when one drug combines and inactivates another. For example, heparin, which decreases the ability of the blood to clot, is a strong acid and can be neutralized by combining with protamine, a strong base.

Additive Effects

When one drug has an effect that is the same as the effect of another drug, the response of both drugs when given together is said to be additive. For instance, if 2 mg of drug A produces the same effect as 2 mg of drug B, then 1 mg of drug A plus 1 mg of drug B will give the same response as 2 mg of drug A or B given alone.

Potentiation

Potentiation, on the other hand, refers to an effect of two drugs which is greater than can be accounted for by an additive effect. Potentiation usually occurs when one drug increases the absorption and distribution or decreases the biotransformation and excretion of other drugs. For example, sulfonamides prevent oral anticoagulants from binding to plasma proteins; this increases the plasma level of free drug available for distribution. The excess anticoagulant can cause a hemorrhage.

Cumulation

Repeated administration of the same drug can cause an accumulation in the body so that the effect produced is greater than occurs with a single dose. Cumulation occurs usually with the longer acting drugs when the doses are given close together. A drug may be given in large doses early in treatment in order to obtain the required blood level that will produce the desired effect. The blood level is then maintained by administering lower doses.

Tolerance and Tachyphylaxis

When certain drugs are administered repeatedly, they produce decreasing responses over a period of time. In order to maintain the same response, increasing doses must be administered. This phenomenon, known as tolerance, is due to: (1) conditions which decrease the amount of drug available at the site of action (enzyme induction), called drug-disposition tolerance; and (2) a decrease in the response of the cell where the drug acts, called *cellular tolerance.* Tolerance is frequently a characteristic of central nervous system drugs such as morphine, alcohol, barbiturates, and amphetamines. The development of tolerance may occur with some drug responses but not with others. For instance, morphine produces drowsiness, analgesia (decreased pain), and a reduction in the size of the pupils ("pinpoint" pupils). After repeated administration the drowsiness and analgesia decrease but the pupillary effect does not change. Tolerance which occurs over a short period of time is termed tachyphylaxis.

Variability of Drug Response

Individuals vary in their responses to the same drug. In any given population a few individuals will respond well to low doses. A few individuals will require high doses for the same response. The largest number of individuals will obtain this same response with doses halfway between these two extremes. This variability exists even after those factors that modify drug activity such as genetic abnormalities, weight, age, disease states, and psychological factors, have been taken into account. The reasons for these differences are not easy to determine but could be attributed to individual variations in receptor sites as well as in the absorption, distribution, tissue storage, biotransformation, or excretion of drugs.

Pharmacogenetics

Sometimes a single gene can affect a pharmacological response by causing an abnormal change in a tissue or enzyme. For instance, the drug succinylcholine, which produces skeletal muscle relaxation, is inactivated in a few minutes by the enzyme cholinesterase found in plasma and liver. However, in some individuals the response produced lasts several hours. These individuals possess an abnormal cholinesterase which can not adequately metabolize succinylcholine. This genetically determined trait does not cause a problem until drugs that are inactivated by cholinesterases are administered.

Weight and Body Shape

A small person who receives the same dose of a drug as a large person will have a more pronounced effect because there will be less fluid for dilution and therefore the drug will be more concentrated at the site of drug activity. In addition, body shape will also affect drug distribution. The body composition of a short fat person is different than that of a tall lean one even though the weight may be the same. The lean person has a higher percentage of body water than the fat person; therefore, a drug ingested by the former will be diluted to a greater extent than one ingested by the latter.

The drug response will be less for the lean person because less drug is present at the site of activity. Very obese persons store lipid-soluble drugs to a greater extent than lean persons because the obese person has a higher percentage of blood flowing to fat tissue and more fat for storage. More drug is required to produce an effect, and the drug is removed from the body at a slower rate.

Various ways are used to calculate drug dosage. The average adult dose is generally calculated for a 70-kg (150-lb) man, and adjustments can be made for persons of other weight by using the formula called *Clark's rule:*

$$\text{Adjusted dose} = \frac{\text{average dose}}{70 \text{ kg}} \times \text{weight}$$

If the average dose of a drug is 100 mg, a 50-kg (110-lb) woman should receive an adjusted dose of approximately 71 mg. This type of adjustment is especially important if the dose which causes a therapeutic effect is close to the dose which causes a toxic effect. Doses can also be calculated on the basis of body surface area. This takes into consideration the body height as well as weight. It is considered a more accurate method of dose determination.[1]

Sex

Women generally need smaller doses than men to obtain the same response. This is usually because women are smaller than men. Distribution of drugs could also be affected since women have a greater percentage of body fat and a lesser percentage of body water and lean tissue than men for equivalent weight.

Age

Drug dosage in children can be reduced relative to the weight of child according to Clark's rule. However, whenever possible it is better

---

[1] D. DuBois and E. F. DuBois, Tables for Determination of Dose by Surface Area, *Arch. Intern. Med.,* **17:**865, 1916.

to utilize a dose that has been determined by practice rather than to rely on a standard formula since a child is not just a small adult. We know that there are differences in drug response in the infant and young child that are due to incomplete development. Many enzymes involved in the biotransformation of drugs are absent or present in small quantities in the newborn. As a result, drug response will be more intense and prolonged even though adjustment has been made for size. In addition there is a danger that drugs will be administered too frequently and that toxic levels will be reached due to cumulation. Also, the blood-brain barrier of infants is more permeable, and large water-soluble molecules are capable of passing into the brain.

Effects of drugs during old age have not been studied extensively, but in general older people are more sensitive to drugs. Although a slower absorption may decrease drug effectiveness, most frequently, impaired biotransformation and excretion enhance the drug response.

Disease States

Physiological changes in the body may alter drug effects. Increased body temperature will increase biotransformation, and changes in pH will affect drug transport. Since drugs are distributed by the fluids of the body, dehydration will result in a higher concentration of drugs in the body while excessive hydration will result in a greater dilution. Patients who are hyperthyroid are unusually responsive to the cardiac stimulant effect of epinephrine. Patients with myasthenia gravis, a disease which causes muscle paralysis, will respond excessively to the muscle relaxant tubocurarine.

Placebo Effect

The influence of other factors on drug response besides the chemical properties of drugs is known as a *placebo effect*. It is the effect that is caused by the mere fact of drug administration. In drug testing, the placebo effect is separated from the chemical effect of a drug by giving an inert substance (a placebo) which looks, feels, and tastes like the drug to a control group and the drug itself to a test group. For example, when a drug used for the relief of pain was tested, it was found that the control group obtained 30 percent reduction of pain while the test group obtained 75 percent reduction. Only 45 percent of the pain reduction can be attributed to the chemical properties of this drug, while 30 percent has to be attributed to other factors.

In the past, the placebo response had been attributed solely to psychological factors. It is probable, however, that at least a part of the placebo effect may have a physiological basis. The recent discovery of substances in the brain that are similar in effects to the analgesic morphine indicate that the placebo effect may be due to a self-releasing of these substances in the placebo responder (see Chap. 5).

Considerable variation occurs in placebo response in different individuals and in the same individual under different conditions. In clinical practice, a good placebo effect will occur especially when a patient is highly motivated to obtain relief from a medication. The person dispensing the drug will contribute to an enhanced effect when he or she demonstrates belief in the drug's effectiveness. Conversely, unpleasant side effects can be augmented by a negative attitude on the part of the patient and clinical personnel.

TERMINATION OF DRUG ACTIVITY

Drug action in the body may be terminated by redistribution, excretion, and biotransformation.

Redistribution

A drug can become concentrated at an active site to a greater extent than other areas of the body. When thiopental, a highly lipid-soluble drug, is administered IV, it is first distributed to organs, including the brain, where there is good blood flow. When a sufficient concentration is achieved in the brain, unconsciousness results. The response to thiopental is immediate since rapid movement occurs from the blood to the brain. At the same time the drug continues to be distributed to other parts of the body where, because of poorer blood flow, more time is required for equilibration to occur. As distribution continues, the blood level falls. In order for equilibration to be maintained between blood and brain, the drug now diffuses back into the circulation and is transferred to other parts of the body. When this occurs, consciousness is gained because of the low concentration of drug in the brain. This process is called *redistribution*. Notice that the drug is still present in the body but is not concentrated at the site of drug activity. Other drugs are distributed in the body slowly enough so that redistribution is not important in terminating activity. These drugs have to be biotransformed or excreted otherwise the drug response would continue indefinitely.

Excretion

The body utilizes various mechanisms by which toxic substances, water, and solutes can be removed from the body. These same mechanisms are utilized for the removal of drugs and drug products.

Drugs must first be present in the bloodstream in order that they may be distributed to excretory organs. As drugs are being removed from the body, the blood level decreases, allowing the molecules present at the site of action and other tissues to return to the blood and also be available for elimination. This process contributes to the termination of drug response. Drugs may be removed from the body by any organ that makes contact with the outside environment. Salivary glands, sweat glands, lacrimal glands, mammary glands, and the placenta excrete insignificant amounts of drugs from the body. However, an amount that is too small to produce an effect in an adult may adversely affect a fetus or nursing infant when present in the placenta or maternal milk.

The Lungs The lungs are an important pathway for the removal of volatile anesthetics. A few other drugs that become volatile at body temperature may also be excreted in this manner. The liquid drug paraldehyde, used to produce sleep, is excreted in large amounts through the lungs. This limits its use because the unpleasant odor of this drug produces an offensive breath, and large doses can irritate and damage lung tissues. Important amounts of alcohol are also removed in this manner. Measurement of alcohol concentration in the breath provides a simple means of detecting whether a driver of a vehicle is inebriated.

The Gastrointestinal Tract Water-soluble drugs taken orally or transported into the gastrointestinal tract by various fluids will be removed through the feces, while lipid-soluble drugs will be reabsorbed.

The liver and biliary system play an important role in transporting drugs into the gastrointestinal tract. Drugs are excreted by the liver through the bile into the small intestines by three secretory processes, the first for anions, the second for cations, and the third for large nonionized molecules like steroids. The first two transport systems are like those described below for the kidney. Since no mechanism exists for reabsorption of ionized molecules, excretion through the feces becomes an important pathway for terminating their activity.

On the other hand, a nonionized drug secreted by the third active process is reabsorbed and returned to the liver by means of the portal vein. The drug is then secreted again through the liver-bile-intestine circuit. Repeated recycling between the liver and the intestines prolongs the action of these drugs.

The Kidneys The most important organ of excretion is the kidney. The amount of drug excreted through this pathway is dependent on filtration, reabsorption, and secretion by the renal tubules.

Filtration In the kidney the plasma is filtered through the glomerulus, a dense network of arterioles and capillaries, into the renal tubules. The high pressure here combined with the porous quality of the capillary membranes enables all the substances in the plasma except the plasma proteins to be filtered. This fluid entering the renal tubule is called the ultrafiltrate of the plasma. Of the plasma that passes through the glomerulus, one-fifth is filtered. Most unbound drugs, small or large, ionized or nonionized, will pass with the filtrate. However, drugs that are bound to plasma proteins will remain in the circulation.

Reabsorption A large proportion of the water that enters the renal tubules is returned to the body. Therefore, drugs present in the tubular fluids become more concentrated than drugs in the plasma. Since lipid-soluble drugs will equilibrate on both sides of cell membranes they will by the process of passive diffusion return to the circulation. Elimination of these lipid-soluble compounds is dependent to a great extent on their biotransformation in the liver to water-soluble compounds which can then be eliminated by the kidney. On the other hand, drugs that are ionized will not be reabsorbed but will be eliminated in the urine. The pH of the urine will affect the elimination of weak acids and bases as previously mentioned. Weak acids will be more rapidly eliminated if the urine is made more alkaline; weak bases will be more rapidly eliminated if the urine is made more acid.

Secretion The walls of the kidney tubules are also capable of actively secreting drugs into the lumen where they can be eliminated. This is done by active transport mechanisms. There is one system which secretes anions (negatively charged molecules) and another which secretes cations (positively charged molecules). The various anions compete with each other for the carrier. For instance, penicillin, an acid (the disassociated molecule is negatively charged) which is highly ionized, is secreted by this system. The drug probenecid, which is also an acid, has a high affinity for the carrier mechanism and effectively blocks the secretion of penicillin. Of course, the penicillin which has been filtered will be eliminated also since it is a charged molecule, and no special mechanism is available for its reabsorption. Other acids which are secreted by this system include aspirin, many diuretics, and sulfonamides. The cationic carrier system transports bases such as naturally occurring histamine, quinine, and quaternary ammonium compounds (see Glossary). The two carrier systems function in a similar manner but do not affect each other. For instance, probenecid will interfere only with the secretion of acids and not bases. How rapidly a particular drug is excreted may depend on filtration alone, filtration and secretion, or filtration and reabsorption.

Biotransformation

The mechanisms by which drugs alter bodily function were discussed earlier in this chapter. However, drugs do not only act on the body, but the body also acts on drugs. This latter process, which produces changes in the chemical structure of drugs, is called *biotransformation*. Sometimes the term *metabolism* is used instead. More frequently, this latter term is reserved for processes that involve substances formed by the body (endogenous), while biotransformation is used to describe the effects on substances that are administered (exogenous). Enzymes combine with and act upon appropriate groups on a molecule, producing products which may be less active, equally active, or more active than the parent product. A product may also have different characteristics or be more toxic than the parent compound. The majority of drugs, however, are changed into compounds that are inactive. Steric fit and binding forces govern the ability of a particular enzyme to combine with a compound in a manner previously described for drug-receptor combinations.

Drug biotransformation takes place in many tissues of the body, including the plasma, the brain and kidney, the walls of the gastrointestinal tract, and also by microorganisms found in the intestines. However, most of drug transformation takes place in the liver. The products of biotransformation are usually more water soluble and less lipid soluble than the parent compound. This facilitates elimination by the kidney since lipid-soluble drugs are reabsorbed by the kidney tubules while water-soluble drugs are excreted. A few drugs are transformed to compounds that are more lipid soluble. The following reactions—oxidation, reduction, hydrolysis, and conjugation—are involved in altering the chemical structure of drugs in the body.

Oxidation   This reaction involves the loss of electrons by a molecule and either the addition of oxygen or a change which results in an increased ratio of oxygen to other atoms in the molecule. Oxidation involves many varied reactions. These include the conversion of alcohols to acids (see below), the addition of oxygen to nitrogen or sulfur, the formation of a hydroxyl group (— OH), the replacement of an amine (—NH_2) group by oxygen, and the removal of a methyl (— CH_3) or ethyl (— C_2H_5) from a nitrogen, sulfur, or oxygen atom. The following are examples of oxidation reaction:

$$CH_3C\,\boxed{H_2OH} \longrightarrow CH_3C\,\boxed{OOH}$$
Ethyl alcohol   Acetic acid

$$CH_3CONH \bigcirc O\,\boxed{C_2H_5} \longrightarrow$$
Phenacetin

$$CH_3CONH \bigcirc O\,\boxed{H} + \boxed{CH_3CHO}$$
Acetaminophen (Tylenol)

Ethyl alcohol is changed to an inactive product, acetic acid. The analgesic phenacetin is changed into a product that is equally effective and less toxic. Both phenacetin and acetaminophen are used therapeutically.

Reduction   This is the reverse of oxidation. The reaction involves a gain of electrons, a loss of oxygen, or a reduction in the ratio of oxygen in the molecule. In the following example chloral hydrate, a sedative-hypnotic drug, is reduced to trichloroethanol:

Chloral hydrate   Trichloroethanol

The product trichloroethanol is also active and more lipid soluble than chloral hydrate.

Hydrolysis   This process involves the splitting of a water molecule (HOH). The hydrogen (H) is added to one part of a molecule and the hydroxyl (— OH) group to the other part. Hydrolysis is involved in the transformation of compounds with ester (— COO—) and amide (— CON—) linkages. Most local anesthetics contain one or the other of these structures. Procaine is transformed in the following manner:

Procaine (ester)

Para-aminobenzoic acid (PABA)   Diethylamino ethanol

The two metabolic products of procaine lack local anesthetic activity.

Conjugation   This is a process by which a drug is combined with various natural substances of the body. These substances include glucuronide, glycine, sulfate, and the methyl group. Many drugs first undergo biotransformation by oxidation, reduction, and hydrolysis before they are conjugated. The conjugation products are nearly always inactive and very water soluble. The glucuronides are strong acids and are secreted by the active transport mechanism of the renal tubules.

Liver Microsomal Enzymes   Most of the enzymes that participate in drug biotransformation, except the liver microsomal enzymes, are also involved in the metabolism of normally occurring substances in the body that are related to the drug structure. These enzymes frequently transform inactive drugs into active compounds and will act upon water-soluble as well as lipid-soluble drugs. Most of the time the products formed are more water soluble than the parent compound, but they can also be more lipid soluble.

The liver microsomal enzymes, on the other hand, nearly always change an active drug into an inactive compound. These enzymes are found in smooth canallike structures in the liver called the *smooth endoplasmic reticulum*. A large proportion of drug oxidation and reduction takes place here, as well as a few hydrolysis reactions. Glucuronide conjugation is the only conjugation reaction found here, and is also involved in inactivating normally occurring compounds like hormones. The other reactions, however, are almost exclusively involved in the biotransformation of foreign substances that are lipid soluble.

Enzyme Induction   The activity of the liver microsomal enzymes can be increased by certain drugs that are biotransformed by these enzymes. This process, called enzyme induction, occurs because these drugs stimulate the formation of new enzymes. Since more enzymes are now available, biotransformation of compounds utilizing this pathway is accelerated.

For instance, when phenobarbital is given over a period of time, biotransformation occurs at a faster rate and larger doses are needed to maintain the same blood levels. Besides increasing its own biotransformation, phenobarbital can also increase the metabolism of other drugs, therefore decreasing their blood levels and therapeutic effectiveness. Enzyme induction is the cause of many drug interactions.

SIDE EFFECTS AND TOXICITY

We have so far considered the way that drugs are taken into the body, reach their sites of action, and are inactivated and removed from the body. The intensity and duration of drug response is dependent on a balance of all these factors. Unfortunately, besides the desired therapeutic response, undesirable results also occur. These are called *side effects*. In most instances this term is synonymous with *toxicity*. A side effect is always unwanted, but a toxic effect is sometimes desirable. For instance, drugs used for the treatment of cancer are especially toxic to rapidly growing cells, and antibiotics are toxic to microorganisms, yet both of these toxic responses are desirable therapeutic effects.

All drugs are capable of producing side effects. These may be trivial, serious, or fatal. Among the more serious side effects of drugs are those which involve damage to the liver, kidney, and bone marrow. The liver and kidney are very susceptible since many drugs become concentrated in these organs.
A side effect may be:

1 Dose dependent. The cardiac drug digitalis will improve cardiac function at the proper dose, but when that is exceeded, disruption of cardiac rhythm occurs. The side effect can be eliminated by decreasing the dose. By increasing the dose cardiac toxicity will occur in all individuals.
2 Dose independent. Allergic reactions (see Chap. 16) and pharmacogenetic responses may occur only in some individuals and may occur even with small doses. Even large doses will not produce a response in nonsusceptible individuals.
3 Inseparable from the therapeutic response. Sometimes a side effect is inseparable from a therapeutic effect. The drug scopolamine relieves motion sickness at the same dose that it also produces the side effect of drowsiness.

4 Interchangeable with the therapeutic effect. Sometimes a response that is a side effect in one situation will be a therapeutic effect in another. The drug atropine produces dry mouth and an increase in heart rate. If it is used to increase the rate of a heart that is beating too slowly, then the dry mouth would be a side effect. On the other hand, if a dentist uses this drug to decrease salivation, any increase in heart rate would be undesirable and therefore considered a side effect.

THERAPEUTIC INDEX

Therapeutic index is a term used to define the relationship between toxicity and effectiveness. In the laboratory, the therapeutic index is defined as the ratio between the LD_{50} and the ED_{50}. The LD_{50} (lethal dose 50 percent) is the dose required to kill 50 percent of animals in a population. The ED_{50} (effective dose 50 percent) is the dose which produces a particular therapeutic effect in 50 percent of the population. The LD_{50} divided by the ED_{50} gives the therapeutic index. The larger the index the safer is the drug. In humans, instead of using the lethal effect, which obviously cannot be determined, the dose which produces toxic effects (TD_{50}) is divided by the effective dose.

$$\text{Therapeutic index} = \frac{LD_{50} \text{ or } TD_{50}}{ED_{50}}$$

ANSWER TO CHAPTER CASE

In this situation we are concerned with the effectiveness of drugs. Aspirin is a mild analgesic whose maximum effectiveness is usually achieved by taking 2 tablets. Additional amounts are unlikely to produce relief and will increase the chance of producing toxic effects. If it were simply a matter of potency, then increasing the dose would be beneficial. More effective analgesics such as codeine or propoxyphene mixtures are likely to be prescribed when aspirin alone is not effective.

QUESTIONS

1 What is the difference between a specific and a nonspecific mechanism of action?
2 What are receptors, and how do they interact with drugs? How do the affinity, intrinsic activity, structural specificity, and agonistic and antagonistic properties of drugs affect receptor activity?
3 How do genetic predisposition, weight, age, and disease states alter the activity of drugs?
4 How can dental personnel enhance a patient's response to medication?
5 How do redistribution, biotransformation, and excretion influence the duration of drug activity?
6 What is meant by induction of liver microsomal enzymes? How does this process affect drug activity and drug interactions?

READING REFERENCES

Blackwell, B., "Patient Compliance," *N. Engl. J. Med.,* **289:**249–252, 1973.

Bourne, H. R., "The Placebo—A Poorly Understood and Neglected Therapeutic Agent," *Ration. Drug Ther.,* **5**(11):1–6, 1971.

Coleman, A. B., and J. J. Alpert (eds.), *Symposium on Poisoning in Children, Pediatr. Clin. North Am.,* **17:**471–758, 1970.

Dikstein, S. (ed.), *Fundamentals of Cell Pharmacology,* Charles C Thomas, Springfield, Illinois, 1973.

Goldstein, A., L. Aranow, and S. M. Kalman, *Principles of Drug Action: The Basis of Pharmacology,* Wiley, New York, 1974, pp. 1–154.

Goth, A., *Medical Pharmacology,* Mosby, St. Louis, 1976, pp. 1–26.

Levine R. R., *Pharmacology, Drug Actions and Reactions,* Little, Brown, Boston, 1973, pp. 17–97.

Part Two

Drugs Prescribed and Used by the Dental Profession

Chapter 3

Autonomic Drugs

While completing a dental prophylaxis, the dental hygienist observes that a patient produces excessive amounts of saliva. This patient is currently taking a drug called neostigmine. Should the hygienist recommend an antisialagogue for future dental appointments? Should she be concerned that the patient is taking neostigmine?

Never fibers serving glands, smooth muscle, and cardiac muscle belong to the *autonomic portion* of the nervous system. This portion is sometimes called the *involuntary* or *vegetative nervous system*. It is an efferent system, that is, its nerve fibers service only outgoing nerve impulses. By contrast there is the somatic portion of the nervous system, which has fibers serving both afferent (incoming) and efferent impulses. The somatic nervous system is concerned with reception of stimuli and with sending commands to skeletal muscle for movement, speech, and posture.

Since this chapter is about the drugs that affect the functioning of the autonomic nervous system, a review of the system is necessary at the start.

An important feature distinguishing the autonomic from the somatic nervous system is shown in Fig. 3-1. In the somatic nervous system, one nerve fiber conducts the nerve impulse from the central nervous system to the

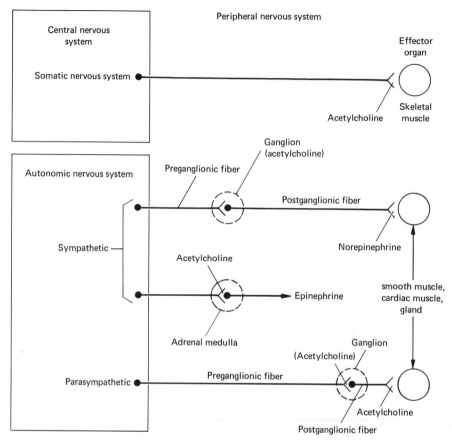

Figure 3-1 The autonomic nervous system and the efferent portion of the somatic nervous system: a comparison. (*From A. Vander, J. Sherman, and D. Luciano, Human Physiology, 2d ed., McGraw-Hill, 1975. Used by permission.*)

effector, which is skeletal muscle. In the autonomic nervous system, a chain of two nerve fibers conducts impulses to the effector organ. There is one exception to this rule, the adrenal medulla, which will be described later.

The place where the two nerve fibers link is called a *synapse*. Synapses are collected in structures known as *ganglia*. Some ganglia are strung out like chains along both sides of the vertebral column. Others are found in the walls of the organs that the nerve fibers supply. Still others are in collections elsewhere.

The fiber over which the nerve impulse travels on leaving the central nervous system is called the *preganglionic fiber*. It carries the impulse to the synapse. The *postganglionic fiber* then carries the impulse to the end of the nerve. Here, a gap similar to a synapse exists between the nerve ending and the effector organ.

The synapse and synapselike areas consist of a gap across which the nerve impulse must be transmitted by way of a chemical. For the nerve fibers considered here, there is no other way for the nerve impulse to cross this gap. The chemical transmitter is released by the nerve fiber carrying the nerve impulse. It crosses the gap and sets off activity in the postganglionic fiber or at the receptor site of the effector organ. The chemical transmitter must then be inactivated so that the impulse stops. This is accomplished by metabolism of the transmitter, by recapture of the transmitter, or by its diffusion away from the receptor organ.

Not all autonomic fibers have the same function. Two major kinds are recognized. Those leaving the cranial (brainstem) and sacral portion of the spinal cord are called *parasympathetic fibers*. Those leaving the cord between these outposts are called *sympathetic fibers*.

Many organs have both sympathetic and parasympathetic nerve supply. The two kinds of fibers often have opposite influences, one being excitatory and the other inhibitory. For example, in the heart, stimulation of the sympathetic fibers increases the rate of the heartbeat while stimulation of the parasympathetic fibers slows the rate. In general, sympathetic stimulation brings about reactions helpful in sudden emergencies ("flight or fight"), while parasympathetic stimulation is concerned with conservation and restoration of energy stores.

NEUROHUMORAL TRANSMITTERS

The transmitter chemicals of the synapse are called *neurohumoral transmitters*. They are summarized in Fig. 3-1. At the synapse between preganglionic and postganglionic nerve fibers, in both the sympathetic and parasympathetic divisions, acetylcholine (ACh) is the neurohumoral transmitter. It is also the transmitter in the synapselike area between postganglionic parasympathetic fibers and their effector organs. Finally, ACh is the transmitter released by a selected group of postganglionic sympathetic fibers. Nerve fibers that liberate acetylcholine are called *cholinergic fibers*. Because the majority of autonomic fibers release acetylcholine, it is considered the major transmitter.

Drugs can be introduced that produce direct effects on the receptor site of the effector organs, without using the autonomic nervous system. If the drug mimics the action of acetylcholine it is called *parasympathomimetic* or *cholinomimetic*.

As shown in Fig. 3-1, the majority of postganglionic fibers of the sympathetic nervous system release norepinephrine (also called noradrenaline and levarterenol). They are called *adrenergic fibers*. The adrenal medulla is a special case. It is supplied by preganglionic nerve fibers. The glandular tissue can be considered its postganglionic fibers. The final product of these fibers, that is, of the gland, is epinephrine, which is released into the bloodstream. Because of this the adrenal medulla is considered an endocrine gland and the epinephrine it releases, a hormone (see Chap. 15).

Epinephrine and norepinephrine are the main transmitters of the sympathetic division. Therefore, drugs which act like epinephrine or norepinephrine are called *sympathomimetic* drugs.

Acetylcholine is usually inactivated by the enzyme acetylcholinesterase. The action of epinephrine and norepinephrine is terminated by dilution in body fluids, recapture by nerve endings, or enzyme metabolism.

Obviously, drugs that mimic ACh, epinephrine, or norepinephrine may have a wide range of effects. Also, drugs altering the inactivation of these transmitters alter the effects produced by them. For example, the level of norepinephrine within adrenergic nerves can be increased when the enzyme involved in its metabolism is inhibited by a drug. Similarly, inhibition of acetylcholinesterase will prolong the effect of ACh. Also, the adrenergic transmitters can be altered by drugs which cause only small amounts to be released from nerve endings. These small amounts, when diluted by body fluids, will have minimal effect.

Some drugs block the effects of the transmitters by preventing them from reaching their receptor sites or by blocking the receptor sites. Other drugs inhibit the synthesis of neurohumoral transmitters in the nerve fiber ending.

Drugs which counteract acetylcholine are called *anticholinergic* or *parasympatholytic* drugs, while those decreasing the effect of epinephrine or norepinephrine are called *antiadrenergic* or *sympatholytic*. The suffix *lytic* means dissolving or loosening.

Two types of receptors are believed to exist in effectors activated by the adrenergic system: alpha (α) and beta (β). The nature of these receptors is unknown, but they have complementary functions. For example, contraction of the smooth muscles of blood vessels (*vasoconstriction*) is due to excitation of alpha receptors, while relaxation of these smooth muscles (*vasodilatation*) is due to excitation of beta receptors.

Most tissues have both alpha and beta receptors with one type predominating. Therefore, response to an adrenergic drug is dependent on the predominant receptor type and nature of the drug. Alpha stimulation will occur with alpha-stimulating drugs in tissues having mainly alpha receptors. If the same drug reaches a tissue with a majority of beta receptors, the response will still be one of alpha excitation since only the alpha receptors are being stimulated. In contrast, responses to drugs exciting both alpha and beta receptors

Table 3-1   Some Functions Mediated by the Autonomic System

Function	Sympathetic response	Parasympathetic response	Comment
Adrenal medulla	Increases secretion of neurohumoral transmitters		
Blood pressure	Increases, usually due to vasoconstriction	No change although local vasodilation	
Digestion	Decreases stomach motility, decreases peristalsis, secretions	Increases stomach motility, increases peristalsis and secretion	
Heart activity	Increase heart rate, increase in force of contraction	Decrease heart rate, decrease in force of contraction	
Liver activity	Increases glycogenolysis, gluconeogenesis	Increases glycogen synthesis	
Respiration	Relaxes bronchial smooth muscle	Contracts bronchial smooth muscle	
Salivation	Increase secretion (thick saliva), vasoconstriction	Increase secretion (thin saliva), vasodilatation	Parotid glands lack sympathetic innervation
Sweating	Increases in palm of hands mainly	Increases in most areas	
Tears		Increase	
Vision	Contraction of radial muscle (mydriasis)	Contraction of sphincter muscle (miosis), constriction of ciliary muscle for near vision	

are dependent on the predominant receptor type. For example, the blood vessels of the skin contain a majority of alpha receptors with the response to stimulation being vasoconstriction. Blood vessels in skeletal muscle contain a majority of beta receptors so that the response to stimulation is vasodilatation.

Some clinically significant actions affected by the autonomic system are presented in Table 3-1. From this table one can see that the sympathetic and parasympathetic systems usually work opposite to each other. Knowledge of the responses to autonomic nerve activity permits anticipation of the action of different drugs on this system and its receptor sites.

DRUGS AFFECTING THE AUTONOMIC NERVOUS SYSTEM

Drugs affecting receptors in this system have one of four effects:

1 Interference with the synthesis or release of transmitters

Table 3-2 Drugs Affecting the Autonomic Nervous System

Drug	Type	Action
Alpha-methyl-*p*-tyrosine	Antiadrenergic	Limits synthesis of norepinephrine
Atropine	Anticholinergic	Blocks effect of ACh at receptor site
Carbachol	Cholinergic	Enhances release of ACh; stimulates cholinergic receptors on effector cell
Hemicholinium	Anticholinergic	Limits synthesis of ACh
Hexamethonium	Anticholinergic	Ganglionic blocking agent which enhances receptor blockage of ACh
Methyldopa	Antiadrenergic	Limits synthesis of norepinephrine (mostly CNS)
Monoamine oxidase inhibitors		Inhibits the inactivation of epinephrine and norepinephrine
Phenylephrine, isoproternol	Sympathomimetic	Occupies same receptor site as epinephrine and norepinephrine and mimics transmitter effect
Physostigmine, neostigmine	Cholinomimetic	Inactivates acetylcholinesterase
Pilocarpine	Cholinergic	Stimulates ACh receptors
Reserpine, guanethidine	Antiadrenergic	Slow depletion of transmitter; latter also blocks release
Tetraethylammonium	Anticholinergic	Enhances release of ACh, blocks ganglia
Tyramine, ephedrine, amphetamine	Adrenergic	Enhances liberation of norepinephrine and epinephrine

2 Enhancement of transmitter release
3 Occupation of transmitter receptor sites
4 Inhibition of transmitter breakdown

Selected drugs and their mechanisms of action are listed in Table 3-2. One should note that drugs blocking the transmitter chemical at the ganglia can exert their effect on ganglia of both divisions of the autonomic system.

THE PHARMACOLOGY OF SPECIFIC DRUGS

To understand the pharmacology of certain adrenergic drugs, one must remember that blood vessels have both alpha and beta receptors. As stated earlier in this chapter, stimulation of alpha receptors excites smooth muscle to contract, resulting in vasoconstriction. Stimulation of beta receptors inhibits contraction, resulting in vasodilation.

Epinephrine Hydrochloride (Adrenalin)

Epinephrine, a catecholamine, is produced endogenously by the adrenal medulla and also synthetically. Epinephrine can stimulate both alpha and beta receptors. Since the alpha receptors predominate in blood vessels of the skin, mucous membrane, and kidneys, epinephrine produces vasoconstriction. However, blood vessels of skeletal muscle have mainly beta receptors, so epinephrine produces vasodilation at this site. Also, stimulation of the heart's beta receptors increases the heart's rate, force of contraction, cardiac output, and oxygen utilization.

The stimulatory effect on the conduction and excitability of the heart results in the production of cardiac irregularities at high doses or when cardiac disease is present. Because of this cardiac effect, epinephrine should not be used in conjunction with general anesthetic agents which make the heart more sensitive to the stimulatory effects of epinephrine. Epinephrine is in local anesthetic solutions at concentrations ranging between 1/50,000 and

1/250,000. A discussion of this usage can be found in Chap. 7, Local Anesthetics.

Stimulation by epinephrine of alpha receptors in the pancreas results in an inhibition of insulin secretion.

Other effects of epinephrine include elevation of blood glucose, lactate, and free fatty acids. In addition it increases oxygen consumption 20 to 30 percent.

Beta receptors are found in the smooth muscle of bronchi. In this tissue, epinephrine inhibits muscle tone with a resultant bronchodilation.

It is the drug of choice for all acute asthmatic attacks as well as other acute allergic reactions. In the case of asthma it stimulates beta receptors in the bronchi with a resultant decrease in resistance in the pulmonary channels. As a result, the asthmatic breathes better. It is available in a $\frac{1}{100}$ dilution for inhalation and $\frac{1}{1000}$ solution for injection in these patients (0.2 to 0.5 mL) in cases of asthmatic attacks.

Also, 0.2 to 0.5 mL of a $\frac{1}{1000}$ solution can be administered parenterally to abate an allergic reaction involving the circulation. The mechanism of vasoconstrictive action of this effect is one of physiological antagonism since the actions of epinephrine are opposite to those of histamine and other chemicals released during an allergic reaction.

Solutions of epinephrine should be stored in dark bottles away from light. Otherwise, decomposition of the solution by light can result, with the solution turning yellow. Such decomposition inactivates the vasoconstrictor and can possibly produce hallucinogenic effects in patients. The dental auxiliary should routinely monitor these solutions to counteract this problem.

The drug is only effective by injection, since oral administration results in its destruction in the gastrointestinal tract and in the liver. Once epinephrine and most adrenergic amines (including norepinephrine) are released in the body, they are metabolized by monamine oxidase (MAO) and catechol-O-methyl-transferase (COMT).

Epinephrine is contraindicated in patients with congestive narrow-angle glaucoma, and in conjunction with cyclopropane and halogenated general anesthetics. It should be used cautiously and in low doses in patients with cardiovascular disease, hypertension, and hyperthyroidism.

Norepinephrine (Levarterenol)

This chemical, a catecholamine, is manufactured by the body and is the principal neurohumoral transmitter of the sympathetic system. Also, it can be made synthetically. It acts mainly on the alpha receptors. It also has a weak effect on the beta receptors in the heart and, in higher doses, produces cardiac effects similar to epinephrine. Its side effects and contraindications are similar to those described for epinephrine. Injection of this drug into soft tissues will result in vasoconstriction with necrosis and sloughing. Because of this it is not recommended for use with local anesthetics. It is available synthetically as Levophed, and its main use is to counter hypotension in shock.

Isoproterenol

Isoproterenol is a synthetic catecholamine derivative of epinephrine which stimulates mainly beta receptors. It is also a stimulant of cardiac muscle. Its cardiac effects result in an increase in rate and contractile force. It relaxes bronchial smooth muscle and is a vasodilator. Its side effects are similar to epinephrine. It is made commercially as Isuprel and is used to treat bronchial asthma and heart block.

Ephedrine

This drug, a noncatecholamine, originally was obtained from plants but is now made synthetically. It stimulates both alpha and beta receptors to a lesser degree than epinephrine. Although its effect on bronchial muscle receptors is less than that of epinephrine, its effect at this site of action is of a longer duration. For this reason asthmatics often use it by inhalation. Patients using ephedrine sprays routinely show side effects similar to those described for epinephrine. Additionally, they may suffer from CNS stimulated insomnia. Motivation of such patients may be difficult. However, if the insomnia is a persistent problem, referral to their physician is in order since this may be the sign of a physical or emotional disorder.

Phenylephrine Hydrochloride (Neo-Synephrine)

This synthetic chemical is similar in structure to epinephrine but is classified as a noncatecholamine. It is a strong stimulator of alpha receptors. It has been used as a vasoconstrictor in local anesthetic solutions but is less potent than epinephrine. Therefore, a larger relative dose is necessary to obtain the same effect. Although it does not affect the heart, its side effects are similar to those described for epinephrine.

It has also been used in opthamology to provide dilation of the pupil of the eye (mydriasis) and as a nasal decongestant. It only has transient decongestant action and when used improperly can produce increased nasal congestion.

Mephenteramine Sulfate (Wyamine)

This synthetic drug is also a noncatecholamine. It is mainly an alpha-receptor stimulator with minimal effects on the heart. However, large doses can depress the heart. This drug directly acts on receptors and indirectly stimulates the release of norepinephrine. It is useful in treating hypotensive emergencies since it has fewer central nervous system effects than most other drugs of its type. The usual dose is 15 to 30 mg given parenterally.

Amphetamines

These drugs are manufactured synthetically and are also adrenergic noncatecholamines. They stimulate alpha and beta receptors and the central nervous system. These drugs are effective orally. Amphetamines are used to treat mental depression, increase "alertness," and to suppress appetite. Side effects include dizziness, increased blood pressure, cardiac palpitations and arrhythmias, increased respiration, increased motor activity and "state of feeling alert," euphoria, and hallucinations. Prolonged use leads to mental depression and fatigue. While these drugs are appetite depressants, the effect is short-lived and their value is questionable. There is also some evidence that these drugs produce gingival hyperplasia. However, the mechanism of this effect is not clear.

Prolonged use of these drugs may lead to addiction. Because of their high abuse potential, prescribing of these drugs is strictly controlled.

Topical Use of Sympathomimetic Amines in Dentistry

Epinephrine and other sympathomimetic amines have been sometimes placed on a bleeding wound to produce local hemostasis. Although the bleeding is stopped temporarily, two serious consequences may occur:

1 The initial vasoconstriction may be followed by a "rebound vasodilation," and bleeding may recur after the patient has left the office.
2 Systemic absorption of the drug occurs, and systemic effects may occur such as increased heart rate, elevated blood pressure, and so on.

Various retraction cords and solutions are available containing epinephrine or other sympathomimetic amines. However, these can also cause systemic effects, and their usage is discouraged for this reason.

In patients with cardiac problems the use of these drugs for hemostasis should be not only discouraged but prohibited. Many substitute methods are available to control bleeding topically, including the application of pressure over the bleeding area. For gingival retraction, a number of nonsympathetic amines are available which are as effective (Chap. 18).

THE DENTAL PATIENT AND AUTONOMIC DRUGS

The characteristics of drugs affecting the autonomic system are important to dental auxiliary personnel since they serve as a model system for understanding the function of nerves, drug interactions, and adverse effects that may occur in patients taking drugs affecting the autonomic system. Also, antisialagogues and vasoconstrictors are drugs used in dentistry which affect this system.

Drugs modifying the sympathetic system are used in the treatment of hypertension, peripheral vascular disease, and specific cardiac problems. Drugs modifying the parasympathetic system are used to treat a number of disorders, as previously discussed. In view of the broad usage of these drugs, many dental patients will be taking them for medical reasons. Therefore, some general considerations will be presented regarding precautions in dental patients taking autonomic affective drugs.

Patients taking antiadrenergic drugs may be more sensitive to positional changes due to inadequate accommodation of blood pressure to changes in position. This effect is called *orthostatic hypotension*. Therefore, abrupt movements of a patient should be avoided.

Parasympathomimetic or sympathomimetic drugs increase salivary secretions. Therefore, preparations are necessary for control of excess fluids during the operative procedure. This is especially true for cholinergic drugs which have a greater effect on salivation than their adrenergic counterparts.

Anticholinergic drugs are useful in dentistry

by reducing secretions (antisialagogue) and for premedication prior to general anesthesia. The two most commonly used drugs are scopolamine and atropine. These drugs block the interaction of acetylcholine with its appropriate receptor in smooth muscle, glands, and the heart. Doses of atropine used in dentistry do not affect the central nervous system. On the other hand, scopolamine has depressant effects on the central nervous system, which accounts for its usefulness as a preanesthetic agent.

Atropine, scopolamine, and related drugs cause dilation of the pupils of the eye and are often used for these properties by ophthalmologists for examination and sometimes therapy. These agents may cause visual disturbances, restlessness, tachycardia, euphoria, skin rashes, fatigue, sweating, acute psychoses, or gastrointestinal disturbances. However, since these drugs are used dentally for short-term medication (as antisialagogues), side effects are usually minimal. Because they counteract the vagus nerve's action of slowing of heart rate, tachycardia may occur. Therefore, they should be used with caution in patients with cardiac problems. They are also not recommended in nursing mothers since these anticholinergic drugs appear in the mother's milk and may adversely affect the infant. Also, they are contraindicated in patients with glaucoma, intestinal obstruction, and prostate problems.

Atropine and related drugs are often used to treat patients with gastrointestinal disorders or peptic ulcers. Therefore, these patients may have abnormally dry mouths (xerostomia), increased dental caries, dental plaque, and gingivitis.

The usual dosage of atropine as an antisialagogue is 0.3 to 1.0 mg, 1 h before an appointment. Propantheline bromide (Pro-Banthine), an atropinelike drug, is also a useful antisialagogue in a dose of 15 mg, 30 min before an appointment. Scopolomine is usually not used as an antisialagogue because of

its depressant effects on the central nervous system. However, as a preanesthetic medication, injectable doses of 0.3 to 0.6 mg are used.

Patients taking anticholinesterase drugs such as neostigmine or physostigmine probably should not be given atropine or atropinelike drugs for reduction of salivary flow (antisialagogue effect). Atropine or similar drugs may interfere with the cholinergic action of neostigmine and physostigmine.

Patients with inadequate salivary flow sometimes have difficulties wearing a removable prosthetic appliance. Pilocarpine, a parasympathetic drug, has been used with limited success to increase salivation in an oral or parenteral dose of 5 mg. Because of the nature of this drug, side effects can be expected as outlined for the parasympathetic system in Table 3-1. The most common complaints of these patients are sweating or vasodilation.

ANSWER TO CHAPTER CASE

Neostigmine is a drug which exerts its effect by inhibition of cholinesterase activity. Therefore, neostigmine produces an effect in the body similar to acetylcholine and is classified as a parasympathomimetic drug. From Table 3-1 one notes that parasympathetic stimulation results in increased secretions of thin saliva which is derived mainly from serous glands.

The hygienist should not recommend an antisialagogue to reduce salivary flow because, although antisialagogues decrease salivary flow, they may interfere with the therapeutic effect of neostigmine on the gastrointestinal tract. Since neostigmine is usually used to treat serious postoperative intestinal complications, the result of counteracting its effect to overcome the side effect of increased salivation could be most detrimental to the patient's health.

One should note that the most common drugs used as antisialagogues are either atropine or related drugs.

The hygienist's main concern regarding neostigmine medication is that this drug is necessary to treat some postsurgical gastrointestinal problems and to be prepared for patients receiving this drug to present with excess saliva.

QUESTIONS

1 What are neurohumoral transmitters? Name two.
2 Name five body functions affected by the autonomic nervous system, and discuss the effect of both the sympathetic and parasympathetic systems on these functions.
3 How can drugs alter the autonomic nervous system?
4 What dental considerations are important in the management of patients taking drugs which alter the autonomic nervous system?
5 What are alpha and beta receptors? Categorize drugs in this chapter as to their effect on these receptors.
6 What are the dangers of applying epinephrine topically on wounds in the oral cavity? List the effects that may occur following its topical application.

READING REFERENCES

Eger, E. I., "Atropine, Scopolamine and Related Compounds," *Anesthesiology,* **23:**365–383, 1962.

Elliott, G. D., and E. Stein, "Oral Surgery in Patients With Atherosclerotic Heart Disease," *J. Am. Med. Assoc.,* **227:**1403–1404, 1974.

Forsyth, R. P., et al., "Blood Pressure Responses to Epinephrine-Treated Gingival Retraction Strings in the Rhesus Monkey," *J. Am. Dent. Assoc.,* **78:**1315–1319, 1969.

Gangarosa, L. P., and F. J. Halik, "A Clinical Evaluation of Local Anesthetic Solutions Containing Graded Epinephrine Concentrations," *Arch. Oral Biol.,* **12:**611–621, 1967.

Katz, B., *Nerve, Muscle and Synapse,* McGraw-Hill, New York, 1966.

Mandel, I. D., et al., "The Effect of Pharmacologic Agents on Salivary Secretion and Composition in Man. I. Pilocarpine, Atropine and Anticholinesterases," *J. Oral Ther. Pharmacol.,* **4:**192–199, 1968.

Antimicrobial Agents

Hello, is this Dr. Brown's office? Yesterday I had gum surgery and Dr. Brown prescribed pills to prevent infection. These nauseated me and I am now having stomach pains. What shall I do? Is this problem related to the medication?

Antimicrobial agents either suppress the growth of microorganisms or destroy them. They are divided into two categories: antibiotics and sulfonamides. In dentistry, antibiotics are more frequently used, and therefore this chapter primarily considers them.

Modern antimicrobiol therapy began when Paul Ehrlich treated syphilis with salvarsan, an organic chemical. Much later, in 1936, sulfonamides were introduced for treating infections. Antibiotics became clinically available in 1941. Since then, numerous antibiotics have become available and new antibiotics are constantly being evaluated.

ANTIBIOTICS

Antibiotics are chemical substances which were originally produced by microorganisms and either retard the growth of microorganisms or result in their death. Now, some antibiotics are chemically synthesized.

An ideal antibiotic should:

1 Be selective and effective against microorganisms without injuring the host
2 Destroy microorganisms (bactericidal action) rather than retard their growth (bacteriostatic action)

41

3 Not become ineffective as a result of bacterial resistance

4 Not be inactivated by enzymes, plasma proteins, or body fluids

5 Quickly reach bactericidal levels throughout the body and be maintained for long periods of time

6 Have minimal adverse effects

Depending on the antibiotic there are several mechanisms of action. They include:

1 Inhibition of bacterial cell wall synthesis

2 Alteration of bacterial cell membrane permeability

3 Alteration of bacterial synthesis of cellular components

4 Inhibition of bacterial cell metabolism

GENERAL CONCEPTS

Certain basic terms and concepts are important in understanding the pharmacology of antibiotics.

Resistance

Microorganisms are sometimes resistant or unaffected by an antibiotic. Resistance can be (1) natural, that is, present before contact with drug, or (2) be acquired and develop during exposure to the drug. The development of acquired resistance is genetic, with a change in the microorganism DNA which is inherited by each subsequent generation. Once resistance develops to an antibiotic, it persists, and a new antibiotic must be found which will destroy the resistant strain.

Microorganisms resistant to a particular drug frequently are resistant to other chemically related antimicrobial agents. This is referred to as cross-resistance. Occasionally, cross-resistance can also occur to two chemically dissimilar drugs.

Antibiotic resistance usually results from inactivation of the antibiotic by bacterial enzymes, development by the bacteria of alter-

nate metabolic pathways unaffected by antibiotics, or by biochemical alterations in the bacteria which prevent the uptake or binding of the antibiotic.

Antibiotic effectiveness can be reduced by inadequate therapy. For example, if a drug is given at a late stage of a disease, it may not control the large numbers of microorganisms.

At other times, no clinical improvement may be seen even when the microorganisms are sensitive to the antibiotic. This may result from too low a dose of antibiotic. This has an additional danger in that low doses only destroy the weaker microorganisms and allow the stronger to survive, multiply, and possibly become drug resistant. The antibiotic thus serves to permit growth of less susceptible microorganisms without the competition of the more susceptible bacteria already destroyed by the antibiotic. This phenomenon is called *selective pressure*. The process of selecting increasingly less susceptible or resistant microorganisms occurs in a stepwise manner. Therefore, it is imperative that an antibiotic concentration which will kill these microorganisms be reached at the site of the infection. This can also occur if drug therapy is not long enough. In view of this, it is important that patients take all the medication prescribed for them and at the intervals at which it is prescribed. Too often, patients prematurely stop taking an antibiotic because they "feel better." Lastly, antibiotics can be ineffective if they do not reach therapeutic levels where the infection is, or are antagonized by interacting with other drugs.

Spectrum of Activity

This term refers to the different types of microorganism affected by an antibiotic. Antibiotics may affect only a few species of microorganisms and have a limited spectrum of activity or affect a wide variety and have a broad spectrum of activity. Broad-spectrum antibiotics are only necessary if an infection is caused by a variety of microorganisms. Often, an infection caused by one microorganism will even respond more readily to a limited spectrum antibiotic directed toward that microorganism.

Superinfections

When patients are receiving antibiotic therapy, suppression of one group of microorganisms may permit the growth of another group of bacteria that are normally present but do not cause disease. In large numbers they can produce a superimposed infection called a superinfection.

Type of Action

Antibiotics are either bacteriostatic or bactericidal. Bacteriostatic antibiotics inhibit the growth and multiplication of microorganisms while bactericidal antibiotics kill or destroy microorganisms (see Fig. 4-1). In general, bacteriostatic antibiotics alter the metabolic pathways or synthesis of cellular components. In contrast, bactericidal drugs interfere with the synthesis or function of either the cell wall, cell membrane, or both.

When two bactericidal antibiotics are given together, they may exert a greater effect than when each is given separately. This is called antibiotic synergism. Sometimes, however, when a bacteriostatic and a bactericidal antibiotic are given together, their effectiveness is negated or reduced. This is called antibiotic antagonism. In the majority of dental infections, combination therapy is not usually necessary. However, in the prophylaxis of patients with a history of rheumatic fever, combination therapy for antibiotic synergism is indicated.

ANTIBIOTICS USED IN DENTISTRY

The most common antibiotics used in dentistry are listed in Table 4-1. The antibiotics in Table 4-1 are listed according to frequency of usage, with the most commonly used listed first. Dosages vary according to the drug used.

Table 4-1   Antibiotics of Use in Dentistry

Antibiotic	Action	
	Bacteriostatic	Bactericidal
Penicillin V		√
Penicillin G		√
Ampicillin		√
Erythromycins	√	
Tetracyclines	√	
Oxacillin, nafcillin		√
Cephalosporins		√
Nystatin	√	
Bacitracin		√
Linomycin	√	
Vancomycin		√
Streptomycin		√

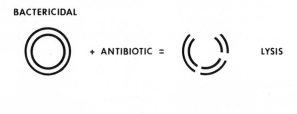

BACTERICIDAL

+ ANTIBIOTIC =   LYSIS

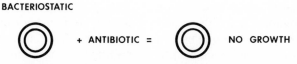

BACTERIOSTATIC

+ ANTIBIOTIC =   NO GROWTH

Figure 4-1   Mode of action of antiobiotics.

However, with oral administration, the initial dose should be double the subsequent doses so that high blood levels are rapidly obtained.

With the most commonly used penicillins, erythromycins, and tetracyclines, the usual dose is 250 mg given 4 times per day.

Penicillin

Penicillin was the first antibiotic used in humans. Although the effects of this mold derivative were discovered as early as 1928 by Sir Alexander Fleming in London, England, therapeutic trials did not take place until 1941. This delay mainly resulted from lack of sufficient amounts for a clinical trial. Difficulties in penicillin production occurred because broth cultures of Penicillium could not be produced rapidly.

Research in the United States resulted in quantity production not only by biosynthetic Penicillium but also by semisynthetic methods.

Types of Penicillin The first discovered penicillin, Penicillin G, is still the most effective penicillin against susceptible microorganisms that do not produce penicillinase. Penicillinase is an enzyme produced mainly by staphylococci which breaks down penicillin and renders it inactive. Newer semisynthetic penicillins do destroy these penicillinase-producing bacteria. Penicillins can be subdivided into several categories.

Category I These penicillins are the best for treating sensitive microorganisms. They are not stable in acid, however, and must be buffered for oral use. Otherwise, they are inactivated by stomach acids.

Category I includes penicillin G (Pentids) and benzathine penicillin G (Bicillin). Both oral and injectable forms are available. Another form of penicillin G is procaine penicillin. It is only available in the injectible form in either an oil or water base and may be used to produce prolonged blood levels. Because prolonged blood levels are produced by it, it can

be injected once every 24 h in order to maintain therapeutic blood levels. These penicillins are effective mainly against gram-positive microorganisms and spirochetes.

Category II These penicillin derivatives are acid stable and are rapidly absorbed orally. While their potency is slightly less than those in Category I, the difference is not clinically significant for dental infections. Because they are well absorbed orally, they are used most often for dental infections. Drugs included are phenethicillin (Maxipen, Syncillin) and penicillin V (Compocillin-Vk, Pen-Vee, Uticillin VK, V-Cillin). Various oral dosage forms are available. They have the same spectrum of activity as drugs in Category I.

Category III These penicillin derivatives destroy penicillinase-producing microorganisms such as staphylococci. Drugs included are methicillin (Staphcillin, Celbenin), oxacillin (Prostaphlin, Bactocill), dicloxacillin (Dynapen, Pathocil, Veracillin), nafcillin (Unipen), and cloxacillin (Tegopen). Methicillin is not acid stable and must therefore be administered only by injection. The others can be given orally and are acid stable.

Category IV These penicillin derivatives are important because of a broader spectrum of activity, including not only gram-positive but also gram-negative bacteria. These antibiotics are called broad-spectrum penicillins. Drugs included are ampicillin (Amcil, Alpen, Pen-A), amoxicillin (Larotid, which is a derivative of ampicillin), and carbenicillin (Pyopen, Geopen). They are acid stable and can be given orally or by injection. Carbenicillin is by injection only.

Mechanism of Action Penicillin is a bactericidal drug which inhibits the synthesis of some bacterial cell walls. Deficient cell walls do not protect bacteria against high osmotic pressure. Thus, fluids enter the cell causing swelling, membrane disruption, and subsequent cell death. Because penicillin acts during the synthesis of cell walls, penicillin is most effective against multiplying bacteria. Because of this, the administration of a bacteriostatic drug in conjunction with penicillin therapy could render the penicillin ineffective.

Dosage Forms Penicillin is available in a number of dosage forms including tablets, liquids, suppository, and injectable preparations. Injectable preparations (parenteral forms) are available with varying degrees of half-life in plasma. For example, crystalline aqueous forms result in high initial levels of penicillin and are rapidly eliminated by the body, in contrast to procaine or benzathine preparations which maintain lower detectable blood levels for as long as 10 to 20 days. Some injectable forms of penicillin combine the crystalline aqueous form with procaine penicillin G when a high initial blood level is required in addition to a prolonged effect. The disadvantage of long-lasting preparations is that difficulties are encountered in controlling allergic reactions to them since they are not rapidly eliminated from the body.

Topical forms of penicillin were once used but are now considered dangerous because topical penicillin frequently resulted in allergic reactions. Therefore, this route of administration is no longer used.

Penicillin is not only used to treat infections but is also used prophylactically in patients with a history of rheumatic fever. For the treatment of infection the usual dosage for drugs in Categories I, II, and IV is 250 mg given 4 times per day. In Category III, the dose varies with the drug, as shown in Table 4-2.

Kinetics Penicillin can be given orally, intramuscularly, or intravenously. Since penicillin absorption following oral administration is influenced by the presence of food in the stomach, more predictable blood levels can be obtained if it is given on an empty

Table 4-2 Dosage of Drugs in Category III

Drug	Dosage
Dicloxacillin	0.125–0.5 g every 6 h
Methicillin	1–2 g every 6 h
Nafcillin	0.25–1 g every 6 h
Oxacillin	0.5–1 g every 6 h

stomach. Alternatively, predictable blood levels are also seen when given parenterally.

Once absorbed, penicillin is widely distributed throughout the body including the saliva and gingival crevicular fluid. It does not pass the blood-brain barrier in normal patients, but during meningitis it does pass through and may be clinically effective. Penicillin is rapidly eliminated from plasma by the kidneys.

Adverse Effects Penicillin toxicity is extremely low and, except for allergic reactions, it is one of the safest drugs known. However, intrathecal injection or topical application on the brain has resulted in convulsive reactions.

The incidence of allergic reactions to penicillin has been estimated at 1 to 5 percent. Topical application, exposure to penicillin powder, and aerosol preparations of penicillin are more likely to lead to penicillin sensitivity and allergic reactions. The oral route is the least likely to cause penicillin allergy. Patients with a general history of drug allergies should be carefully evaluated since they may be more prone to hypersensitivity reactions to penicillin. Also, a careful history of previous penicillin therapy must be taken to ascertain if hypersensitivity occurred, that is, rash, itching, swelling, and so on.

Various procedures have been attempted to determine if a person is allergic to penicillin. The most promising test to date uses small amounts of penicillin combined with various penicillin derivatives in an intradermal injection. These preparations have been labeled MDM and BPL (Pre-Pen). However, some patients who have tested negative to this skin test have had allergic reactions to penicillin. Therefore, although these are the best tests available, they do not guarantee that a negative response is definitely a sign of lack of hypersensitivity to penicillin.

Whenever a patient is given penicillin, the dental auxiliary must monitor the patient for signs of hypersensitivity and have the proper emergency drugs readily available should they be required. The most common signs of antibiotic hypersensitivity are rash, itching, fever, swelling, and eosinophilia.

The Prophylaxis of Patients with Rheumatic Fever History

Certain patients with a history of rheumatic fever should be premedicated with an antibiotic prior to dental procedures which elicit gingival bleeding. Although penicillin is the antibiotic of choice for this procedure, other antibiotics are also useful. For this reason, this topic is dealt with at the end of this chapter.

Cephalosporins

These antibiotics are structurally related to penicillin and are named because they are semisynthetically derived from a mold,

Cephalosporium acremonium. Cephalosporins are effective against most gram-positive microorganisms, including staphylococci, and are also effective against *Proteus mirabilis, Esherichia coli, Klebsiella,* and *Enterobacter.*

Various Cephalosporins The cephalosporins available are summarized in Table 4-3. These antibiotics, however, are not usually advantageous over other antibiotics for treating dental infections except that they may be safe for use in patients with penicillin allergies. However, there have been reports of cross-hypersensitivity between cephalosporins and penicillin.

Mode of Action Cephalosporins are bactericidal and inhibit bacterial cell wall synthesis in a manner similar to penicillin.

Kinetics Most cephalosporins are widely distributed throughout the body. However, they do not easily cross into the cerebrospinal fluid and are therefore not indicated in meningitis. Most of the administered dose is excreted unchanged in the urine within 4 to 6 h of administration.

Table 4-3 The Cephalosporins

| Name | | | | |
Generic	Trade	Antibacterial spectrum	Adult dose	Route
Cephadrine	Anspor, Velosef	Gram-positive, gram-negative	0.25–0.5 g every 6 h 2–4 g daily	po, IM, IV IM, IV
Cephalexin	Keflex	Gram-positive and not all staphylococci	0.25–0.5 g every 6 h	po
Cephaloglycin	Kafocin	Urinary tract pathogens	0.25–0.5 g every 6 h	po
Cephaloridine	Loridine	Gram-positive, gram-negative	0.5–1 g every 6 h	IM, IV
Cephalothin	Keflin	Gram-positive, gram-negative	0.5–3 g every 6 h	IM, IV
Cephapirin	Cefadyl	Gram-positive, gram-negative	0.5–1 g every 6 h	IM, IV
Cephazolin	Ancef, Kefzol	Gram-positive, gram-negative	0.25–0.5 g every 8 h	IM, IV

Adverse Effects   The incidence of hypersensitivity reactions is almost as high as with penicillin. Although patients allergic to penicillin may not be allergic to the cephalosporins, the possibility of an allergic reaction to cephalosporins is higher than in other patients. Also, cephalosporins can lead to increased hemolysis of red blood cells. Because of this, tests for hemolysis should not be performed in patients taking cephalosporins. On occasion, renal damage has also occurred with some of these drugs, as well as local pain and tissue sloughing at the site of injection. Other side effects include neutropenia, superinfections (especially with *Pseudomonas* and *Enterobacter* species) and thrombophlebitis following intravenous injection.

Erythromycin

This drug is classified as a macrolide antibiotic. It is one of the safer antibiotics in use today and often is a satisfactory alternate for penicillin, particularly in patients who are allergic to penicillin.

Salts of Erythromycins   A number of erythromycins are available and are summarized in Table 4-4. All have a similar spectrum of activity and differ mainly in their route of administration.

Topical preparations are available but should not be used because of an increased possibility of hypersensitivity. The highest plasma concentrations of oral erythromycin are attained with the estolate form. However, the most rapid plasma levels of active drug are reached with the stearate form. The estolate form of erythromycin, on rare occasion, produces an allergic reaction in the liver resulting in cholestatic hepatitis. This disorder only occurs after 10 days of treatment. It seldom occurs after treatment of infections of dental origin since erythromycin is usually prescribed for shorter durations of time.

Mechanism of Action   Erythromycin is bacteriostatic or bactericidal, depending on the dose given and infection. Usually with dental infections, low doses are bacteriostatic and high doses are bactericidal. These drugs act by inhibiting protein synthesis.

Dosage and Dosage Forms   The dosage forms include liquids, tablets, capsules, ointments, and suppositories. Erythromycin base is destroyed by gastric juices and must be protected with a buffer, a protective coating which is acid resistant (enteric coated), or in the ester form.

Dosage varies according to the route of ad-

Table 4-4   Various Erythromycins

Generic name	Trade name	Route of administration
Erythromycin	E-Mycin, Ilotycin, Robimycin, RP-Mycin	po, rectal
Erythromycin estolate	Ilosone	po
Erythromycin ethylsuccinate	Erythrocin Ethyl Succinate, EES 400, Pediamycin	po, IM
Erythromycin gluceptate	Ilotysyn Gluceptate	IV
Erythromycin lactobionate	Erythrocin Lactobionate	IV
Erythromycin stearate	Bristamycin, Erythrocin Stearate, Ethril, Pfizer-E	po

Table 4-5 Dosage of Erythromycins

Route of administration	Dose
Intramuscular	5–8 mg/kg body weight daily
Intravenous	15–20 mg/kg body weight daily
Oral	0.25–1 g every 6 h

ministration and is summarized in Table 4-5. In cases of severe infection the oral dose can be doubled. However, the daily dose of this drug should not exceed 4 g.

Spectrum of Activity Erythromycin is effective against most gram-positive microorganisms sensitive to penicillin G. They are also effective against infections due to *Staphylococcus aureus* but not as effective as the "anti-staphylococcal penicillins." In general, its antibacterial spectrum lies between penicillin and the tetracylcines.

Bacterial resistance has been reported to appear relatively early in patients receiving the drug over a prolonged period of time.

Kinetics Erythromycin rapidly diffuses throughout the body, and all tissues except the brain contain higher concentrations than those found in plasma. As with penicillin, it passes into cerebrospinal fluid in patients with meningitis.

This antibiotic is concentrated in the liver and is excreted in bile, urine, and feces. Although the kidneys assume some significance in removal of this drug from the body, nonrenal mechanisms are more important. A large amount can be found in bile and only about 15 percent in urine. During pregnancy erythromycin passes the placental barrier but does not appear to harm the fetus.

Adverse Effects The main side effects after oral administration result from irritation of the gastrointestinal tract. Irritation, including nausea, vomiting, and abdominal pain, can be minimized if the patient takes this drug with food.

As stated earlier, cholestatic hepatitis has also been associated with the use of the estolate form. Symptoms of this disorder include nausea, vomiting, and abdominal pain followed by jaundice, fever, and a disturbance in white blood cells.

The incidence of hypersensitivity reactions to erythromycin is low and includes fever, eosinphilia, and skin eruptions.

Tetracycline

The tetracyclines are broad-spectrum antibiotics which were initially obtained from soil microorganisms. They are useful in a number of dental infections and are often used in place of penicillin or erythromycin.

Various Tetracyclines Seven basic types of tetracyclines are currently in use. They are similar chemically and therefore possess a similar antibacterial spectrum and have cross-hypersensitivity. When resistance or hypersensitivity occurs to one tetracycline, it will also occur to all in this group. The tetracyclines are summarized in Table 4-6. Topical opthalmic preparations are available, but their use in the oral cavity is questionable since topical application results in an increased incidence of sensitization. Although topical sensitization is theoretically possible, this has not been widely reported for tetracyclines.

The first tetracyclines developed were chlortetracycline, oxytetracycline, tetracycline, and demeclocycline. The next group of tetracyclines developed were doxycycline, methacycline, and minocycline. All these agents have a similar spectrum of activity. However, minocycline appears to be the most effective in treatment of meningococcal infections. The newer tetracyclines can be administered in smaller doses since they are more rapidly absorbed and more slowly excreted. From Table 4-6, it can be noted that most of the tet-

Table 4-6 Various Tetracyclines

Generic name	Trade name	Route of administration	Affected by metal ions
Chlortetracycline HCl	Aureomycin	po, IV	+
Demeclocycline HCl	Declomycin	po	+
Doxycycline and salts	Vibramycin	po, IV	−
Methacycline HCl	Rondomycin	po	+
Minocycline HCl	Minocin, Vectrin	po, IV	−
Oxytetracycline and salts	Terramycin	po, IM, IV	+
Tetracycline and salts	Achromycin V, Panmycin, Robitet, SK-Tetracycline, Tetracyn, Sumycin, Tetrex	po, IM, IV	+

racyclines are affected by metal ions except for doxycycline and minocycline. This interaction has been observed with dairy products and antacids due to their calcium content. The tetracyclines bind to calcium in the gastrointestinal tract and cannot be absorbed, so minimal therapeutic benefits can be expected. A similar interaction has been reported with products containing iron, magnesium, and aluminum. Therefore, patients should be told to refrain from these products for at least 1½ h prior to or following administration of the medication by the oral route (see Fig. 4-2).

Mechanism of Action The tetracyclines are bacteriostatic drugs which retard the growth of susceptible bacteria by inhibiting protein synthesis. Since they all have the same mechanism of action, resistance to one implies resistance to all tetracyclines.

All tetracyclines can block the antibacterial effect of penicillin. Penicillin is most effective

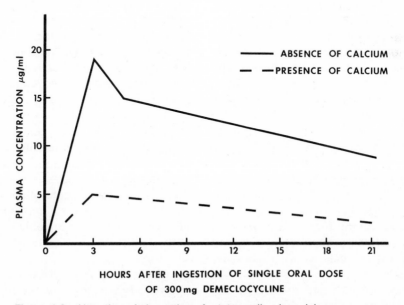

Figure 4-2 Alteration of absorption of a tetracycline by calcium.

on multiplying, growing bacteria while tetracyclines exert their effect by slowing down
the rate of bacterial growth and multiplication.
Therefore, concomitant administration of
these drugs is contraindicated.

Dosage and Dosage Forms   The oral dosage
forms include tablets, chewable wafers, capsules, liquids, and ointments. The adult dosage
for tetracycline, oxytetracycline, and chlortetracycline is 250 to 500 mg given 4 times per
day. The adult dosage for demeclocycline and
methacycline is 150 mg 4 times per day, and
that for doxycycline and minocycline is 100
mg 2 times per day.

Spectrum of Activity   The tetracyclines are
broad-spectrum antibiotics which are effective
against a number of oral gram-negative and
gram-positive cocci and bacilli. They are also
effective against a few viruses, treponemata,
mycoplasma, chlamydia, and rickettsia. Also,
minocycline may be effective against staphylococci not affected by other tetracyclines.

Kinetics   These drugs are most often administered orally since injections are usually
painful. Peak plasma levels are slowly attained
so the daily recommended dosage is usually
doubled the first day of therapy. These antibiotics pass into most body fluids and tissues.
They can also pass through the placenta and
occur in low doses in the milk of lactating
mothers. However, no adverse effects on the
newborn have been reported when the child
receives low doses in the mother's milk. This
antibiotic also passes into gingival crevicular
fluid and is therefore in intimate contact with
plaque in the gingival crevice.

They have an affinity for and are found in
higher concentrations in rapidly growing and
metabolizing tissue such as liver, tumors,
bone, and teeth.

Tetracyclines are excreted mainly by the
kidneys and can be recovered from the urine
in the unchanged form. Treatment with tet-

racyclines can also adversely alter the normal
oral and intestinal flora resulting in gastrointestinal problems, including diarrhea. Some
patients have also developed monilial infections of the gastrointestinal tract, the oral cavity, and vagina due to alteration of the flora.

Adverse Effects   The side effects associated
with tetracycline therapy are varied. A number of side effects have been related to the use
of outdated tetracyclines, and side effects also
are more common in pregnant patients (in addition to the tooth-staining problem). These
side effects and toxicities are summarized in
Table 4-7. From Table 4-7 one notes that these
drugs are contraindicated in all females in the
childbearing age range who *may* be pregnant.
In these females, the risks involved in therapy
are too high for the therapeutic value possibly
associated with dental usage.

In one animal study, tetracyclines were
found deposited in damaged areas of the heart,
particularly regions containing calcified deposits. Whether these agents are therefore
contraindicated in humans with a history of a
cardiac infarct is questionable. Further investigations to clarify this are needed; however,
no additional studies since 1962 have been reported. Although the incidence of allergy is
low, allergy to one tetracycline usually means
allergy to all other tetracyclines.

Regarding teratogenesis, the effects on formation of hands and limbs is not established.
Other side effects associated with tetracycline therapy are rare and include lym-
phoepithelioma and simulated lupus erythematosus.

Regarding the discoloration of teeth, one
should note that this is a permanent discoloration which is only correctable by covering the
tooth with restorative materials.

Comments on Tetracycline Uses
*Main Indications for Nondental Condi-
tions*   Since their introduction in 1948, tetracyclines have been widely used. This wide-

Table 4-7 Side Effects and Toxicities*

Tetracyclines

Blood urea nitrogen	Elevation of blood urea nitrogen occurs mainly in patients taking diuretics or presenting initially with a high blood urea nitrogen. Nausea, vomiting, and their sequelae are associated with this rise.
Bone	Possible retardation of growth and development—may be transient.
Gastrointestinal tract	Overgrowth with monilial microorganisms has been reported on a number of occasions in conjunction with tetracycline therapy. However, some articles question this statement. Alteration in absorption of vitamin K may occur leading to inadequate formation of prothrombin and subsequent bleeding problems.
Liver	Lethal hepatic toxicity has been reported in conjunction with use in pregnancy and in nonpregnancy in presence of renal dysfunction, shock, and sepsis. Abnormal liver function tests have been reported (due to high dose in presence of renal dysfunction).
Renal	Azotemia. Also, renal disorders have been reported following administration during pregnancy. A Fanconi-type syndrome has been associated with the use of outdated or degraded tetracycline. Therefore, they should be kept only until their expiration in a sealed container and stored away from UV light and moisture. Nephrogenic diabetes insipidus has been reported in conjunction with administration of demethylchlortetracycline.
Skin	Photosensitivity (especially with demeclocycline), rash, oncholysis. Seldom seen with chlortetracycline, minocycline, and tetracycline.
Teeth	Permanent discoloration, dysgenesis due to administration of tetracycline during the last trimester of pregnancy or the first 7 years of life.
Teratogenesis	These agents may be potential teratogens, and result in malformed hands and limbs. Do *not* use in females of childbearing age range who have missed one or more menstrual periods.
Vertigo	Reported with the use of minocycline.

* Taken from the *J. Periodontol.* **40**:157, 1976.

spread use has led to frequent antibiotic resistance. A number of gram-negative bacilli now carry factors conferring resistance to tetracyclines and to other drugs; this has decreased their effectiveness.

Tetracyclines remain the drug of choice for a variety of rarely occurring infections.

Possible Indications for Dental Conditions Tetracyclines have been suggested for treatment of various oral conditions.

Acute Necrotizing Ulcerative Gingivitis For treatment of ANUG, antibiotics are not usually necessary, and their indiscriminate use is undesirable and unsound. They do not suppress the acute symptoms of ANUG any better than initial debridement. Therefore, their only indication for use is in severe cases with systemic involvement. When ANUG does not respond to initial debridement, systemic disorders may be prevalent and the condition may have been misdiagnosed as ANUG. Obviously, antibiotic use in this case would be to no avail.

Periodontal Abscesses A periodontal abscess will respond to local drainage at least as well as the response to tetracyclines. Therefore, unless there is the possibility of cellulitis, antibiotic therapy is usually not necessary. When antibiotic therapy is indicated, a better response can be obtained with a penicillin.

Adjunct to Periodontal Surgery A number of clinicians, including this author, use tetracyclines to improve the healing of periodontal surgery and minimize postoperative discomfort and infection. However, this is only clinical opinion and not based on clinical studies since they are lacking. A few studies have been reported which suggest that postoperative discomfort is decreased by antibiotics following periodontal surgery.

Clinical studies on humans indicates that tetracyclines result in enhanced bone formation or reattachment. In addition, animal studies have suggested beneficial effects of antibiotics in terms of early crestal bone repair and reversal of a unique periodontal syndrome in the rice rat. Clinical studies with tetracyclines should be encouraged since they are effective against many microorganisms found in periodontal pockets. Their value may be in diminishing the pathogenic potential of these microorganisms. Since plaque is dynamic, a bacteriostatic drug would retard growth of certain microbial components of plaque. Therefore, by reducing these pathogens before and following surgery, an enhanced surgical response could be expected. This hypothesis is supported by studies in our laboratories and elsewhere which have shown tetracyclines in the gingival crevicular fluid following oral administration. Therefore, they become an integral part of the crevicular milieu and may further exert an effect on plaque and gingival health. They have also been shown to be present in saliva.

Periodontal Dressings Tetracyclines have been incorporated in periodontal dressings with a resultant lack of a foul taste in the mouth. However, undesirable tissue reactions occurred, including stomatitis and moniliasis. Since this is a topical application of tetracycline, the possibility of sensitizing patients is increased, along with the possibility of developing resistant strains. In general the use of antibiotics topically in this manner is contraindicated.

Prevention of Subacute Bacterial Endocarditis Tetracyclines are not drugs of choice for the prevention of subacute bacterial endocarditis. As early as 1962, McCormick and colleagues showed that 15 to 19 percent of group A streptococci are resistant to tetracyclines, whereas none were resistant to penicillin or erythromycin. Because of studies such as this, the American Heart Association and the American Dental Association recommend that the first drug of choice for the prevention of subacute bacterial endocarditis is penicillin, and the second drug of choice is erythromycin.

Lincomycin and Clindamycin

These antibiotics were discovered in 1962 in soil samples from Lincoln, Nebraska. Their use should be reserved for patients who cannot take penicillin or erythromycin. Since their adverse effect can be severe, they are seldom used in dental patients.

Types of Antibiotics in This Category Lincomycin (Lincocin) and its semisynthetic derivatives, clindamycin hydrochloride (Cleocin) and other salts, have a similar spectrum of activity. Clindamycin is better absorbed and more potent than lincomycin but has more frequent adverse effects.

Mechanism of Action These antibiotics inhibit bacterial protein synthesis, and are usually bacteriostatic, but in high doses, bactericidal.

Spectrum of Activity Their antibacterial spectrum is similar to the erythromycins. Because of their ability to penetrate bone, however, they are particularly useful in treating osteomyelitis involving alveolar bone.

Kinetics Lincomycin is only partially absorbed from the gastrointestinal tract, while clindamycin is almost completely absorbed. These drugs are excreted in feces, urine, and bile, with the biliary route being the most important.

Both drugs are widely distributed in body tissues, including bone. They also cross the placental barrier. Although lincomycin will pass through inflamed meninges as in meningitis, clindamycin does not.

Dosage and Dosage Forms These drugs are available as capsules, liquids, and injectable preparations. The oral dose for Lincocin is 500 mg and for clindamycin it varies with the salt prescribed. For the HCl form it is 150 to 300 mg, for the palmitate HCl form it is 8 to 12 mg/kg, and the phosphate form is for injection only. All oral doses are given 3 to 4 times per day.

Adverse Effects The incidence of diarrhea with these drugs is high. However, a more serious problem is the development of a severe hemorrhagic colitis which has sometimes been fatal. Therefore, serious consideration should be given to using this drug. Other side effects include glossitis, stomatitis, nausea, vomiting, skin rashes, vaginitis, and changes in blood cells. The incidence of hypersensitivity reactions to these drugs is low.

Vancomycin

Vancomycin (Vancocin), discovered in 1956, is a glycopeptide with an unknown chemical structure. Information is presented on it since it is useful in both preventing and treating bacterial endocarditis. The only commercially available derivative is Vancocin Hydrochloride.

Mechanism of Action Vancomycin is bactericidal and exerts its effect by inhibiting cell wall synthesis.

Dosage and Dosage Forms It is available as an aqueous solution for oral use and in injectable form for intravenous use. The oral dose is 0.5 to 1 g every 6 h and 2 g daily divided into two to four doses.

Spectrum of Activity This drug is bactericidal for gram-positive bacteria. Cross-resistance with other antibiotics has not been reported.

Kinetics It is poorly absorbed following oral administration. Therefore, the intravenous route is preferred. It penetrates most body fluids, including cerebrospinal fluid, when the meninges are inflamed. Its main route of excretion is via the kidney. The drug is poorly absorbed through oral mucosa, and some studies have reported improvement in gingivitis following topical application.

Adverse Effects Side effects are severe. Therefore it should be restricted to bacterial endocarditis prophylaxis, and gram-positive infections where no other antibiotic will work.

The untoward effects include phlebitis and pain at the injection site, deafness, toxic changes in the kidney, anaphylaxis, skin rashes, and fever. No adverse effects have been reported from the topical route of administration.

Nystatin

Nystatin (Mycostatin, Nilstat), a polyene antibiotic, was discovered in 1954 and is an excellent antibiotic for the treatment of fungal infections.

Mechanism of Action This drug binds to the covering membrane of susceptible fungi altering the permeability of the cell membrane leading to cell death. The drug is both fungistatic and fungicidal.

Dosage and Dosage Forms This antibiotic is available as tablets, or liquid for oral or vaginal use, and as an ointment and cream for topical and vaginal use. The dose for each form is summarized in Table 4-8.

Prosthetic appliances from patients with oral lesions are sometimes immersed in solutions of nystatin for 24 h to kill fungi attached to the prosthesis.

Kinetics This drug can be given orally but is poorly absorbed from the gastrointestinal tract. Also, it is not absorbed from skin and mucous membranes. It is not given parenterally. When taken orally, large amounts are found in feces. It exerts its main effect via the topical route in most cases.

Adverse Effects Adverse effects are rare and include nausea, vomiting, and diarrhea following ingestion. However, no adverse effects have been reported via the topical route. Hypersensitivity reactions have not occurred nor has resistance.

Table 4-8 Dosage of Nystatin

Form	Dosage
Oral liquid	400,000 to 600,000 units held in mouth and then swallowed, 4 times daily
Oral tablets	500,000 to 1,000,000 units 3 times daily
Topical	100,000 units applied twice daily
Vaginal form	100,000 to 200,000 units daily

Streptomycin

Streptomycin, discovered in 1949, is an antibiotic useful to dentistry only in the prophylaxis of certain patients with a history of complications from rheumatic fever and will only be discussed in this respect. It is also useful in the treatment of tuberculosis and bacterial endocarditis. Because of its severe toxicity, the drug has limited usefulness.

Mechanism of Action Streptomycin is bactericidal, inhibiting bacterial protein synthesis.

Spectrum of Activity It is effective against gram-positive, gram-negative, and acid-fast microorganisms. Unfortunately, bacterial resistance develops rapidly, limiting its usefulness.

Dosage and Dosage Forms It is available only in the injectable form. The dosage for the intramuscular route, which is applicable to dental situations, is 15 to 25 mg/kg body weight divided into two daily doses.

Kinetics Since it is not absorbed from the intestinal tract, the injectable route must be used. It distributes throughout plasma and all extracellular fluids before being excreted mainly unchanged by the kidneys.

Adverse Effects Severe eighth nerve damage is common, causing loss of both balance and hearing. Its use can also cause blood disorders and severe kidney damage. Allergic reactions occur, ranging from rashes to shock.

Bacitracin

Bacitracin, discovered in 1943, is sometimes used topically for dental infections. It is effective against gram-positive cocci and bacilli, *Actinomyces,* and *Fusobacterium.* Rarely, hypersensitivity reactions have been reported after topical application. It is available as an ointment containing 500 units per gram for topical use and often is combined with other topical antibiotics such as neomycin and polymyxin, which have some broad-spectrum properties. It has been placed in some periodontal dressings, but its value is questionable. It is not used parenterally since kidney damage is common following such usage.

Sulfonamides

The first sulfonamide was synthesized in 1908 as para-aminobenzoicsulphonamide but was not used as an antibacterial agent until 1936. Since that time many sulfonamides have been synthesized. Although they are effective in some infections of dental origin, antibiotics are more effective and safe. Therefore, sulfonamides are indicated in those infections of dental origin where antibiotics cannot be used. The sulfonamides are contraindicated for topical application to oral mucosa because they are highly allergenic. However, they are sometimes used topically for minor eye infections and acne.

Mechanism of Action   The sulfonamides are bacteriostatic. Since the sulfonamides are structurally similar to paraaminobenzoic acid, they interfere with its uptake by bacteria. Para-aminobenzoic acid is important to bacterial metabolism since bacteria utilize this acid to make folic acid, which is essential to the vitality of most microorganisms.

Dosage and Dosage Forms   The sulfonamides are available as tablets, liquids, creams, and vaginal suppositories. They are usually given orally, but parenteral forms are also available. The dose varies with the product and condition being treated.

Spectrum of Activity   The sulfonamides are effective against many gram-positive and some gram-negative bacteria. They are also effective against some large viruses of trachoma and lymphogranuloma venereum. They are mainly used to treat lower urinary tract infections.

Kinetics   Once the sulfonamides enter plasma, they are rapidly concentrated in urine. Some are excreted unchanged, whereas others are metabolized in the liver. The sulfonamides can be classified as short, intermediate, and long acting on the basis of duration of effect in the body.

Many bacteria develop a high degree of resistance to sulfonamides during therapy. Once resistance to one sulfonamide develops, a resistance to all others also occurs (cross-resistance). Because the sulfonamides concentrate in urine, crystals may form in the urinary tract as a complication of therapy. Therefore, sulfonamides are usually administered with large amounts of fluid and in combination with other sulfonamides to decrease the concentration of any one agent.

Adverse Effects   A number of adverse effects are associated with sulfonamide therapy, the most common being allergic reactions. The most frequent allergic reactions may be detected as urticaria, rash, fever, pruritus, dermatitis, and photosensitivity. Less frequent allergic reactions include Stevens-Johnson syndrome, erythemia nodosum, and exfoliative dermatitis. Sensitivity to one sulfonamide usually indicates sensitivity to all sulfonamides.

Other adverse effects include nausea, vomiting, diarrhea, headache, dizziness, vertigo, tinnitus, and mental depression.

Sulfonamide therapy may result in toxic effects in the urinary tract due to the formation of sulfonamide crystals in urine. Adequate urinary volume is important to minimize this effect. Also, since some sulfonamides are not soluble in alkaline media, agents such as

Table 4-9 Suggested Antibiotic Prophylaxis for Dental Procedures*

Procedure	Mitral valve prolapse syndrome	Most congenital heart disease† rheumatic or other acquired valvular heart disease, idiopathic hypertrophic subaortic stenosis	Prosthetic heart valves
Dental examination with minimal gingival trauma and adequate dental hygiene; simple filling of dental caries above the gingival margin	*Adults:* Penicillin, 2.0 g po 1 h prior to the procedure, followed by 500 mg po every 6 h for eight doses.¶** *Children:* Same as adult dosage. However, reduce each dose by 50% for children under 30 kg.¶**	*Adults:* Aqueous penicillin G, 1,000,000 units, plus procaine penicillin G, 600,000 units, IM, in addition to streptomycin (1 g) 30 min prior to the procedure. Repeat daily for the 2 days following the procedure or give 500 mg penicillin V every 6 h for eight doses.** *Children:* Aqueous penicillin G, 30,000 units/kg, plus procaine penicillin G, 600,000 units, IM, in addition to streptomycin, 20 mg/kg, IM, 30 min prior to the procedure. Follow with 500 mg (oral) penicillin V every 6 h for eight doses. For children less than 30 kg, the dose of penicillin should be 250 mg every 6 h for eight doses.** Or *Adults:* Penicillin, 2.0 g po 1 h prior to the procedure, followed by 500 mg po every 6 h for eight doses.¶** *Children:* Same as adult dosage. However, reduce each dose by 50% for children under 30 kg.¶	*Adults:* Vancomycin, 1 g IV over 30 min, given ½ h prior to the procedure and then 500 mg of erythromycin every 6 h for eight doses. *Children:* Vancomycin, 20 mg/kg IV over 30 min, given as above. Single dose should not exceed the adult dose, and the total daily dose should not exceed 45 mg/kg per 24 h. This is followed by erythromycin (10 mg/kg) every 6 h for eight doses. Or *Adults:* Aqueous penicillin G, 1,000,000 units, plus procaine penicillin G, 600,000 units, IM, in addition to streptomycin (1 g) 30 min prior to the procedure. Repeat daily for the 2 days following the procedure or give 500 mg penicillin V every 6 h for eight doses.** *Children:* Aqueous penicillin G, 30,000 units/kg, plus procaine penicillin G, 600,000 units, IM, in addition to streptomycin, 20 mg/kg, IM, 30 min prior to the procedure. Follow with 500 mg (oral) penicillin V every 6 h for eight doses. For children less than 30 kg, the dose of penicillin should be 250 mg every 6 h for eight doses.**

Table 4-9 Suggested Antibiotic Prophylaxis for Dental Procedures* (Continued)

Procedure	Mitral valve prolapse syndrome	Most congenital heart disease† rheumatic or other acquired valvular heart disease, idiopathic hypertrophic subaortic stenosis	Prosthetic heart valves
All other dental procedures, for example: dental extraction(s)‡, drainage of dental abscess, extensive gingivitis and poor dental hygiene with other dental procedures, cleaning with calculus removal below gingival margin, filling of caries below gingival margin, application of orthodontic appliances§	Same as above Or *Adults:* Aqueous penicillin G, 1,000,000 units, plus procaine penicillin G, 600,000 units, IM, in addition to streptomycin (1 g) 30 min prior to the procedure. Repeat daily for the 2 days following the procedure or give 500 mg penicillin V every 6 h for eight doses.** *Children:* Aqueous penicillin G, 30,000 units/kg, plus procaine penicillin G, 600,000 units, IM, in addition to streptomycin, 20 mg/kg, IM, 30 min prior to the procedure. Follow with 500 mg (oral) penicillin V every 6 h for eight doses. For children less than 30 kg, the dose of penicillin should be 250 mg every 6 h for eight doses.**	Same as above Or *Adults:* Vancomycin, 1 g IV over 30 min, given $\frac{1}{2}$ h prior to the procedure and then 500 mg of erythromycin every 6 h for eight doses. *Children:* Vancomycin, 20 mg/kg IV over 30 min, given as above. Single dose should not exceed the adult dose, and the total daily dose should not exceed 45 mg/kg per 24 h. This is followed by erythromycin (10 mg/kg) every 6 h for eight doses.	Same as above

* These are examples of many commonly performed procedures, as it is impossible to mention all circumstances. Physicians and dentists must individualize depending upon the patient and the procedure if not covered here or in the text.

** For patients allergic to penicillin, substitute erythromycin for penicillin or use the following: *Adults:* 1 g erythromycin 1½ to 2 h prior to the procedure, followed by 500 mg every 6 h for eight doses. *Children:* Same as adult dose. However, under 30 kg body weight, give 20 mg/kg initially and 10 mg/kg every 6 h for eight doses.

† For example, ventricular septal defect, tetralogy of Fallot, aortic stenosis, pulmonic stenosis, complex cyanotic heart disease, patent ductus arteriosus, or systemic to pulmonary artery shunts.

‡ Does not include exfoliation of deciduous teeth.

§ Does not include adjustments of orthodontic appliances.

¶ This regimen should not be used in those patients who are receiving daily *oral* penicillin for prevention of recurrent attacks of rheumatic fever, since they have been shown to harbor penicillin-resistant organisms in their oral cavities.

sodium bicarbonate are given in conjunction with therapy to make urine more alkaline.

Blood dyscrasias have also occurred with sulfonamide therapy. Clinical signs associated with these are sore throat, fever, pallor, or jaundice. These symptoms should be watched for in patients on long-term therapy, and periodic blood counts are indicated during such therapy. These drugs cross the placenta and are excreted in milk. Therefore, since sulfonamides can cause problems in infants, they should not be given to pregnant or lactating females.

ANTIBIOTIC MANAGEMENT OF THE PATIENT WITH VARIOUS CARDIAC PROBLEMS

Patients may have histories of cardiovascular problems that require antibiotic prophylaxis.

The occurrence and extent of bacteremias following dental procedures vary with the extent of the procedure and the amount of trauma and health of the gingival tissues. Prophylactic antibiotic therapy is recommended for dental procedures that are likely to cause gingival bleeding to minimize the risk of bacteremias leading to cardiac infection (subacute bacterial endocarditis).

Streptococcus viridans, a microorganism found in the gingival crevice, has an affinity for diseased heart valves or weakened cardiac tissues. This microorganism can lodge in heart tissues and produce bacterial endocarditis, a life-threatening disease. Therefore, these patients must be premedicated with antibiotics, as outlined in Table 4-9. The question of prophylactic antibiotics in a patient who has a history of rheumatic fever but no signs of cardiac damage is left to the judgment of the dentist. If the dentist is certain that a physician has examined the patient with such a history and has found no sign of cardiac damage, prophylactic therapy should not be necessary.

Further discussion of this topic can be found in Appendix F.

ANSWER TO CHAPTER CASE

Certain antibiotics are sometimes used after periodontal surgery. If a tetracycline or an erythromycin were prescribed, a side effect of these drugs is gastrointestinal upset, nausea, and, sometimes, diarrhea. This problem can obviously be overcome by stopping the medication. Before the medication is stopped, the patient should be told to take it with food and never on an empty stomach. However, when this advice is given in relation to tetracycline medication [with the exception of doxycycline (Vibramycin) and minocycline (Minocin, Vectrin)] the concomitant food intake should not include metal-containing products since metals such as iron and calcium bind tetracycline in the gastrointestinal tract. The result of this binding is that the tetracycline administered cannot be absorbed from the gastrointestinal tract into the bloodstream in amounts large enough to have a therapeutic effect.

QUESTIONS

1 Define an antibiotic and name the four most commonly prescribed in dentistry.
2 List the four possible mechanisms of action of antibiotics.
3 What is the most common side effect associated with penicillin therapy?
4 Compare the spectrum of activity of erythromycins, penicillins, and tetracyclines.
5 What are the most common side effects of tetracyclines?
6 How can tetracycline therapy result in permanent discoloration of teeth?
7 What is the value of antibiotic therapy in the treatment of acute necrotizing ulcerative gingivitis?
8 Which patients should be premedicated with antibiotics prior to dental procedures which result in gingival bleeding? Discuss the use of these antibiotics.

READING REFERENCES

Archard, H. O., and W. C. Roberts, "Bacterial Endocarditis After Dental Procedures in Patients with Aortic Valve Prosthesis," *J. Am. Dent. Assoc.,* 72:648–652, 1966.

Ariaudo, A. A., "The Efficacy of Antibiotics in Periodontal Surgery: A Controlled Study with Lincomycin and Placebo in Sixty-eight Patients," *J. Periodontol.,* 40:150, 1969.

Baer, P. N., C. F. Sumner, and G. Miller, "Periodontal Dressings," *Dent. Clin. North Am.,* **13:**181–191, 1969.

Ciancio, S. G., "Tetracyclines and Periodontal Therapy," *J. Periodontol.,* **43:**155–159, 1976.

Sabath, L. D., "Drug Resistance in Bacteria," *N. Engl. J. Med.,* **280:**291–294, 1969.

Stahl, S. S., "The Healing of a Gingival Wound in Protein-Deprived, Antibiotic-Supplemented Adult Rats," *Oral Surg.,* **17:**443, 1964.

Tedesco, F. J., R. W. Barton, and D. H. Alpers, "Clindamycin Associated Colitis," *Am. Intern. Med.,* **81:**429–433, 1974.

"Tetracycline in Breast Milk," *Br. Med. J.,* **4:**568, 1969.

Weinstein, L., Antimicrobial Agents, Penicillins and Cephalosporins, in L. S. Goodman and A. Gilman (eds.), *The Pharmacological Basis of Therapeutics,* 5th ed., MacMillan, New York, 1975.

Analgesics

Mr. Thompson is scheduled for the extraction of a lower right incisor. The dentist plans to prescribe an analgesic for the patient. She asks you about the patient's medical history, and you reply that he has an ulcer. What type of analgesics should not be prescribed?

Analgesics are drugs that have the ability to reduce or abolish pain. They can be divided in relation to their therapeutic effects into mild, moderate, and strong analgesics. These classifications are obviously arbitrary since pain cannot be that strictly categorized.

The drugs classified as *mild analgesics* are used to treat pain that ranges from mild to moderate. They include the salicylates, the aniline derivatives, and propoxyphene (Darvon), a weak member of the narcotic family.

The *moderate analgesics* treat pain that ranges from moderate to moderately severe. The weaker members of the narcotics such as codeine are included in this group, as well as varying combinations of codeine or propoxyphene with the salicylates and aniline derivatives.

All *strong analgesics* are drugs that are functionally similar to morphine, the major narcotic found in opium. Generally, dentists in the United States prescribe mild to moderate analgesics since they are usually effective against pain of dental origin. However, dentists should not hesitate to prescribe a strong analgesic if severe pain is anticipated. One of the greatest disservices a dentist can render patients is to prescribe the wrong analgesic or no analgesic in the presence of postoperative pain.

Table 5-1 Analgesics Used in Dental Treatment of Mild to Moderate Pain

| Drug | Dose, mg | | Administration |
	Adult	Children	
Aspirin	300–600	65/kg	po every 3–4 h
Acetaminophen (Tylenol)	325–650	150–300 (6–12 years) 60–120 (1–6 years) 60 (under 1 year)	po every 4 h maximum daily adult dose 2.4 g; maximum daily child dose 1.2 g
Propoxyphene HCl (Darvon)	65	—	po every 3–4 h
Propoxyphene napsalate (Darvon-N)	100	—	po every 4 h
Various mixtures of aspirin and acetaminophen with phenacetin and caffeine			

It is important to remember that analgesics are most effective when given *prior to the onset of pain rather than afterwards*. In view of this, if postoperative pain is expected, the dentist should give patients analgesics while they are still ''protected from pain'' by a local anesthetic.

The various analgesics discussed in this chapter are outlined in Tables 5-1, 5-2, and 5-3.

MILD ANALGESICS

The salicylates are prototypes of mild analgesics and will be discussed extensively, while the aniline derivatives will be discussed only as they differ from the salicylates. These two groups are also referred to as ''antipyretic'' analgesics in order to differentiate them from the narcotics. Propoxyphene is classified

Table 5-2 Analgesics Used in Dental Treatment of Moderate to Moderately Severe Pain

Drug	Dose, mg	Administration
Pentazocine HCl (Talwin)	Adult 50–100	po every 3–4 h
Pentazocine lactate (Talwin)	Adult 30	IM every 3–4 h
Oxycodone (mixture—see text)	Adult 1 tablet Percodan Children 1 tablet Percodan-Demi	1 h preoperatively, then every 6 h
Codeine	Adult 30–60	po every 4 h
Various mixtures of codeine or propoxyphene with aspirin, phenacetin, and/or acetaminophen		

Table 5-3 Analgesics Used in Dental Treatment of Moderately Severe to Severe Pain

Drug	Dose, mg	Administration
Morphine	Adult 10	SC or IM every 3 h
Hydromorphone (Dilaudid)	Adult 2	po or parenterally every 4–5 h
Meperidine (Demerol)	Adult 50–100; children 25 (under 16 years)	po or parenterally every 4 h
Methadone (Dolophine)	Adult 2.5–10	po, SC, IM every 4 h
Anileridine (Leritine)	Adult 25–50	po or IM every 4–6 h
Fentanyl citrate (Sublimaze)	Adult 0.5–0.1	IM; same dose IV every 2–3 min for preoperative and postoperative pain

here because of its weak analgesic effects, but it should be kept in mind that it is pharmacologically similar to the other narcotics.

Salicylates

The bark of the willow tree was known from ancient times for its ability to diminish fever. After its active ingredient, salicin, was identified in the early 1800s, a group of compounds was synthesized that are chemically related to this substance. Three of these compounds, aspirin or acetylsalicylic acid, sodium salicylate, and salicylamide, are useful for their analgesic, antiinflammatory, and antipyretic effects. Aspirin is the most common and most potent salicylate used systemically. Sodium salicylate is less potent than aspirin and more potent than salicylamide, whose clinical effectiveness has been questioned.

Other salicylates, because of their irritant qualities, are used only for their topical effects. Salicylic acid is used as a keratolytic agent, while methyl salicylate is used in salves and ointments as a counterirritant.

Analgesia The salicylates are useful for the relief of mild to moderate pain. They are effective in the treatment of headaches, arthralgia (joint or neural pain), and muscular ache, but are not effective against visceral pain. The analgesic effect is due to both a central and a peripheral component. Decrease in the synthesis of prostaglandins appears to be involved in both the central and the peripheral analgesia, as well as the antiinflammatory and antipyretic actions of the salicylates. In the central nervous system, salicylates reduce the levels of prostaglandins in nerve terminals, and this appears to be involved in blockage of transmission in certain nerves. The hypothalamus is the probable site of central analgesic action. No other sensation besides pain appears to be affected, nor do these drugs produce drowsiness or mental disturbances in analgesic doses.

The peripheral analgesic response occurs at the site where pain originates. Although more evidence is needed, it appears to be produced in the following manner: During the pain response certain chemicals like bradykinin are released from injured tissues and stimulate pain receptors in the area. The prostaglandins, another class of chemicals rapidly synthesized by inflamed tissues, enhance this sensation of pain. The salicylates have a blocking effect on the action of bradykinin and also prevent the synthesis of the prostaglandins. As a result the sensation of pain is decreased.

Antipyresis The term "pyretic" in Greek means fever; therefore an antipyretic drug is one which decreases fever. The salicylates are able to return body temperatures to normal in a feverish person, but do not decrease normal body temperatures. The control of body temperature takes place in the hypothalamus, which acts like a thermostat for the body. It maintains a constant body temperature by establishing a balance between heat production and heat loss. In fever, the thermostat is set higher. During viral or bacterial infections, chemicals called pyrogens which are derived and released from white blood cells (polymorphonuclear leukocytes) stimulate the synthesis of prostaglandins in the brain. In turn the action of prostaglandins on the hypothalamus is equivalent to resetting the thermostat at a higher level. In a manner similar to that described for the analgesic effect, the salicylates inhibit the synthesis of prostaglandins and prevent the pyretic effect.

The lowering of the hypothalamic thermostat by the salicylates results in heat loss due to increased sweating and increased vasodilatation of cutaneous tissues. The evaporation of sweat cools the body, while cutaneous vasodilatation causes a shift of blood from the warmer, deeper parts of the body to the cooler surface where heat is lost to the environment. Reduction of fever by salicylates should be reserved for when the fever is approaching dangerous levels or when considerable physical discomfort is evident. Body temperature must not be allowed to climb to 106°F (41°C) since this high level of heat produces lesions in the brain and other parts of the body. Body temperatures below 104°F need not be treated. At least in some instances it appears that a rise in body temperature may be beneficial. Fever

is known to cause destruction of gonococcal and syphilitic organisms and may also increase the ability of the body to prevent bacterial invasion. It is possible that some benefit is derived from fever in many diseases. Also, when a fever is reduced and the related discomfort is relieved, an underlying disease may be ignored because the person feels better. One must also consider that salicylates only treat the symptoms: they do not affect the disease process itself. High body temperature that is due to dehydration, exercise, or excessive environmental heat is not reduced by salicylates.

Antiinflammatory Effects The salicylates have the ability to reduce inflammation. Various chemical substances that participate in the inflammatory reaction include histamine, the kinins, 5-hydroxytryptamine, and prostaglandins. (See Chap. 16.) Prostaglandins not only contribute directly to inflammation but also potentiate the inflammatory effects of the other mediators. Salicylates, by blocking the synthesis of prostaglandins, not only block their direct effects but decrease the effects of the other mediators as well. Salicylates also block the response of the kinins.

The antiinflammatory effects of the salicylates are particularly important in treating diseases where inflammation is part of a degenerative process which damages or destroys the tissues involved. In rheumatoid arthritis and rheumatic fever, they reduce joint pain and swelling and slow down the accompanying deterioration of tissues. However, the disease process is not affected, and cardiac as well as other complications are not decreased.

The antiinflammatory effect produced by the salicylates is significant only at fairly high doses, 3.6 to 6.0 g daily. The analgesic doses of aspirin usually used in dentistry, 300 to 600 mg every 3 to 4 h, which adds up to 2.4 to 3.6 g daily, may have contributing antiinflammatory effects, especially at the upper dose level. However, increasing the dose to produce a greater antiinflammatory response does not usually produce additional relief and will increase the frequency and severity of side effects.

Uricosuric Effects   A prime factor in the production of gout is the overproduction or decreased elimination of uric acid. Because of the high blood levels of uric acid, deposits of this chemical occur in joints as urate crystals and produce inflammation.

At one time salicylates were used to treat this disease, but now more effective uricosuric agents like allopurinol (Zyloprim), probenecid, (Benemid), and sulfinpyrazone (Anturane) are used for chronic treatment; the antiinflammatory drug colchicine (Colbenemid) is used for acute attacks. Salicylates in large doses (over 5 g per/day) increase the renal excretion of uric acid; however, in low doses they produce an opposite effect, a decrease in uric acid excretion. Even small analgesic doses of salicylates should not be given at the same time as other uricosuric agents because they antagonize the uricosuric effect of these drugs.

Inhibition of Platelet Adhesiveness and Coagulation   Small breaks in capillaries cause platelets to aggregate and clump together. The clumped platelets fill in the breaks and prevent bleeding. Aggregated platelets also contribute to the formation of clots when injury is more extensive. Aspirin in doses as small as 300 mg prevents the adhesion of platelets to each other and decreases the formation of clots. This ability to prevent clot formation is being studied in the prevention of venous and coronary thrombosis (clot formation in veins or the coronary circulation) and pulmonary embolism (a clot which becomes dislodged from a larger blood vessel and becomes lodged in a smaller one in the pulmonary circulation). Because aspirin inhibits platelet adhesiveness it can, in analgesic doses, cause bleeding in patients on anticoagulant therapy and with bleed-

ing tendencies. Since aspirin has a tendency to cause bleeding from the gastric mucosa, there is a special danger of blood loss from this area. Sodium salicylate has a much weaker effect than aspirin on platelet aggregation.

In larger doses (generally over 6 g/day, but this effect has also been reported at doses as low as 2 g) salicylates decrease the formation of prothrombin (a coagulating factor) in a manner similar to that of the oral anticoagulants. However, this effect is usually small and rarely of clinical significance. More importantly, the salicylates decrease the plasma protein binding of oral anticoagulants, thereby increasing the free, active blood level of the anticoagulants. This effect, which results in increased or prolonged bleeding, occurs when doses greater than 3 g/day are used.

Respiratory and Metabolic Effects and Disruption of Acid-Base, Water, and Electrolyte Balance   Salicylates are able to affect respiration and to increase the production of carbon dioxide (CO_2) in the body. Since CO_2 is equivalent to an acid, loss of CO_2 produces alkalosis, and retention produces acidosis. Stimulation or depression of respiration by salicylates will affect the CO_2 level.

In high therapeutic doses, such as are used for the treatment of arthritic conditions (5 g or more), salicylates stimulate respiration by increasing the production of CO_2, which in turn produces stimulation of the respiratory centers of the brain. At this dose level the increased respiration results in the elimination of the excess CO_2 that is being produced. Therefore, no change occurs in acid-base balance. If, however, the increased respiratory response is depressed by drugs like morphine, the excess CO_2 will be retained and acidosis will develop.

Higher doses of salicylates (approximately 12 g) further increase respiration by direct stimulation of the respiratory centers. Excessive loss of CO_2 due to the marked increase in ventilatory rate results in alkalosis. The kidney will compensate by removing bicarbonate (loss of base). This will decrease the severity of the aklakosis and return the body pH toward normal. The loss of bicarbonate (negatively charged ion) is accompanied by the loss of sodium and potassium (positively charged ions) and water. Further increase in dosage (above 12 g in adults and less in children is definitely in the toxic range) leads to depression of the respiratory centers. In this instance, retained CO_2 leads to respiratory acidosis. High doses also produce a metabolic acidosis caused by: (1) the acidity of the salicylates, (2) the disruption of carbohydrate metabolism which results in increased production of organic acids, and (3) impairment of renal function which decreases the elimination of strong acids. All the respiratory and metabolic effects are of prime importance when poisoning with the salicylates occur. (See Side Effects and Toxicity; Overdosage.)

Absorption, Distribution, Biotransformation, and Excretion   Salicylates are weak acids that are well absorbed from the stomach and intestines. Buffered aspirin is absorbed at a somewhat faster rate than unbuffered aspirin, but the differences are minimal. Absorption is improved when salicylates are taken with a full glass of water rather than just a few mouthfuls. Distribution and elimination are strongly affected by the pH of tissues. Biotransformation to salicylic acid, an active product, occurs in the gastrointestinal tract, the plasma, and liver. Salicylic acid is excreted unchanged and as conjugated products of glycine and glucuronic acid. In basic urine, up to 85 percent of salicylic acid is excreted unchanged, while in acid urine this may be as low as 5 percent.

Therapeutic Uses   The most important use of the salicylates in dentistry and medicine is for the alleviation of pain. These drugs also have important antiinflammatory and an-

tipyretic effects. They are used to reduce inflammation, fever, and pain in rheumatoid diseases and to decrease fever and discomfort due to colds and other infections.

Side Effects and Toxicity   The most common side effects of salicylates are the results of irritation of the gastric mucosa. These include nausea, vomiting, gastrointestinal discomfort, and the loss of small amounts of blood from gastrointestinal mucosa. Large therapeutic doses stimulate a center in the brain called the chemoreceptor trigger zone (CTZ) which also produces nausea and vomiting. Salicylates will aggravate existing peptic ulcers and may contribute to the formation of new ones. Disturbances of carbohydrate metabolism can cause hypoglycemia in certain diabetics which can result in loss of therapeutic control of the diabetes.

Overdosage   Since over 12,000 tons of aspirin are sold in the United States each year, it is not surprising that toxic effects due to overdosage and accidental poisoning occur frequently. Children are the frequent victims of the careless handling of these drugs. Mild toxicity called salicylism, which usually occurs after prolonged treatment with large doses, is characterized by nausea, vomiting, diarrhea, dimness of vision, hearing loss, drowsiness, tingling in ears (tinnitus), sweating, fever, thirst, and hyperventilation.

More severe intoxication in adults is usually due to ingestion of a single large dose. Severe disturbances of acid-base balance occurs. Alkalosis when present will increase the excitability of the central nervous system and produce lightheadedness, numbness and tingling of the extremeties, and numbness around the mouth. Development of acidosis will depress the central nervous system and lead to coma. Delirium, hallucinations, and convulsions may precede the coma. Hypoglycemia is present, and potassium deficit may occur. Fever (the opposite of the therapeutic antipyretic effect) is present and is especially severe in children. Various types of skin eruptions may occur. Hemorrhages can result from damage to the gastric mucosa and interference with the clotting mechanism. Loss of water due to loss of electrolytes, as well as from fever and sweating, can cause severe dehydration. (Also see Respiratory and Metabolic Effects, and Disruption of Acid-Base, Water, and Electrolyte Balance.)

Treatment consists of adjusting the acid-base balance, administration of glucose to counter the hypoglycemia, and replacement of fluids and electrolytes. It is especially important to counter the acidosis since an acidotic patient will retain higher levels of salicylates in tissues, and increasing the pH results in increased elimination by the kidneys. Treatment of salicylate poisoning is frequently unsatisfactory, and death may result.

Allergic Reactions These can occur with all the salicylates but are most frequently the result of aspirin administration. Skin rashes and asthmatic attacks occur most frequently, while angioedema accompanied by laryngeal swelling is not uncommon. Death may result from asthma and laryngeal swelling because of interference with respiration.

Salicylates produce allergic reactions most frequently in persons who have a history of allergic diseases, especially asthma, and caution should be exercised when prescribing for these patients.

Acetylsalicylic Acid (Aspirin) All the effects described above for the salicylates apply to aspirin. It can be administered either orally or as a suppository (see Table 5-1).

Sodium Salicylate Sodium salicylate is similar to aspirin but it is less potent. Unlike aspirin, sodium salicylate does not decrease platelet adhesiveness. It is available as tablets containing 300 to 600 mg of drug.

Salicylamide Salicylamide is no longer an official drug. It is less effective than aspirin or sodium salicylate. Its effects are unreliable and its use is not recommended.

Topical Uses of Salicylates Two other salicylates, salicylic acid and methyl salicylate, are too irritating to be used systemically but have limited use when applied topically.

Salicylic Acid This drug is used as a keratolytic agent. It is employed as a wart and corn remover and for the treatment of athlete's foot.

Methyl Salicylate This drug is useful as a counterirritant for the treatment of painful muscles and joints. Systemic poisoning resulting in death has occurred due to absorption from the skin. Poisoning with this drug is common in children.

Aniline Derivatives

The two aniline derivatives used therapeutically are phenacetin and acetaminophen. These drugs are similar to the salicylates in analgesic and antipyretic effects. They are also able to decrease prothrombin levels and increase bleeding tendencies with prolonged use of large doses. However, they do not have any effect on platelet adhesiveness. Unlike the salicylates, the antiinflammatory effect is too weak to be useful in the treatment of rheumatoid diseases. These drugs do not cause gastrointestinal ulceration or bleeding or affect respiration and acid-base balance. They do not produce a uricosuric effect.

Poisoning is as harmful with these drugs as with salicylates. Liver and kidney damage can be produced with both drugs, while methemoglobinemia and destruction of red blood cells occurs mainly with phenacetin. Seventy-five to eighty percent of phenacetin is converted to acetaminophen in the body. Most of the pharmacological effects are due to acetaminophen, but phenacetin itself is also active. Minor biotransformation products of both compounds are responsible for many of the toxic effects of these two drugs.

Acetaminophen (Tylenol, Tempra) Acetaminophen is becoming as popular as aspirin for its use as an analgesic and antipyretic. It is well tolerated when proper analgesic doses are used. The main advantage when compared to aspirin is the fact that it does not produce or aggravate peptic ulcers or cause gastrointestinal disturbances or bleeding.

Side Effects and Toxicity Allergic reactions are rare but can be serious. Urticaria, laryngeal edema, and agranulocytosis have been reported.

Overdosage Ingestion of excessive amounts can cause liver necrosis which is potentially fatal. Necrosis of the kidney tubules, hypoglycemia, and thrombocytopenia can also occur. The ability to cause methemoglobinemia is minimal when compared to phenacetin and is rarely of significance. Prolonged administration of full analgesic doses can potentiate the hypoprothrombic effects of anticoagulants. This drug should not be administered for more than 10 days without consulting a physician. The total dose consumed in 1 day should not exceed 2.4 g. It should not be administered to children under 3 years of age, unless authorized by the dental practitioner or physician.

Phenacetin This drug is no longer official. It is rarely used alone but is primarily employed in analgesic mixtures. It has the same therapeutic effects as acetaminophen but differs to some extent in toxicity. Like acetaminophen, excessive amounts can cause liver and kidney necrosis and hypoglycemia. Overdosage or chronic use can produce a significant amount of methemoglobinemia and hemolysis of red blood cells. Central nervous system effects such as sedation, restlessness, excitement, and euphoria have been noted with phenacetin. The average adult dose is 300

mg, and the total dose per day should not exceed 2.4 g.

Propoxyphene (Darvon)

This drug is listed here for convenience because of its mild analgesic action. However, it should be remembered that it is related in structure and function to methadone, a strong narcotic. At the usual 65-mg dose it is probably equivalent to aspirin in analgesic potency. However, when used with the salicylates or aniline derivatives, the analgesic effect is potentiated, and the combination is useful in treating moderate to moderately severe pain.

Propoxyphene should not be used with alcohol because excessive sedation could result. It also should not be used with other drugs that produce sedation unless prescribed by a dentist or physician who is aware that the two types of drugs are being used together. Propoxyphene has a low addiction liability when compared to stronger narcotics, but it resembles them when large amounts are taken. Like other narcotics, the pharmacological and toxic effects can be reversed by narcotic antagonists. Also, chronic use during pregnancy will produce physical dependency and withdrawal symptoms in the newborn. Propoxyphene has become a seriously abused drug in the United States and is frequently involved in suicide attempts. It is best not to prescribe it in excessively large amounts. In usual analgesic doses the most frequent side effects are nausea, vomiting, dizziness, and sedation. These effects are less prominent when a patient is lying down. Less frequently occurring reactions include headache, weakness, euphoria or dysphoria, and gastrointestinal and minor visual disturbances.

Moderate Analgesics

Drugs in this category are the less potent members of the narcotic group. Codeine is the classic example. In addition, combination of weak narcotics with the antipyretic analgesics potentiate the analgesic effects and keep side effects at a minimum. Combinations are more effective than weak narcotics used alone for the treatment of moderately severe pain. The increased analgesic effect occurs because the narcotics at this level primarily decrease the subjective components of pain, while the antipyretic analgesics raise the pain threshold. (For details on narcotic effects refer to the section on morphine.)

Codeine   This drug is a natural substance found in opium. It has approximately one-twelfth the potency of morphine. The mechanisms of action, pharmacological, and toxic effects of codeine are similar but much weaker than morphine. Codeine is very effective when given orally. The fact that codeine is less potent is important because in the doses given it has less addiction potential and produces few side effects. In dentistry codeine is used when analgesics stronger than aspirin or acetaminophen are required. Codeine is frequently used along with aspirin. These two types of drugs enhance each other's analgesic effect. Codeine may be used with a sedative to produce sleep in the presence of pain. Codeine is also used for its antitussive (anticough) effects.

Oxycodone (Percodan)   This drug is a semisynthetic. It is less potent than morphine when taken alone. Like codeine it is effective when taken orally. In available doses it resembles codeine in analgesic effect. It is available as an analgesic only in combination with other drugs. Percodan contains 4.9 mg of oxycodone, 224 mg of aspirin, 160 mg of phenacetin, and 32 mg of caffeine. Percodan-Demi is the same as Percodan except that the dose of oxycodone is 2.4 mg.

Pentazocine (Talwin)   This drug, which possesses both narcotic effects and weak antagonistic activity, was developed for the express purpose of producing an analgesic with lowered addiction liability. It is effective as an analgesic but too weak to be used as an antagonist. Pentazocine appears to be similar in potency to codeine, and the side effects in therapeutic doses are similar to other narcotics. Unlike the narcotics that do not have antagonistic effects, respiratory depression does not increase as rapidly when increasing doses are given. In doses above 60 mg effects such as anxiety, nightmares, and hallucinations have been reported. These are effects which occur with other weak antagonists and not with narcotics. This drug should be used with caution in persons who have received other narcotics since it may precipitate withdrawal symptoms. The addiction potential is low, approximating that of propoxyphene.

STRONG ANALGESICS

Morphine is the prototype of "strong" analgesics. Confusion exists concerning the terminology used to classify drugs that are related to morphine in structure and function. Some classify all these drugs as narcotics. Others only classify as narcotics the strong analgesic drugs that are potentially very addicting and are included in Schedule II of the Controlled Substances Act of 1970 (see Chap. 22). They classify the milder drugs that are not subject to this control and have a low potential for addiction as nonnarcotics. The first classification will be used here because these drugs act in a similar manner and differ mainly in potency; therefore, all agents related to morphine in structure and function will be referred to as narcotics.

Evidence indicates that a specific receptor exists in nervous tissue of the central and peripheral nervous systems that mediates the various effects of the narcotics. Although the chemical formulas of some of the synthetic narcotics appear to be unrelated, they have a three-dimensional structure in common that would account for action on a similar receptor. Recently, substances called enkephalins have been identified in brain tissue. These naturally occurring or endogenous compounds resemble the narcotics in their effects and are probably the natural chemical mediators that activate the narcotic-sensitive receptors of nervous tissue. It can be postulated that these natural substances modify pain by interacting with these receptors and that the narcotics produce their effects by the same pathway.

The effect of narcotics on pain is twofold. They have in common with the antipyretic analgesics the ability to raise the threshold of pain. In addition they alter the subjective component of pain, the suffering that pain causes. Suffering varies considerably among individuals and is related to a person's history and general ideas concerning pain. At the lower dose range these agents affect the reaction to pain to a greater extent than the pain threshold. Patients will say that they still feel the pain but do not mind it.

Narcotics in therapeutic doses also produce respiratory depression, drowsiness, and mental clouding. Usually euphoria is present, but dysphoria occurs occasionally. In the euphoric ("high") state, there is an increased sense of well-being, bodily comfort, and absence of pain or distress, while restlessness, anxiety, and discomfort characterize the dysphoric state. Patients receiving these drugs should be warned that driving a car or using heavy machinery could be hazardous. The sedative effects are enhanced by other drugs which depress the central nervous system. Development of physical and psychological dependence is prominent with the more potent members of this group.

Opium

Opium is the dried milky fluid that is obtained from the unripe capsules of the poppy. It contains two commonly used narcotics, morphine and codeine, as well as many other pharmacologically active nonnarcotic alkaloids.

Opium is a preparation known since ancient times and used for both medical and religious purposes. Even 6000 years ago the ancient Sumarians appeared to understand the psychological effects of opium since they referred to the poppy as the "joy" plant.

Morphine and Its Pharmacological Effects

Morphine is the prototype drug for narcotic analgesics. Its effects are discussed in detail below. The other drugs will be discussed briefly, pointing out how they differ from morphine. Many drugs have been synthesized that are analogs (structurally related) of morphine; however, none are superior in analgesic effects.

Many of the pharmacological effects of morphine are due to actions on the central nervous system (CNS), whereas a few are the results of activity on smooth muscle.

Analgesia and Other CNS Effects All forms of pain can be relieved by morphine. It is, however, more effective against dull, chronic pain than sharp, intermittent pain. Analgesia is usually accompanied by drowsiness, decreased physical activity, and difficulty in thinking. There is a tendency to fall asleep when the environment is quiet. Some patients experience euphoria. Occasionally a patient may experience excitement and delirium as well as dysphoria.

Effects on Respiration Morphine has a potent effect on the respiratory centers of the brain. It decreases the sensitivity of these centers to stimulation by carbon dioxide. Some degree of respiratory depression occurs even with small therapeutic doses. This effect is dose dependent and becomes greater with increasing doses until respiratory arrest occurs. Death from overdosage is generally due to respiratory failure. Accumulation of carbon dioxide may be the cause of cerebral vasodilatation and increased cranial pressure that occur after administration.

Gastrointestinal Effects   Morphine is able to produce nausea and vomiting by an action on the chemoreceptor trigger zone in the medullary area of the brain. This generally happens upon first administration but rarely occurs with subsequent doses. This is because morphine also depresses the vomiting center, which no longer responds to stimulation from the chemoreceptor trigger zone. Morphine increases the tone but decreases the propulsive activity of the gastrointestinal tract. This results in delayed absorption of food and constipation. There is also a tendency to ignore the normal sensations that trigger the defecation reflex. Therefore, drugs in this category are very effective in treating diarrhea.

Effect on Pupils   Morphine produces constriction of the pupil of the eye due to a CNS effect. Little tolerance develops to this effect, and morphine addicts typically have constricted pupils.

Effects on the Urinary Tract   Morphine produces urinary retention sometimes accompanied by an increase in desire to urinate. Urinary retention is caused by an increase in the tone of the urinary sphincter which makes urination difficult and an increase in the release of the antidiuretic hormone which decreases the formation of urine.

In contrast, the ability of morphine also to increase the tone of the detrusor muscle of the urinary bladder produces a desire to urinate. However, this sensation may be ignored because of the central effects of this drug. Increased tone of the ureters also occurs, yet morphine produces relief in ureteral colic because of its analgesic effects. Morphine and other strong narcotic analgesics should be used with caution in patients with prostatic hypertrophy since the difficulty in urination which is present in this condition is aggravated by these drugs.

Physical Dependence and Withdrawal Symptoms   When morphine is administered several times daily, with doses totaling 10 mg, for 1 or 2 weeks, withdrawal of the drug produces mild symptoms of discomfort. With increasing doses, more frequent doses, or administration for a longer period of time, the symptoms of withdrawal become increasingly severe. Symptoms are also more severe when withdrawal is abrupt.

Severe withdrawal produces the following symptoms: yawning, restless sleep, dilated pupils, goose flesh, irritability, tremors, sneezing, lacrimation, anorexia, abdominal cramps, nausea, vomiting, diarrhea, chills, sweating, increased heart rate and blood pressure, muscle and bone pain, muscle spasms, kicking movements, weakness, and depression.

The major symptoms subside after a period of 7 to 10 days. However, it takes many more weeks before all physiological and psychological parameters return to normal.

The administration of morphine at any time during either the immediate or the prolonged abstinence period results in a reversal of all these symptoms.

Tolerance   After approximately 1 week of daily use, tolerance develops to the analgesic, respiratory depressant, sedative, euphoric, and emetic effects of morphine. Tolerance develops equally to the toxic effects, and morphine addicts can tolerate many times the dose that would be lethal in a normal individual. Tolerance does not develop to any extent to pupillary constriction or to constipation.

Psychological Dependence   Many factors contribute to the development of psychological dependence. The increasing tolerance which occurs after repeated injections of morphine leads to the administration of increasing doses in order to maintain the desired analgesic or euphoric effects. Increasing doses result in greater physical dependence. The physical dependence initially stimulates drug-seeking behavior in order to reduce or prevent the symptoms of withdrawal. However, later, even when complete withdrawal has taken place, other factors contribute to compulsive drug use. There is the desire to experience again the euphoric effects of the drug or to eliminate the pain and anxiety which previous experience demonstrated would be relieved by the drug. In some individuals, an intense euphoria or relief of distress increases the drug dependency. The social environment also plays a role. Drug addicts who return to an environment where drug use is prevalent and socially acceptable will have their drug dependency reinforced.

Therapeutic Uses Morphine is used as a preanesthetic drug and for the treatment of moderately severe to severe pain. It has an important use in the treatment of postoperative pain and the pain of terminal illnesses.

Morphine relieves the dyspnea (difficult and labored breathing) caused by pulmonary edema of acute left ventricular failure. It is not known whether this effect is due to improved respiration because of decreased pain and reduced anxiety or to direct cardiovascular effects.

Dosage, Absorption, and Biotransformation Morphine is well absorbed by the subcutaneous (SC) and intramuscular (IM) routes which are normally used. Occasionally it is given by the intravenous (IV) route for a more rapid effect. The oral route is not used since it is less effective. The usual dose is 10 mg per 70 kg body weight. Most of the drug is conjugated in the liver to the glucuronide.

Side Effects and Toxicity Therapeutic doses may produce nausea, vomiting, drowsiness, sedation or excitement, dizziness, euphoria or dysphoria, and a decrease in physical activity and mental functions. Physical dependency and withdrawal symptoms will occur after chronic use. Psychological dependency may develop. Chronic use during pregnancy will cause withdrawal symptoms in the newborn. Allergic reactions are rare and usually are manifested as skin rashes and urticaria. Anaphylactoid reactions have been reported after administration of morphine IV.

Overdosage High doses of morphine will produce severe respiratory depression which leads to cyanosis, a fall in blood pressure, and coma. The patient will appear asleep or in a stupor and have pinpoint pupils. Convulsions may occur in infants and children. A narcotic antagonist will rapidly reverse all these effects as long as tissue damage has not occurred. Narcotic antagonists must be used with care in morphine addicts since these drugs will precipitate withdrawal.

Contraindications Morphine produces bronchoconstriction and should not be administered to asthmatics. Great caution must be exercised if these drugs are to be used in patients with severe respiratory difficulties such as those associated with diseases like emphysema. It should not be used in patients with neurotic or hysterical tendencies since it can produce excitement and delirium in these persons. Morphine can increase intracranial pressure and is contraindicated in patients with jaw fractures and other head injuries.

Drug Interactions Great care must be taken when morphine is used with the phenothiazines, monoamine oxidase inhibitors, and tricyclic antidepressants, since these drugs intensify the depressant effects of morphine.

Semisynthetics

These compounds are synthesized by modifying the basic structure of morphine. They differ from morphine mainly in their potency.

Hydromorphone (Dilaudid) This drug is 5 times more potent than morphine. It has a rapid onset of action and short duration. The adult dose is 2 mg orally (po) and 1 mg SC.

Oxymorphone (Numorphan) Potency is 10 times greater than morphine. The adult dose of 1 mg SC is comparable to 10 mg of morphine.

Hydrocodone (Dicodid) Potency of this drug is between morphine and codeine. It is used primarily to relieve cough but is probably no better than other narcotics in producing this effect. The adult antitussive dose is 5 to 10 mg po.

Synthetic Narcotics

The pharmacological and toxicological actions produced by these drugs resemble those of morphine. Although the chemical structures of these drugs do not resemble that of morphine, they are similar in both three-dimensional aspects and reactive sites.

Meperidine (Demerol) This drug is approximately 10 times *less* potent than morphine when given SC. It is also effective when absorbed po. It provides effective analgesia against moderately severe pain. Since it is less potent, it produces fewer side effects. In equivalent analgesic doses meperidine produces less constipation than morphine and in toxic doses may sometimes produce tremors, muscle twitches, and seizures. The adult dose is 50 mg, and the dose for children under 16 is 25 mg. Promethazine hydrochloride potentiates the effects of meperidine, and these two drugs are sometimes used together.

Methadone (Dolophine) Methadone is somewhat more effective than morphine when administered SC, but unlike morphine it is effective po. It produces less sedation than morphine when used infrequently. However, repeated administration may produce marked sedative effects. Methadone is used to suppress withdrawal symptoms for an extended period of time in narcotic-dependent individuals. Euphoria is less prominent with methadone, and psychological dependence

does not develop as frequently as it does with morphine. Methadone is used for the treatment of moderately severe to severe pain. The usual adult oral dose is 2.5 mg. For severe pain, 5 to 10 mg may be used. It may be administered po, SC, or IM.

Anileridine (Leritine) This drug is similar to meperidine but it is more potent. The usual adult dose is 25 mg IM or po. For severe pain 50 mg may be used.

Fentanyl Citrate (Sublimaze) Fentanyl is a potent narcotic with a rapid onset and short duration of action. It may be used IV and will produce a peak effect in 3 to 5 min. The duration of analgesia is approximately 1 h. Fentanyl is especially useful for surgery of short duration which is performed in outpatients. The IV dose is 0.05 to 0.1 mg every 3 min until the desired effect is achieved. The IM dose is 0.05 to 0.1 mg.

Narcotic Antagonists

Naloxone (Narcan) This narcotic antagonist is able to reverse completely all the effects of narcotics as long as it is administered before any secondary damage has occurred (for example, tissue damage due to lack of oxygen, dehydration, acid-base imbalance). Naloxone is also capable of reversing the pharmacological effects of drugs like pentazocine that have dual agonistic and antagonistic narcotic actions. Since naloxone has little or no narcotic action of its own, it is preferred for narcotic antagonism. Naloxone is used for the treatment of narcotic overdosage; however, in addicts it must be used with care because it can precipitate withdrawal symptoms. When narcotics are used as preanesthetic medication and during surgery, naloxone can produce a rapid reversal of effects when the operation is over. In oral surgery this is useful in facilitating early discharge of ambulatory patients.

Naloxone may be administered by IV, IM, or SC routes. The usual adult dose is 0.4 mg which can be administered at approximately 3-min intervals.

Nalorphine (Nalline)   This drug is a partial agonist. When it is used alone, it has the effects of a weak morphine; however, it is also capable of antagonizing the effects of morphine and other narcotics. Since the agonist effects are too weak to be useful therapeutically, the drug is used as a narcotic antagonist. It will not antagonize the effects of other partial agonists that have significant analgesic activity. (See Moderate Analgesics: Pentazocine.)

ANSWER TO CHAPTER CASE

Aspirin or drug combinations containing any of the salicylates may aggravate ulcers and should be avoided. Besides producing pain the ulcers may perforate and severe bleeding result. Acetaminophen (Tylenol) should be prescribed for this patient.

QUESTIONS

1 How do the narcotic analgesics differ from the nonnarcotic analgesics?
2 What category of analgesics produce physical and psychological dependence, the development of tolerance, and withdrawal symptoms? Define these terms.
3 What type of drugs are effective against severe pain?
4 Is aspirin frequently effective in treating pain of dental origin?
5 When is the best time to administer an analgesic to a dental patient?
6 What adverse reactions can be produced by analgesics that contain aspirin, phenacetin, acetaminophen (Tylenol), codeine, or propoxyphene (Darvon)?

READING REFERENCES

Allen, G. D., and R. A. Meyer, "An Evaluation of the Analgesic Activity of Meperidine and Fentanyl," *Anes. Prog.,* **20:**72–75, 1973.

Boyer, T. D., and S. L. Rouff, "Acetaminophen Induced Hepatic Necrosis and Renal Failure," *J. Am. Med. Assoc.,* **218:**440–441, 1971.

Council on Dental Therapeutics, *Analgesics in Accepted Dental Therapeutics,* American Dental Association, 1977, pp. 131–148.

Hoon, J. R., "Bleeding Gastritis Induced by Long-Term Release Aspirin," *J. Am. Med. Assoc.,* **229:**841–842, 1974.

Jaffee, J. H., and W. R. Martin, "Narcotic Analgesics and Antagonists," in L. S. Goodman and A. Gilman (eds.), *Pharmacological Basis of Therapeutics,* Macmillan, 1975, pp. 245–283.

Miller, R. R., A. Feingold, and J. Paxinos, "Propoxyphene Hydrochloride: A Critical Review," *J. Am. Med. Assoc.,* **213:**996–1006, 1970.

Nelson, J. E., and P. C. Bourgault, "Current Concepts of Analgesic Action," The Fourth Symposium of the Pharmacology, Therapeutics and Toxicology Group of the International Association for Dental Research, 1978.

Weiss, H. J., "Aspirin—A Dangerous Drug?" *J. Am. Med. Assoc.,* **229:**1221–1222, 1974.

Sedatives, Hypnotics, and Tranquilizers

A patient reports to the dental office for her semiannual prophylaxis. She is wearing a maxillary partial denture. Her medical history states that she is taking tranquilizers daily and has done so for 6 months. You note that areas under the partial denture are red but not painful. Can this redness be possibly related to her drug therapy?

The dental situation can produce anxiety, excitement, and fear in a patient. Frequently, this can be alleviated if the dentist and the dental auxiliaries appear confident and carefully explain the procedure and the degree of discomfort that can be expected. When this approach fails, various groups of drugs can be administered in order to quiet the patient.

Production of moderate sedation is achieved with oral administration of drugs classified as sedative-hypnotics, the antianxiety drugs (minor tranquilizers), and the sedative-antihistamines, as well as inhalation of nitrous oxide.

Many of these same drugs, plus the narcotics and the major tranquilizers, are given intravenously (IV) alone or in combination to produce deep sedation when severe anxiety exists or when prolonged or traumatic procedures are required. Deep sedation should be administered by personnel qualified to give general anesthesia since there is danger that the patient may become unconscious.

PATIENT CARE AND PRECAUTIONS

Nitrous oxide inhalation and oral administration of the various sedatives and antianxiety drugs provide the least potent method of assuring adequate operating conditions with minimal upset of the patient's bodily function and daily routine. (Nitrous oxide and IV sedation are discussed in Chap. 8.)

Sedative effects by oral administration may usually be achieved by prescribing a drug for 1 or 2 days before an appointment or by administering a single, usually larger dose at an appropriate time so that the peak effect of the drug is achieved at about the same time that the dental procedure begins. All these drugs are capable of producing drowsiness and lack of coordination. Patients should be warned that *these and other effects can be dangerously enhanced if alcohol or other sedative drugs are ingested at the same time.* Serious central nervous system depressant effects can produce unconsciousness and respiratory depression which can threaten life. Another problem involves the driving of a motor vehicle or working with heavy machinery, which may become hazardous under the influence of these drugs.

When these drugs are given at the lower end of the dose range in the manner that a physician prescribes sedative drugs, it is not necessary that a patient be driven to and from the office. However, he should be queried as to whether he has taken this type of medication before and what effect it had on him. He should be warned of the possible side effects. The first dose should be taken at home and the patient should observe his responses. If no side effects occur, then it should be safe for the patient to drive himself to the office. On the other hand, if the dose administered is in the upper end of the dose range (diazepam, 10 mg), the patient should be driven to and from the dental office. He should be warned to avoid driving and not to operate heavy machinery for the rest of the day. He should also be warned if the drug is capable of producing residual effects for several days afterward. During this time period, in some individuals, driving and the use of heavy machinery could be

hazardous. In addition, during this time period ingestion of alcohol or other central nervous system (CNS) depressants could enhance these side effects.

Among the disadvantages of oral administration is the difficulty of obtaining the proper dose response since a standard dose may be inadequate in some patients but produce drowsiness in others. It is difficult to increase the dose within the time period allowed, and the appointment may have to be cancelled. Control is lost when a drug is being self-administered by a patient. Frequently, the prescribed dose will not be taken in the proper amount and at the proper time. This is especially true for children when they receive liquid medication (frequently prescribed because it is administered with greater ease). They may spill or spit some of it out, and as a result the dose received may be inadequate. The patient should receive detailed instructions about taking a drug, and the importance of following these exactly should be pointed out.

BARBITURATE SEDATIVES AND HYPNOTICS

The barbiturates have been in use for sedation and to induce sleep since the early 1900s. They are still good and safe drugs but are presently used less than the antianxiety drugs diazepam (Valium) and chlordiazepoxide (Librium).

The barbiturates are classified according to their duration of action—ultrashort, short to intermediate, and long. They are capable of producing all levels of CNS depression, from light sedation to coma and death. They differ from each other primarily in onset and duration of action, which is due primarily to variations in the fat solubility of these agents.

For moderate sedation, these drugs are used in low enough doses so that anxiety and fear are lessened, the patient is relaxed, muscle tone is reduced, and the patient is capable of better cooperation. The same drugs, called *hypnotics,* given in larger doses, are used to produce sleep.

Effects of Lipid Solubility

The barbiturates that are highly lipid soluble enter the CNS without delay producing a rapid onset of action. Those that are less lipid soluble pass into the CNS more slowly and therefore take longer to achieve a response. The highly lipid soluble drugs are also metabolized more rapidly producing a brief duration of action. The less lipid soluble drugs are metabolized slowly and excreted partly unchanged resulting in a longer duration of action. In addition, the ultrashort-acting barbiturates which are administered IV will, because of high lipid solubility, redistribute from the brain to other parts of the body. This terminates the drug response even though the active drug is still present in the body.

Pharmacological Effects

CNS The barbiturates produce their effects because neurons at different levels of the CNS become inactive. At sedative-hypnotic doses the main effect is on the reticular activating system, that part of the brain which sends arousal signals to the cerebral cortex. At increasing doses there is progressive depression of other parts of the brain resulting in unconsciousness, followed by respiratory depression, coma, and death.

Excitement and Analgesia Inhibition of inhibitory neurons may lead to a state of excitement and delirium. This tends to occur most frequently at lower dose levels, in children, when a hypnotic dose is not followed by sleep, or in the presence of moderately severe pain or psychological disturbances. These drugs have no analgesic action of their own, but sometimes clinically mild to moderate pain may be relieved due to the general sedative effects. However, this action is not reliable. These drugs should only be given with analgesics in the presence of moderate to severe pain. Actually, at low dose levels pain can sometimes be enhanced.

Anticonvulsant Activity All barbiturates are capable of inhibiting convulsions at doses that produce CNS depression approaching unconsciousness. The ultrashort-acting barbiturates are sometimes used IV for this purpose. Some barbiturates like phenobarbital will prevent convulsions at doses that produce little or no sedation. These are used in the treatment of epilepsy.

Other Effects The barbiturates decrease the tone and motility of the gastrointestinal tract. Phenobarbital is frequently used in sedative doses to relieve various gastrointestinal symptoms. These drugs have little effect on respiration and the cardiovascular system in sedative and hypnotic doses. Generally, the only changes seen are those that can be attributed to decreased activity and sleep.

Metabolism and Excretion

The barbiturates are mostly biotransformed by oxidation and conjugation in the liver microsomal system. Almost complete biotransformation of the ultrashort and intermediate drugs occurs, but only 50 percent of phenobarbital is transformed. The rest is excreted unchanged. Excretion is an important pathway for removal of long-acting barbiturates.

Administration and Therapeutic Uses

This depends on onset and duration of action. The ultrashort-acting barbiturates are used IV to produce general anesthesia. All the others may be used for daytime sedation and to produce sleep. (See Table 6-1.) The long-acting barbiturates are usually preferred for daytime sedation over several days since it is easier to maintain a constant blood level. The short-acting drugs are preferred to produce sleep since these are usually metabolized by the time awakening occurs. These drugs can be used in dentistry before a dental procedure

Table 6-1 Barbiturates

Classification	Name	Sedative dose	Hypnotic and preoperative dose
Long acting	Phenobarbital (Luminal)	15–30 mg 2–4 times daily	100 mg 1–2 h before procedure
Short to intermediate acting	Amobarbital (Amytal); pentobarbital (Nembutal); secobarbital (Seconal)	30–60 mg 2–4 times daily	100 mg ½–1 hr before procedure
Ultrashort acting	Thiopental (Pentothal); methohexital (Brevital)	IV for general anesthesia; individual adjustment in dosage needed	

and to produce sleep the night before and after an appointment. An analgesic should also be given when pain is present after treatment. The sedative-hypnotics are usually given po but may also be administered intramuscularly (IM) and IV. However, they are too irritating to be injected SC. Because the barbiturates are frequently used to commit suicide, only a few days' supply should be prescribed at one time.

Side Effects and Toxicity

In sedative and hypnotic doses, these drugs produce few side effects. Drowsiness and loss of coordination sometimes occur and may endanger the person who drives or uses heavy machinery. Symptoms resembling a hangover may rarely occur following awakening after a hypnotic dose. Allergic reactions consisting of skin eruptions, urticaria, and angioedema are seen infrequently. The serious allergic reactions of exfoliative dermatitis and liver damage are extremely rare but have been reported.

Barbiturate Overdosage Overdosage with these drugs leads to respiratory paralysis, cardiovascular depression, and renal shutdown. Treatment is directed toward maintenance of respiration and circulation. Sodium bicarbonate and osmotic diuretics are given to increase drug excretion. In addition, the osmotic diuretics help maintain kidney function by increasing excretion by the kidney. CNS stimulants like doxapram (Dopram) are sometimes used in emergencies.

Drug Dependence Prolonged use of these drugs results in the development of physical and psychological dependence and tolerance. After continuous use, withdrawal results in the production of anxiety, tremors, excitement, and convulsions. However, these problems do not develop from the short periods involved in the use of these drugs in dentistry. The main danger involves the possibility of inadvertently prescribing these drugs to an addict.

Drug Interactions

All drugs which depress the CNS have an additive effect when used together. Serious CNS depression can occur if this is not taken into consideration. The drugs in this category include the general anesthetics, the sedative-hypnotics, alcohol, the tranquilizers, the antidepressants, and the narcotic analgesics.

The barbiturates stimulate the synthesis of liver microsomal enzymes and therefore decrease the activity of drugs whose biotransformation depends on these enzymes. By this process barbiturates decrease their own activity, the activity of anticoagulants, phenytoin (diphenylhydantoin, Dilantin), and tricyclic antidepressants. On the other hand, the monoamine oxidase (MAO) inhibitors will enhance the effects of barbiturates by inhibiting their metabolism.

Contraindications and Precautions

The only known absolute contraindication to the barbiturates is the disease porphyria. Patients with this disease have an abnormal amount of porphyrins in the blood. Barbiturates stimulate the production of porphyrins and aggravate this disease. The long-acting barbiturates should be used with caution in the presence of kidney disease, while the others should be used with caution in the presence of liver disease. The potential for drug dependency and the narrow range between the therapeutic doses and the toxic doses are serious disadvantages of the barbiturates. Oversedation can occur easily. These drugs are frequently used to commit suicide, and death can occur rapidly from overdosage (1 g or more).

MISCELLANEOUS SEDATIVES AND HYPNOTICS

These drugs have similar effects to the barbiturates and can be used when barbiturates are contraindicated. Prolonged administration of these drugs can lead to physical and psychological dependence, the development of tolerance, and withdrawal symptoms upon termination. The pharmacology of these drugs is not known as well as that of the barbiturates. This can be a disadvantage in case of overdosage.

Chloral Hydrate

Chloral hydrate is similar in onset and duration of action to the short-acting barbiturates. It is a good sedative-hypnotic for every kind of patient but is frequently preferred for children, debilitated patients, and the elderly. The excitement phase appears less frequently with this drug than with other sedative-hypnotics. It is irritating to the gastric mucosa and can produce nausea and vomiting. This can be prevented by administering chloral hydrate with large amounts of fluids. Chloral hydrate is contraindicated in patients with known hepatic or renal and circulatory impairment, and it can potentiate the effects of oral anticoagulants when the initial dose of chloral hydrate is administered to a patient on anticoagulant therapy. This effect is not seen with repeated administration of chloral hydrate.

Other Sedative-Hypnotics

Many other agents are used for sedative and hypnotic effects. These include the following: (1) Glutethimide (Doriden) is a drug resembling the short to intermediate barbiturates in therapeutic doses. However, overdosage causes greater hypotension than the barbiturates and produces the atropinelike effects of mydriasis, dry mouth, and loss of function of the gastrointestinal tract and the urinary bladder. This drug is similar to the barbiturates in producing increased synthesis of liver microsomal enzymes. For this reason glutethimide will also decrease the activity of oral anticoagulants, phenytoin, and the tricyclic antidepressants. It is also contraindicated in porphyria. (2) Propriomazine (Largon) is a potent sedative and adjunct to anesthesia and analgesia and may be used to promote sleep. The use of other depressants should be cut at least in half in the presence of this drug. (3) Ethchlorvynol (Placidyl) produces sleep in 15 min to 1 h. Duration of effect is approximately 5 h. It is contraindicated in porphyria and decreases the activity of oral anticoagulants.

ANTIANXIETY DRUGS (MINOR TRANQUILIZERS)

Considerable overlap occurs in classification of antianxiety drugs and the sedative-hypnotics. There is even greater difficulty in trying to differentiate between the effects of the two groups. In this section the two major groups of antianxiety drugs, the benzodiazepines and propanediols, will frequently be compared to the barbiturates in order to point out their advantages and disadvantages. Both the antianxiety drugs and the sedative-hypnotics are used in a similar manner therapeutically. They can be used for the treatment of overexcitement and anxiety that is due to either a stressful situation or to a neurosis. They are effective when used orally (po) for preoperative sedation, parenterally for deep sedation, as preanesthetic sedatives, and to produce sleep.

The antianxiety drugs, especially the benzodiazepine derivatives, have distinct advantages over the barbiturates. Reduction of anxiety with the antianxiety drugs occurs at doses which produce fewer undesirable CNS side effects, such as drowsiness and ataxia and loss of coordination, than are seen with the barbiturates. Less mental and physical impairment also occurs when the antianxiety drugs are used for oral preoperative sedation. In addition, the safety range between the therapeutic doses and the toxic doses is much greater with the antianxiety drugs when compared to the barbiturates. Because of this, suicide attempts with drugs like chlordiazepoxide rarely result in death even though they are used frequently for this purpose. This is in contrast to the barbiturates, where death is a common sequela of poisoning.

The antianxiety drugs also produce skeletal muscle relaxation by means of action on the CNS. This central muscle relaxant effect is prominent when these drugs are administered parenterally. However, this relaxant effect has not been demonstrated to be greater than that which is produced with the barbiturates when administered po. All these drugs will produce some degree of muscle relaxation that is related to their sedative effects.

The Benzodiazepines

Diazepam (Valium) and chlordiazepoxide (Librium) are the most popular antianxiety drugs presently in use in the United States. Other popular benzodiazepine derivatives include oxazepam (Serax) and clorazepate (Tranxene). Flurazepam (Dalmane) is a related drug that is used primarily as a hypnotic. The various benzodiazepines have similar pharmacological effects but vary mainly in potency, onset, and duration of action.

Pharmacological Effects When the benzodiazepines were administered to animals, they produced an increase in spontaneous and exploratory activity. Behavior which had been motivated because of punishment was suppressed, while behavior that was suppressed due to punishment was restored. Other symptoms of stress and apparent frustration were lessened. Although meprobamate (Miltown) and the barbiturates can also produce these effects, they only do so at doses that also produce drowsiness and ataxia. These effects on behavior appear to be analogous (although unproven) to reduction of anxiety in humans. In the clinical situation reduction of anxiety by the benzodiazepines occurs at doses that produce fewer side effects than those which are produced by the barbiturates.

Generally, in both animals and humans, hostility and aggressive behavior is reduced. However, paradoxically, in certain instances and in certain individuals this behavior is increased. This is similar to the release of hostile behavior that is observed occasionally in persons under the influence of alcohol. It appears that this is due to the suppression of related anxiety which was preventing the latent hostility from being expressed.

These clinical and animal behavioral effects can also be equated with certain actions of these drugs on brain structures. The spread of activity originating in both the limbic system and the reticular formation is suppressed. The limbic system is the old part of the brain which is involved in emotions, and the reticular formation is an area related to awakening or arousal. Both these areas are affected by the benzodiazepines and the barbiturates. However, the limbic system, the area which one would expect to be associated with anxiety, appears to be more sensitive to the benzodiazepines than to the barbiturates. Suppression of the reticular formation occurs at higher doses and is equated with the CNS symptoms of ataxia and drowsiness. The barbiturates affect both the limbic system and the reticular formation within a narrower dose range.

The manner by which the benzodiazepines produce skeletal muscle relaxation is not completely known but appears to involve several sites. These drugs facilitate the action of neurons which have an inhibitory effect on skeletal muscle. This occurs both at the level of the brainstem and the spinal cord. In addition, these drugs can directly depress motor nerve and muscle function.

The benzodiazepines have strong anticonvulsant activity. They are effective in aborting seizures caused by electric shock, analeptic drugs, local anesthetics, and epileptic seizures. They are also effective in suppressing the so-called night terrors, the severe nightmares that sometimes occur during sleep.

Diazepam (Valium) In medicine diazepam is used primarily for the treatment of neurotic anxiety. It is most effective for this purpose when the therapeutic dose used is close to the dose which produces sedative side effects such as drowsiness. For this reason the dosage must be individualized.

Diazepam is more potent than chlordiazepoxide in its central muscle relaxant and anticonvulsive properties. It is used clinically to treat muscle spasticity that accompanies various diseases such as cerebral palsy, multiple sclerosis, and Parkinson's disease. Due to various advantages of the benzodiazepines mentioned previously, these drugs are preferred for treating these conditions. However, their superiority over barbiturates and other sedatives in producing muscle relaxation has not been demonstrated when these drugs are administered by the oral route. However, when diazepam is used IV it is very effective in treating muscle spasticity due to various causes. It is also an excellent drug for aborting repetitive convulsive seizures. Diazepam, like other benzodiazepines, is useful in the treatment of insomnia caused by excessive anxiety. It is the major drug used for the treatment of night terrors.

In dentistry, diazepam and other benzodiazepines are usually preferred to barbiturates when used as sedatives. A successful regime to reduce stress and anxiety and relax a patient before an operative procedure involves using 5 mg of diazepam the night before, 5 mg upon arising, and 10 mg 2 h before the dental procedure. This regimen helps assure a more complete and uniform response. This is due to several factors: a good night's sleep insures a more relaxed patient in the morning; since the drug is long-acting the patient will already be fairly relaxed by the time the preoperative dose is taken; this will contribute to a more uniform sedative effect since stress and anxiety which are present preoperatively contribute to the poor absorption of drugs that are administered po at this time. Diazepam may also be administered as a preanesthetic sedative for techniques utilizing ultrashort-acting barbiturates such as methohexital (Breuital).

Diazepam is used IV for dental procedures lasting approximately 1 h. It produces good sedation, muscle relaxation, and amnesia for events that happen after the injection and not for those that precede it. Amnesia occurs in about 10 min and lasts approximately 45 min. This occurs without much effect on the level of consciousness or the cardiovascular and pulmonary systems.

Diazepam may be administered IM, but absorption by this route is slow and erratic. When diazepam is administered po the peak blood level occurs in approximately 2 h, and distribution to all tissues is rapid. Biotransformation is slow and takes about 1 to 2 days. Two active metabolites are formed in the liver, oxazepam and desmethyldiazepam.

Oxazepam, the major metabolite, has a half-life of 3 to 21 h and is excreted in the urine as the glucuronide. Biotransformation of desmethyldiazepam occurs very slowly over a period of days. The slow metabolism of diazepam and the accumulation of active metabolites may produce residual effects that last for several days. It is especially important that the patient be warned that residual effects can make driving and the operation of machinery hazardous and that additive effects with alcohol and other CNS depressants can occur during this time period.

Physical dependence and tolerance can occur, but only after using large doses for a prolonged period of time. Because of the long life of diazepam and its active metabolites, withdrawal symptoms may be delayed a week or more after administration of the last dose. Psychological dependence does not develop as frequently as with the barbiturates, even when larger doses are used, probably because this drug produces much less euphoria. Diazepam is capable of producing cleft palate in newborn mice when administered to the mother in high doses during pregnancy. For this reason it should not be administered to pregnant women since it is not known whether this effect occurs in humans.

The most common side effects of diazepam are the results of CNS depression and include lightheadedness, dizziness, drowsiness, muscle weakness, and ataxia. These effects are more likely to occur in debilitated and elderly people and after IV administration. Diazepam causes localized pain when injected IV or IM. The pain may be induced either by the propylene glycol vehicle or by the precipitated particles in the solution injected. Intravenous administration should be done with care since an extravascular injection will lead to sloughing of tissues. Phlebitis (inflammation of veins) occurs occasionally after IV injection. Postural hypotension may sometimes occur after IV sedation. Other side effects include xerostomia, skin rashes, nausea, impairment of sexual function, and menstrual irregularities. A few cases of blood dyscrasias and jaundice have been reported. Diazepam is suspected of having anticholinergic effects, and for this reason it should be used with caution in patients with glaucoma or prostatic hypertrophy. (See Chap. 3.)

Chlordiazepoxide (Librium) This drug is similar in antianxiety and sedative effects to diazepam but is less effective as a central muscle relaxant and anticonvulsant. It is the chief drug used to alleviate the symptoms of alcohol withdrawal, although other benzodiazepines are equally effective. In dentistry, chlordiazepoxide is as effective as diazepam as a preoperative sedative, but absorption is slower, requiring 4 h for the peak effect. Intramuscular administration is slow and erratic. Intravenous administration also achieves reliable sedative effects, but diazepam is usually preferred for this purpose. The biological half-life varies between 6 and 30 h. Biotransformation occurs in the liver to form two active metabolites, desmethylchlordiazepoxide and demoxepam. The long biological half-life and the active metabolites may produce residual effects, and repeated dosage will result in drug cumulation.

This drug should not be administered to pregnant women since studies indicate that fetal abnormalities may be related to consumption of chlordiazepoxide in the first 3 months of pregnancy. Drowsiness, ataxia, and lethargy are the most frequently occurring side effects. They are especially prevalent in the aged or debilitated patient. Rash, nausea, and changes in sexual drive also occur. *Agranulocytosis* (decreased number of white blood cells) can occur and is characterized by weakness, fever, and sore throat. If these symptoms occur, the drug should be withdrawn and differential white blood cell counts should be made. Likewise, if jaundice is observed, liver function tests should be ordered. Chlordiazepoxide resembles diazepam in the development of dependence, tolerance, and withdrawal symptoms. Precautions for using heavy machinery and for additive sedative effects with other drugs are the same as for diazepam.

Oxazepam (Serax)   This drug is the major metabolite that results from biotransformation of diazepam. Pharmacological and toxicological effects are similar to those of diazepam and chlordiazepoxide. Oxazepam is available in oral preparation only and has a half-life of 3 to 21 h. It is excreted as a conjugation product of glucuronic acid. No cumulative or residual effects have been reported. This drug does not appear to have any active metabolites. The same precautions used in prescribing other benzodiazepine derivatives should be used with this drug.

Clorazepate (Tranxene)   This drug is the newest member of the benzodiazepine family. It is similar in its effects and precautions to other benzodiazepines. Biotransformation results in the formation of the same active metabolite, desmethyldiazepam, that is formed from diazepam. Clorazepate produces long-lasting and cumulative effects. Several studies indicate that it may be superior to diazepam in the reduction of neurotic anxiety and the feeling of muscular relaxation.

Flurazepam (Dalmane)   Only oral preparations are available for this drug. Flurazepam is used primarily as a hypnotic. Its pharmacological and toxicological effects as well as precautions are similar to the effects of other benzodiazepines. Rapid biotransformation results in the formation of an active metabolite. Biotransformation of this metabolite is very slow, with a half-life of 50 to 100 h. Residual and cumulative effects result.

The Propanediols

The second group of antianxiety drugs are derivatives of propanediol and include meprobamate (Miltown), phenaglycodol (Ultran), tybamate (Solacen), and ethinamate (Valmid).

Meprobamate (Miltown)   This antianxiety drug was initially developed in the hope of producing a product with marked central muscle relaxant properties. However, like all central muscle relaxants, meprobamate, administered po, has not been demonstrated to be superior to the sedative-hypnotics in this respect. Meprobamate is primarily used orally as a daytime sedative for the treatment of anxiety and as a hypnotic. Like the benzodiazepines it produces an antianxiety effect at doses that produce little mental or physical impairment. There is also a wide safety margin between therapeutic doses and toxic doses.

In dentistry, meprobamate, 400 mg 4 times per day, has been used as an antianxiety agent in order to facilitate acceptance of new prosthetic appliances by patients. It also appears to relieve apprehension and anxiety in dental patients when 400 mg is administered the night before an operative procedure. The peak effect is reached in 2 to 3 h, and the half-life is 10 h. The usual daytime sedative dose is 200 to 400 mg taken 1 to 3 times per day. Few side effects occur at these doses. The most common are drowsiness and ataxia. There have been isolated reports of aplastic anemia as well as other blood dyscrasias. Various types of allergic dermatitis have been reported, and hypotension occurs occasionally, especially in the elderly. Like the barbiturates, meprobamate is contraindicated in porphyria. The lethal dose of meprobamate is approximately 40 g, and poisoning resembles barbiturate overdosage. Development of drug dependence, tolerance, and withdrawal symptoms occurs at high doses and resembles the actions of barbiturates.

Other Propanediols These drugs are also frequently classified as sedative-hypnotics. Phenaglycodol is similar in action to meprobamate. Few significant adverse side effects have been reported. The usual adult dose for anxiety is 300 mg every 6 to 8 h.

Tybamate (Solacen) resembles meprobamate but has a shorter onset and duration of action. Its half-life is approximately 3 h. The fact that physical dependence has not been reported is probably due to its short duration of action.

Ethinamate (Valmid) is weaker than meprobamate and is used in a similar manner. It has a duration of action of approximately 4 to 5 h.

SEDATIVE-ANTIHISTAMINES

These drugs are frequently classified either as sedative-hypnotics or antianxiety drugs, but since they have distinct characteristics they are best placed in a separate group. (See Chap. 16.) They are good antihistamines but are used most frequently to produce sedation. Poisoning with antihistamines can lead to both CNS depression and coma and CNS excitement, hallucinations, and convulsions. Children are particularly susceptible to the excitement phase. Habituation is rare with these drugs.

Hydroxyzine (Atarax, Vistaril)

This drug is used for preoperative and postoperative sedation. It produces mild sedation.

It is less effective than the sedatives or antianxiety drugs. Like other antihistamines, increasing the dose may not increase the sedative effects but may lead to CNS stimulation. This drug also possesses antiemetic and atropinelike effects. Antihistamines in this chemical category (piperazines) are known to cause fetal deformities in animals and should not be used by pregnant women. This drug should only be administered po and IM.

Promethazine (Phenergan)

Promethazine is a phenothiazine derivative (see major tranquilizers, below) with potent antihistamine activity. It produces a light sleep from which a person can be easily aroused. Promethazine is used along with meperidine as a preanesthetic medication in surgery. It is useful in treating postoperative nausea and vomiting. Headache, nausea, dry mouth, dizziness, and drowsiness are the most common side effects reported. The therapeutic aspects of the nonbarbiturates are summarized in Table 6-2.

THE MAJOR TRANQUILIZERS (ANTIPSYCHOTIC DRUGS)

The primary use of the major tranquilizers is in the treatment of the mental diseases called psychoses. These are disorders of mental functioning serious enough to impair severely the ability of an individual to handle the normal demands of life. They are characterized by a distortion of reality frequently accompanied by hallucinations and delusions. Under the influence of these drugs, psychotic behavior tends to decrease and the ability to function improves. The major tranquilizers produce mental and physical slowing, an indifference to incoming stimuli, and an emotional quieting. This triad of actions is referred to as the neuroleptic syndrome, and these drugs are also called *neuroleptics*.

The major tranquilizers are rarely used in

Table 6-2   Nonbarbiturates

Drugs	Doses	Oral administration route unless otherwise stated
Diazepam (Valium)	Adult 2–10 mg; children 1–2½ mg Elderly and debilitated 2–5 mg 5–10 mg	For sedation 3–4 times daily IM or IV preoperatively inject IV 5 mg (1 mL) per minute
Chlordiazepoxide (Librium)	Adult 15–40 mg; elderly and debilitated 10–20 mg; children over 6 years 10–20 mg Adult 50–100 mg	For sedation once daily IM preoperatively
Flurazepam (Dalmane)	15–30 mg	For hypnosis
Hydroxyzine (Vistaril)	Adult 25–100 mg Children under 6 years 50 mg Children over 6 years 50–100 mg Adults 25–100 mg Children 0.5 mg/kg body weight	Sedation 3–4 times daily Sedation daily in divided doses Sedation daily in divided doses IM preoperatively
Chloral hydrate	Adult 250 mg; children 25 mg/kg body weight (capsule or syrup) Adult 500 mg to 1 g Children 50 mg/kg body weight (maximum 1 g)	3 times daily after meals for sedation 15–30 min 30–45 min preoperatively or before sleep
Promethazine (Phenergan)	Adult 25–50 mg; Children 12.5–25 mg	1–1½ h preoperatively and before sleep
Ethchlorvynol (Placidyl)	500–1000 mg 15 min preoperatively or before sleep	For hypnosis
Ethinamate (Valmid)	500–1000 mg 20 min preoperatively or before sleep	For hypnosis

general dental practice but are administered IV along with other drugs to produce deep sedation. Like the antianxiety drugs and the sedative-hypnotics the major tranquilizers produce sedation and drowsiness, but increasing the dose does not produce general anesthesia. Usually, a patient can be easily aroused even when drowsy from having received large doses. In medicine, tolerance to the sedative effects develops after chronic administration over a period of 2 weeks.

The phenothiazines, especially chlorpromazine (Thorazine), are the most commonly used major tranquilizers. Many of the phenothiazines have antiemetic effects. Chlorpromazine is especially effective in this regard. Nausea and vomiting from various drugs, diseases, or operative procedures are controlled, but nausea and vomiting due to motion sickness are not affected. The phenothiazines produce adrenergic blockade which leads to lowered blood pressure and postural hypotension. Patients being treated with these drugs should arise slowly from the dental chair to prevent fainting due to a drop in blood pressure upon arising. These drugs stimulate the extrapyramidal system of the brain which leads to symptoms resembling

Parkinson's disease. This stimulation is manifested as muscle spasms in various parts of the body, including the muscles of the head and neck, and muscular rigidity. Therefore, when a patient taking phenothiazines complains of vague facial and neck pain, this must be considered. Also, if the muscles are in spasm, dental procedures cannot be carried out until these are controlled. These dental procedures include: occlusal adjustment, bite registration, and quadrant dentistry where occlusal relationships are important.

If a patient is taking this medication, he or she can be managed by lowering of the dose in conjunction with the patient's physician until the dental procedures are completed. An occlusal bite plate can be made to minimize traumatic occlusal forces related to facial muscular spasms. This patient might appear to be a bruxer. The phenothiazines lower the threshold to convulsions; in other words, convulsions can be produced more easily in patients on these drugs. When used for a prolonged period of time, they can reduce the number of circulating leukocytes (*leukopenia*). This leukopenia may be a forewarning of a more serious agranulocytosis. If this occurs, postoperative healing will be poor and the wound may become infected due to altered defenses of the body. A complete blood picture should be obtained before surgery. It has been suggested that these patients should be medicated postoperatively with antibiotics when surgical procedures are carried out.

Long-term therapy with these drugs has also been reported to result in both xerostomia and monilial infections. The latter problem, when it occurs, is usually seen on edentulous ridges covered by prosthetic appliances. It may present as an area of reddened mucosa which may or may not be covered by noncontinuous white spots. The lesion is usually painless, and a member of the dental team is often the first person to detect its presence. This infection responds well to therapy with an antifungal antibiotic such as nystatin (Mycostatin, Chap. 4).

The phenothiazines also have atropinelike effects, and a patient may complain of dry mouth. Due to disruption in temperature control a patient does not adapt readily to changes in environmental temperature. In a hot environment patients are readily subject to heat stroke and will easily become cold in a chilly environment. They may also feel drowsy or weak. Other side effects include palpitations, faintness, nasal stuffiness, and ejaculatory disturbances. Jaundice occurs as the result of an allergic reaction. Long-term administration may result in abnormal pigmentation in areas of the skin exposed to the sun (phototoxicity). Although these drugs may produce many side effects, they are generally very safe to use. Death from overdosage is extremely rare.

There are three types of phenothiazines which differ from each other mainly in the degree of various side effects. Problems and care of the patient in the dental office will vary according to these differences. The aliphatics produce moderate extrapyramidal effects, good sedation, hypotension, and a higher frequency of agranulocytosis than other antipsychotic drugs. The piperazines produce more extrapyramidal effect and less sedation and hypotension than the aliphatics. The piperadines produce more phototoxicity and fewer extrapyramidal symptoms than the others.

Other groups of major tranquilizers also differ mainly in their side effects. The butyrophenones produce more extrapyramidal effects than the phenothiazines but produce less sedation and hypotension. Two butyrophenone derivatives are used in the United States. Haloperidol is used primarily in psychiatry, while droperidol is used in anesthesia for its neuroleptic and antiemetic effects (see Chap. 8). The thioxanthines are similar to the phenothiazines but are weaker in both antipsychotic effectiveness and adverse effects.

ANSWER TO CHAPTER CASE

Patients taking tranquilizing agents such as phenothiazines or meprobamates often are predisposed to oral monilial infections. This is especially noted under full or partial dentures. It is likely that this patient is taking phenothiazine tranquilizers and the area of redness is due to a monilial infection. This condition responds well to treatment with an antifungal agent such as nystatin (Mycostatin).

QUESTIONS

1 How do drugs that are classified as sedatives, hypnotics, and minor and major tranquilizers differ from each other?
2 What types of drugs when given together have an additive effect in producing depression of the central nervous system? When is this additive effect desirable, and when is it dangerous for the patient?
3 What are the advantages of prescribing a drug like diazepam (Valium) instead of barbiturates?
4 What kind of dental problems occur in patients who are being treated with major tranquilizers?
5 What problems are encountered when drugs that depress the central nervous system are prescribed?

READING REFERENCES

AMA Drug Evaluations, *Sedatives and Hypnotics,* 2d ed., Publishing Sciences Group, Acton, Mass. 1973, p. 306.

Foreman, P. A., "Control of Anxiety/Pain Complex in Dentistry, Intravenous Psychosedation with Techniques Using Diazepam," *Oral. Surg.,* **36:**337–349, 1974.

Forney, R. B., and F. W. Hughes, *Combined Effects of Alcohol and Other Drugs,* Charles C Thomas, Springfield, Ill., 1968.

Garrattini, S., et al., *The Benzodiazepines,* Raven, New York, 1973.

Greenblatt, D., and R. I. Shader, "The Clinical Choice of Sedatives and Hypnotics," *Arch. Intern. Med.,* **77:**81–100, 1972.

Saxes, I., "Associations Between Oral Clefts and Drugs Taken During Pregnancy," *Int. J. Epidemiol,* **4:**37–44, 1975.

Chapter 7

Local Anesthetics

Mr. Martin reports that, after receiving an injection of Novocaine, there was severe itching and redness at the injection site. Should your office be concerned about this reaction? Which anesthetics could probably be used safely for Mr. Martin?

Local anesthetics are the most frequently used drugs in dentistry. Their main purpose is to prevent the pain that occurs during dental procedures. These drugs are capable of producing loss of sensation and motor activity when introduced into an area of the body adjacent to nerves controlling these functions. As a local anesthetic penetrates the nerve membrane, the ability of the nerve to conduct an impulse ceases and all function is lost. The drug interferes with the movement of sodium through pores in the neuronal membrane, a process that is necessary for normal conduction.

In dentistry, local anesthetics are used topically, by infiltration, and to produce block anesthesia. Anesthetics applied topically and by infiltration anesthetize nerve endings in the area that contact occurs. In block anesthesia the anesthetic is delivered to the area adjacent to a nerve. Anesthesia will be produced in areas innervated by this nerve, which may be some distance from the site of injection.

Additionally, in medicine, local anesthetics are used to produce spinal anesthesia. This type of injection produces analgesia and complete muscular relaxation without loss of consciousness. Spinal anesthesia is most frequently used for operations of the lower extremities.

STRUCTURE

The major anesthetics are divided into esters and amides. All the esters listed in Table 7-1 except cocaine are derivatives of para-aminobenzoic acid (PABA). It is important to know the structure since ester-type drugs produce more allergic reactions than amides. Cross-sensitivity occurs among the esters, and they should be replaced by amides when allergy is suspected. In addition, esters that are derivatives of PABA will interfere with the antibacterial effect of sulfonamides.

IONIZATION FACTORS

Local anesthetics are weak bases that are poorly soluble in water. The base is usually prepared in the form of an acid salt in order to get it into solution. Even though the injected solution is acidic, it rapidly becomes alkaline because of the buffering ability of the tissues; that is, bases present in the fluid of the tissues remove the excess hydrogen ions injected.

The anesthetic, at the pH of the tissue, is partially converted to its nonionized form, which can then penetrate the nerve membrane. Part of the anesthetic is converted to the ionized form within the nerve. This ionized form, interacting with the inner surface of the neuronal membrane, produces the anesthetic effect. The presence of inflammation in the tissues injected causes a lowering of tissue pH (more acidic) which in turn causes a decrease in the formation of the nonionized base. Fewer molecules penetrate the nerve, reducing the effectiveness of the anesthetic (see Chap. 1).

ANESTHETIC EFFECT IN A MIXED NERVE

When a local anesthetic is applied to a mixed nerve it will penetrate more rapidly the small and the unmyelinated fibers, while the large and the myelinated fibers will be penetrated more slowly. If a mixed nerve contains fibers that innervate all types of body activity, the loss of function will occur in the following order:

1 Autonomic functions
2 Pain
3 Cold
4 Warmth
5 Touch
6 Deep pressure
7 Proprioception (sense of movement and of position of the body)
8 Skeletal muscle tone and activity

Table 7-1   Major Anesthetics Used in Dentistry

Structure	Drug	Systemic toxicity*	Injectable	Topical
Amides	Lidocaine	2	X	X
O	Mepivacaine	2	X	
‖	Prilocaine	1.7	X	
—NHC—				
Esters	Procaine	1	X	
O	Propoxycaine	8–10	X	
‖	Tetracaine	10	X	X
—C—O—	Benzocaine	Low		X
	Cocaine	High		X
Miscellaneous	Dyclonine	Low		X

* The number 1 is assigned to the least toxic agent, procaine. All the other drugs are compared to it.

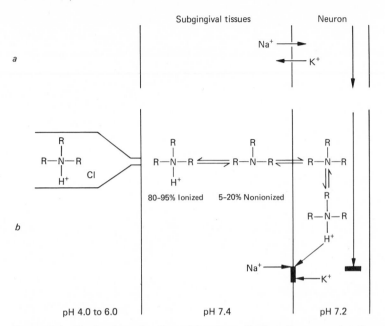

Figure 7-1 Mechanism of action of local anesthetics. R represents other molecules in the local anesthetic structure; H = hydrogen; N = nitrogen; Cl = chloride. (a) Normal conduction. The vertical arrow represents a nerve impulse. The horizontal arrows indicate the movement of sodium (Na$^+$) into the neuron and potassium (K$^+$) out of the neuron, a necessary process for propagation of a nerve impulse. (b) Normal conduction. Demonstrates the injection of the hydrochloric acid salt of a local anesthetic. In the subgingival tissues, 5 to 20 percent become nonionized at the pH of the tissues. Only the nonionized form penetrates the neuron to become partly ionized within the neuron. The ionized form interacts with the inner surface of the neuronal membrane and produces conformational changes in the membrane. The changes prevent the movement of Na$^+$ and K$^+$, thereby blocking conduction of the nerve impulse. (See Chap. 1.)

Local anesthesia as it is used in dentistry usually results in loss of pain, temperature, and touch sensations. Usually pressure is not affected and nerves to skeletal muscles are not present. However, very rarely, block anesthesia which is poorly administered may affect the facial nerve which contains motor fibers to the skeletal muscles of the face. Reversible paralysis of half the face on the side injected will result.

QUALITIES OF AN IDEAL LOCAL ANESTHETIC

Many good anesthetics are available but they still fall short to some extent of the characteristics of an ideal anesthetic. The ideal anesthetic should produce good and reversible anesthesia every time without producing any local or systemic side effects. It should penetrate tissues easily and act quickly and for a sufficient length of time. It must be stable in solution and capable of being sterilized. Most of these criteria can be met by many anesthetics in present use except that all of them are capable of producing side effects.

TOXICITY

Local anesthetics as they are used in dentistry are remarkably safe drugs. However, side effects do occur and can sometimes be serious. These are more likely to occur in young children and the elderly. Adverse effects may be due to the local anesthetic itself or to the vasoconstrictor that is usually present. The local anesthetic will cause stimulation of the central nervous system (CNS) if a sufficient amount of drug is absorbed from the injection site. Excitement and tremors may proceed to convulsions if the blood level is sufficiently high. Excessive stimulation of the CNS is followed by respiratory and cardiovascular depression and loss of consciousness. Lidocaine is more likely to cause depression of the CNS that is not preceded by stimulation.

Local anesthetics can also produce cardiovascular depression. This is usually seen with very high concentrations that are not obtained in dentistry. However, in a few rare individuals, small amounts have caused cardiac arrest. Allergic reactions occur rarely and consist mostly of dermatitis, asthmatic attacks, and serious anaphylactic reactions. Contact dermatitis sometimes occurs in personnel who frequently handle local anesthetics. Allergic reactions occur mostly with the ester type of agent.

Systemic effects that are due to vasoconstrictors include anxiety, excitement, headache, dizziness, tachycardia, chest pain, hypertension, and gastrointestinal disturbances.

Systemic effects are mostly due to overdosage or inadvertant injection into a blood vessel. Fainting as a result of the injection procedure is the most frequently seen undesirable effect of local anesthetic administration. This is not due to the pharmacological effects of the drug, but is a psychological response to the fear or pain of injection. This response may be confused with the chemical effects of the injected drugs.

PREVENTION OF ADVERSE EFFECTS

Adverse effects can be avoided in many instances by taking the following precautions:

1 Take a careful history. If an adverse reaction has occurred previously, substitute another drug.

2 Aspirate before administration in order to avoid an intravascular injection.

3 Inject the smallest amount of the least toxic drug possible in order to produce good anesthesia. (The maximum dose listed under each drug refers to a healthy, average-sized person.)

4 Inject slowly.

5 Avoid repeated injections into the same site over a prolonged period of time. The vasoconstrictor will cause a decrease in blood flow to the area. Edema, tissue damage, and delayed healing will result because the tissues will not be receiving a sufficient amount of oxygen.

TREATMENT OF ADVERSE EFFECTS

The administration of oxygen for the treatment of convulsions ensures that tissues will be properly oxygenated and that the brain will be protected from hypoxia. Recurrent convulsions should be treated with ultrashort-acting barbiturates or diazepam (Valium). Care must be taken that bodily injury or aspiration of vomitus does not occur. If cardiac or respiratory arrest occurs, cardiopulmonary resuscitation should be initiated (see Chap. 18). Vasopressor drugs such as metaraminol may be given intravenously (IV) for treating extreme hypotension. Epinephrine is the drug of choice for treating allergic reactions (see Chap. 18).

METABOLISM

The ester-type drugs like procaine are hydrolized by the cholinesterase of the plasma and liver. In rare individuals loss of consciousness may occur because of a genetic deficiency of plasma cholinesterase (see Chap. 2). The amide-type drugs like lidocaine are first oxidized and then hydrolyzed by the liver microsomal enzymes.

VASOCONSTRICTORS[1]

The vasoconstrictors present in local anesthetic solutions constrict the blood vessels in the area where the solution is injected. Blood flow in and out of the area is decreased. As a result the local anesthetic remains at the site of injection and comes in contact with the tissues to be anesthetized for a longer period of time. This intensifies and prolongs the anesthetic effect. In addition, since the anesthetic leaves the site of injection and enters the circulation at a slower rate of speed, less of the drug is available to produce unwanted systemic effects. The toxicity of the local anesthetic is therefore decreased.

Procaine by itself causes vasodilation and should always be used with a vasoconstrictor. Lidocaine, mepivacaine, and prilocaine may be used without one, since they cause little or no vasodilatation.

TOPICAL ANESTHETICS

Some local anesthetics are applied directly to the oral mucous membranes in order to produce surface anesthesia. These topical anesthetics are used prior to infiltration or block anesthesia in order to prevent the pain of injection. However, anesthesia just below the surface is poor, and pain can be elicited as the needle penetrates to deeper layers. Topical anesthetics are also used to relieve the pain of oral ulcers, wounds, and injuries. Since these drugs are more rapidly absorbed from abraded surfaces, care must be taken to prevent toxic effects. Generally, topicals that are potent and well absorbed are more likely to produce toxic reactions (see tetracaine). These agents are also used to decrease an excessive gag reflex. However, when this protective mechanism is no longer operating, there is danger of the patient aspirating saliva and foreign substances placed in the mouth.

[1] See also Chap. 3.

Surface anesthetics are also useful in reducing pain in postextraction sockets and for removal of sutures. Chlorobutanol, a compound that possesses both local anesthetic and antiseptic properties, is used in combination with clove oil and cinnamon to treat nearly exposed pulp and to alleviate the pain of pulpitis. Dental hygienists may use topical anesthetics to decrease the pain and discomfort produced during instrumentation for probing, exploring, scaling, root planing, and gingival curettage whenever the pain is not severe enough to require a local anesthetic. Tetracaine is very effective but is more likely to produce systemic toxicity. It is best not to use it on abraded tissue. Lidocaine hydrochloride prepared in an aqueous solution is more effective but potentially more toxic than the nonaqueous lidocaine base. The lidocaine base as well as benzocaine and dyclonine may be applied to lacerated tissues. These latter drugs are poorly absorbed and are therefore less effective as well as less toxic. Occurrence of systemic toxicity after topical application of benzocaine or dyclonine are extremely low. Since these last three agents penetrate tissue poorly, they are effective only where they are applied. This means that before root planing and curettage the topical must be applied to the soft tissues within the sulcus where the instruments will come in contact. A syringe and bent needle will facilitate application into the sulcus. Topical anesthetics are also used with surgical dressings after gingival curettage and after periodontal surgery.

The majority of topical anesthetics are capable of sensitizing tissues so that repeated administration of any of these compounds, either applied topically or given by injection, may produce allergic reactions in susceptible individuals. Dental professionals should avoid touching these compounds since repeated handling can result in the development of allergic contact dermatitis. Drugs used for topical anesthesia are listed in Table 7-1.

MAJOR LOCAL ANESTHETICS USED IN DENTISTRY

All these drugs are prepared as the hydrochloride acid salt.

Lidocaine (Xylocaine)

Lidocaine is presently the anesthetic used most often. It produces profound anesthesia of long duration. Although it is twice as toxic as procaine, the amounts used in dentistry do not make it a greater hazard. Little vasodilation occurs so less vasoconstrictor is needed. Some patients experience a sedative effect. Although CNS stimulation can occur, CNS depression without stimulation is more likely to occur because of overdosage. Lidocaine is used topically as well as for infiltration and block anesthesia. When used alone, do not exceed 10 mL of a 2% solution. Lidocaine is used IV in the treatment of cardiac arrythmias and to reduce severe itching and pain.

Mepivacaine (Carbocaine)

This anesthetic is comparable to lidocaine in potency and duration. Although related chemically, this drug does not produce the sedative effect of lidocaine. Mepivacaine is sometimes used without a vasoconstrictor as a 3% solution. Maximum dosage should not exceed 200 mg when used alone.

Prilocaine (Citanest)

Prilocaine is similar to lidocaine when used with a vasoconstrictor. It is a little less toxic then lidocaine but is used in a concentration double that of lidocaine. Prilocaine may be used without epinephrine for short dental procedures.

Procaine (Novocaine)

A 2% solution of procaine with a vasoconstrictor produces adequate anesthesia for most dental procedures. It is less suitable for the removal of vital pulps or when long duration of anesthesia is needed. It is the least toxic of local anesthetics and is not effective topically. It is frequently used with more potent anesthetics such as tetracaine or propoxycaine. Dosage should not exceed 20 mL of a 2% solution. Procaine was the principal drug used between 1905 and 1950 but has now largely been replaced by lidocaine.

Propoxycaine (Ravocain)

This drug is approximately 7 to 8 times more potent and 8 to 10 times more toxic than procaine. It is usually added in small amounts to procaine solution to increase effectiveness and duration.

Tetracaine (Pontocaine)

This drug is a highly potent and potentially toxic agent. For injection it is usually used in small amounts with procaine to increase effectiveness. It is a very effective topical anesthetic but because of rapid absorption and toxicity, the amount used should not exceed 20 mg (1 mL of a 2% solution) and it should be applied to a limited area.

Benzocaine (Ethylaminobenzoate)

Benzocaine is used as a topical anesthetic only. It is used in ointments and powders mostly on oral lesions and wounds. Since it is poorly absorbed, it does not produce systemic effects. It is sometimes used in combination with tetracaine in order to improve its effectiveness.

Cocaine

Cocaine, an alkaloid found in the coca plant, was the first local anesthetic used. It is a powerful CNS stimulant. Cocaine is sniffed or taken IV for its euphoric effects. Psychological dependence develops. It falls into Schedule II of controlled drugs.

Cocaine is a very good local anesthetic but it is no longer used for injection because less toxic agents are available. It is a very effective topical anesthetic but is rarely used in dentistry because of its abuse potential and toxicity. Crystals of cocaine are sometimes used to produce anesthesia for the removal of vital pulp.

Dyclonine (Dyclone)

This topical anesthetic is not an amide or an ester. It may be of use if sensitivity to other anesthetics exists. Anesthesia is slow and may require up to 10 min before an effective level is achieved.

COMPOSITION OF LOCAL ANESTHETICS

Many local anesthetic solutions contain, besides a local anesthetic and a vasoconstrictor, either methylparaben or propylparaben as antibacterial preservatives and an antioxidant such as metabisulfite which prevents the decomposition of the vasoconstrictor. The parabens occasionally cause allergic reactions which can mistakenly be attributed to the local anesthetic itself. Cross-sensitivity exists between the parabens. A patient who is sensitive to one paraben will usually be sensitive to all the others. Fortunately, various preparations of ester-type local anesthetics do not contain these preservatives and can be used in case hypersensitivity to these compounds is supected. If a patient is suspected of being allergic to a particular preparation, it is best to switch to a preparation where none of the compounds contained in it could produce cross-sensitivity. Skin allergy tests for these chemicals as well as tests for local anesthetics and most drugs are not reliable. In addition, the test itself can either sensitize the patient or produce an allergic response.

The bisulfite antioxidants have rarely been reported as causing allergic reactions such as dermatitis or stomatitis. If this compound is suspected, then a local anesthetic without a vasoconstrictor should be used.

CARE OF LOCAL ANESTHETIC CARPULES

It is frequently the responsibility of dental auxiliaries to maintain the stock of local anesthetic Carpules. All local anesthetic containers should be periodically checked for expiration date, and dated Carpules should be eliminated. One should also discard Carpules where a change in color from a clear colorless solution to one with a pink or brownish tint has occurred, since this indicates decomposition of the vasoconstrictor.

Prior to use, the aluminum-sealed end of the dental cartridge should be disinfected. The cartridges should be placed in about 1 in of solution for at least 10 min and should not be left in the solution overnight. Either 91 percent isopropyl alcohol or 70 percent ethyl alcohol can be used. Rubbing alcohol and quaternary ammonium compounds (benzalkonium chloride) are not recommended. Solutions of rubbing alcohol cause a breakdown of the rubber stopper, and benzalkonium chloride destroys the aluminum of the caps. Cartridges should not be autoclaved or stored at temperatures of 104°F or over for more than 48 h since heat tends to break down the vasoconstrictor. Any Carpule with cracks or chips, air bubbles larger than 2 mm, or extruded plunger should be discarded.

ANSWER TO CHAPTER CASE

First, it should be ascertained whether Mr. Martin had indeed received an injection of Novocaine, since laypersons frequently call any local anesthetic by that name. The severe itching and redness was probably the result of an allergic reaction. Injection of the same drug could cause a similar or more severe reaction. Since Novocaine is an ester-type drug, other drugs that are structurally related are also likely to produce an allergic response and should not be used. A local anesthetic, such as lidocaine (Xylocaine), that has an amide structure should be administered instead to this patient.

QUESTIONS

1 What local anesthetic is most frequently used in dentistry?
2 What class of local anesthetics exhibit cross-allergenicity?
3 How do local anesthetics produce their effects?
4 While a mixed nerve is being anesthetized, loss of function will occur in a regular order. Where does pain fit in this order? Is this useful?
5 What adverse reactions can be produced by local anesthetics? How can these reactions be prevented or minimized?
6 What is the purpose of combining vasoconstrictors and local anesthetics?

READING REFERENCES

Adriani, J., "Clinical Pharmacology of Local Anesthetics," *Clin. Pharmacol. Ther.,* **1:**645–673, 1960.

AMA Drug Evaluations, *Local Anesthetics,* Publishing Sciences Group, 1973, p. 206.

Council on Dental Therapeutics, *Accepted Dental Therapeutics,* American Dental Association, 1977, pp. 93–111.

Goodman, L. S., and A. Gilman (eds.), *Pharmacological Basis of Therapeutics,* Macmillan, 1975, pp. 379–403.

Laden, E. L., and D. A. Wallace, "Contact Dermatitis Due to Procaine: A Common Occupational Disease of Dentists," *J. Invest. Dermatol.,* **12:**299–306, 1949.

Munson, E. S., and I. H. Wagman, "Diazepam Treatment of Local Anesthetic-Induced Seizures," *Anesthesiology,* **37:**523–528, 1972.

Schiano, A. M., and R. C. Strambi, "Frequency of Accidental Intravascular Injection of Local Anesthetics in Dental Practice," *Oral Surg.,* **17:**178–184, 1964.

Chapter 8

General Anesthetics and Nitrous Oxide

A five-year-old child is being administered nitrous oxide while three badly decayed teeth are being filled. Near completion of the procedure, you note that his breathing has almost stopped and he appears cyanotic. What are the possible reasons for this problem? What precautions should be taken in patients receiving nitrous oxide?

Dental procedures must sometimes be performed under general anesthesia either because the operation is extensive or traumatic or the health and well-being of the patient require it. General anesthesia is administered under the supervision of a qualified oral surgeon with the help of an anesthetic assistant and a surgical assistant. Although there are various stages to general anesthesia (see below) the term itself means that a state of unconsciousness has been produced. General anesthetics cause a decrease in activity of the central nervous system (CNS). A state of depression ensues which deepens with increasing drug con-

centration in the CNS. If a sufficient amount of a potent drug is administered, the depression will first produce sedation, followed by sleep, unconsciousness, coma, and finally death. Alcohol, the sedative-hypnotics, and the antianxiety drugs act in a similar manner but are used in low enough dosage so that only sedation or sleep is produced. Some gases, like nitrous oxide, when properly administered with sufficient oxygen and without other agents, do not in the usual healthy patient reach a sufficient concentration in the brain to produce deep depression. However, this concentration can produce surgical anesthesia in a patient in profound shock or in one who is severely debilitated.

OBJECTIVES OF GENERAL ANESTHESIA

General anesthesia is produced so that dental or medical operational procedures can be facilitated with the least amount of discomfort for the patient. The objectives sought include:

1 A complete abolition of pain
2 The production of a state of unawareness which will prevent the patient from feeling fear and anxiety during the operation
3 Prevention of noxious reflexes which might interfere with performance of the operation
4 Good muscular relaxation since it is difficult for the surgeon to operate in an area where muscle relaxation is poor

In order to achieve these objectives, several drugs with different characteristics are frequently combined.

INHALATION ANESTHETICS

There are two types of inhalation anesthetics: (1) gases and (2) liquids that can easily be vaporized at room temperatures. Both types produce their effects in the same manner.

The Absorption, Distribution, and Elimination of Inhalation Anesthetics

An inhalation anesthetic moves from the breathing apparatus to the mouth, reaches the lung, and is absorbed from the pulmonary membrane into the bloodstream, where it is distributed to the brain and the rest of the body. When the anesthetic is removed from the breathing apparatus, its movement is reversed and most of the gas is eliminated unchanged through the respiratory tract.

Anesthesia is dependent on the following criteria:

1 The development of partial pressure of the volatile drug in the brain: This in turn is dependent on the partial pressure in the blood, the alveoli, and the inspired air. It is the pressure of the gas which is the driving force in moving the anesthetic from one body compartment to another.
2 The solubility of gas in blood and tissue: The more soluble gases will reach a higher concentration in the brain and will therefore be more potent.
3 Blood flow: Since anesthetics reach the brain by means of the circulation, anesthetic levels will be affected by blood flow through the lungs, the systemic circulation, and the brain.
4 Pulmonary ventilation: Any change in respiration will affect the flow of inhalation anesthetic to the lungs and alter the anesthetic state.

Concentration Effects At the beginning of anesthesia, there is no gas present in the lung and therefore no opposing partial pressure to slow its entry. Any gas present in the inspired air will move rapidly to the lungs and other body compartments until the partial pressure builds up. If at induction time a higher concentration of volatile anesthetic is administered, there will be a more rapid saturation of tissues and a more rapid onset of anesthesia.

Double-Gas Effect This effect is related to the concentration effect. If a low concentration of a potent anesthetic is administered at the same time as a high concentration of a weak anesthetic, the rapid movement of the weak anesthetic into the body tissues will pull in larger amounts of the potent anesthetic than would occur if this anesthetic were given alone. This double-gas effect also facilitates a rapid induction.

Diffusion Hypoxia When an anesthetic gas is removed, the effect that occurs is like the concentration effect except that it is in the opposite direction. When the partial pressure of an anesthetic gas is removed from the inspired air, the gas that was held under pressure in the tissues rushes out and fills the lungs. If the anesthetic is weak and therefore present in large amounts it will take up so much space in the lungs upon emergence that necessary oxygen will be displaced. Inhalation of oxygen will be insufficient, and a hypoxic state will ensue. In order to prevent this effect, oxygen must be administered upon removal of the anesthetic until emergence has occurred.

Potent Anesthetics Anesthetics like ether that are very soluble in body tissues will take a long time before reaching equilibration. Many molecules will dissolve in body tissues leaving less of the anesthetic available for distribution to the brain. Only after many body tissues are saturated does the level in the brain rise sufficiently to produce an effect. Although onset of anesthesia and equilibration is slow, a greater concentration of drug in the brain is eventually reached. As a result these anesthetics are capable of progressively depressing the CNS until all the stages of anesthesia are passed through. Coma and death will ensue if anesthesia is continued at the same partial pressure. Emergence from anesthesia also occurs slowly with these compounds.

Weak Anesthetics Anesthetics like nitrous oxide that are poorly soluble in body tissues must be administered in much higher concentration which produces higher partial pressure. Because of poor solubility, the tissues become rapidly saturated, and the partial pressure builds up rapidly in the brain until it is equal to that of the blood and the inspired air. At this point, no greater anesthetic effect can be achieved. Weak anesthetics can only produce full anesthesia when administered in a concentration approaching 100%. This concentration is incompatible with life since not enough oxygen can be taken in. When admin-

istered with sufficient oxygen, only the first or second stage of anesthesia is usually reached. Emergence from anesthesia occurs rapidly with these poorly soluble drugs.

Toxicity Halothane, methoxyflurane, and enflurane can precipitate dangerous cardiac arrhythmias when vasoconstrictors like epinephrine are administered.

Malignant hyperpyrexia, a condition characterized by fever of unknown origin, acidosis, high blood levels of potassium, and muscle contractions, has been reported with both inhalation and intravenous (IV) anesthetics. Since this condition is inherited, the health history should include questions concerning the possible occurrence of this trait in family members.

Long-term exposure to low concentrations of inhalation anesthetics poses a danger to operating room personnel. It has been reported that these persons may be more susceptible to liver and kidney disease, cancer, and spontaneous abortions. Their offspring are more likely to have congenital abnormalities. The possible danger of chronic exposure can be minimized by improved ventilation and evacuation systems in hospitals and dental offices.

Stages and Planes of General Anesthesia

The progress of anesthesia from light sedation to respiratory paralysis was first described for ether anesthesia. The signs that appear as anesthesia deepens have been divided into the following stages and planes according to Guedel. Although these are completely true only for ether anesthesia, they are frequently referred to in relation to other anesthetics.

Stage 1 Analgesia
       Plane 1 Normal memory and sensation
       Plane 2 Moderate amnesia, partial analgesia
       Plane 3 Amnesia and analgesia
Stage 2 Delirium: Excitement, struggling, in-

creased muscle tone, possibility of vomiting, involuntary defecation and urination, increased blood pressure and heart rate, dilated pupils, unconsciousness

Stage 3 Surgical anesthesia

Plane 1 Light surgical. Patient appears in a quiet sleep, loss of eyelid reflex, pupils constricted

Plane 2 Moderate surgical. Loss of postpharyngeal, laryngeal, and corneal reflexes, pupils constricted, some skeletal muscle relaxation occurs

Plane 3 Deep surgical. Intercostal muscle paralysis, good skeletal muscle relaxation, pupils dilated, pupillary light reflex disappears

Plane 4 Respiratory and circulatory failure. Pupils maximally dilated, paralysis of diaphragm

When surgical anesthesia is desired, stage 1 and stage 2 are passed through as rapidly as possible.

Nitrous Oxide

In dentistry, nitrous oxide is used to produce light analgesic and sedative effects which occur in stage 1 of general anesthesia. The signs and symptoms which have been observed during this period have been described in great detail. Blood pressure and respiration are normal throughout this stage.

There are three planes of nitrous oxide analgesia and sedation:

Plane 1 Slight amnesia; elevation of pain threshold; elimination of fear; relaxed patient; may experience tingling in fingers, toes, lips, or tongue. Some of the symptoms described for this stage may be due to a placebo effect.

Plane 2 Reduced rate of winking; patient is capable of maintaining open mouth; patient follows directions slowly; moderate amnesia and analgesia; patient relaxed, euphoric; feeling of warmth; headiness, or drowsiness; voice changes character, and patient is unconcerned with surrounding activities.

Plane 3 When this plane is reached, there is danger of slipping into stage 2; sometimes body and mandible may be rigid; patient may stare, look angry or sleepy; mouth tends to close; patient no longer follows directions; complete analgesia and amnesia occurs; patient is mostly unaware of surroundings; may experience hallucinations and fear.

At one time nitrous oxide was used mostly for its analgesic effect, and the patient was kept deep in plane 3. Many problems occur at this plane since muscular rigidity sets in and the patient does not follow orders and may experience fear and excitement. At the present time plane 2 is used most frequently because the patient is relaxed and feels well. Since analgesia is incomplete, nitrous oxide must be combined with local anesthetics for most dental procedures.

This poorly soluble weak anesthetic (25%) is nonflammable, nonirritating, and has a pleasant smell. It must be administered with a minimum of 20% oxygen. Although 80% nitrous oxide–20% oxygen may be used for induction, no more than 65% nitrous oxide should be used for maintenance. At this concentration most patients will remain in the first stage of anesthesia. In dentistry the mixture used for sedation is usually no greater than 50% nitrous oxide and 50% oxygen. Effective sedation can be produced in some individuals with concentrations of nitrous oxide as low as 15%. Nitrous oxide also is used in combination with IV anesthetics and other volatile anesthetics for general anesthesia.

Nitrous oxide sedation is beneficial for cardiac patients since it reduces stress and provides a higher concentration of oxygen than would be available in the inspired air. Patients suffering from asthma or epilepsy are also good candidates since stress in these patients will frequently trigger an attack.

Nausea and vomiting may occur occasionally and are most frequently associated with high intake or prolonged administration. Dizziness is sometimes present. Although patients normally recover rapidly from the effects of nitrous oxide and are capable of driving themselves home they must be supervised to make sure that they are ready. A rare patient may have residual effects.

Nitrous oxide is contraindicated in patients with whom communication is difficult since cooperation is required. This usually includes very young children and retarded persons. Nasal obstruction that is severe enough to prevent easy inhalation is an absolute contraindication to nitrous oxide since effective amounts cannot be inhaled.

Precautions Nitrous oxide as it is used for light sedation is very safe. However, when used with other CNS depressants the possibility of entering stage 2 and stage 3 of anesthesia exists. Only qualified anesthetists should deal with this level of anesthesia. Great precautions or a fail-safe system should ensure that no mixup between oxygen and nitrous oxide tanks occur. Several deaths have occurred because patients were mistakenly given pure nitrous oxide instead of oxygen following surgery. The patients became cyanotic and died of respiratory failure. Immediate removal of the nitrous oxide and administration of oxygen could have prevented these deaths.

Ether (Ethyl Ether)

Ether, the major drug used for general anesthesia for over 100 years, is a potent anesthetic with a high degree of safety. It has the advantages of producing good analgesia and muscular relaxation while the respiratory and the cardiovascular systems are well maintained during surgical anesthesia. However, induction is slow, and the drug is flammable and irritating to mucous membranes. Because of the last two characteristics ether is rarely used in modern operating rooms but is of great value where proper equipment is lacking.

Halothane (Fluothane)

This potent anesthetic is a nonflammable, widely used, and reliable agent. A 3% concentration is used to produce a rapid induction, and a 0.5 to 1.5% concentration is used for maintenance. Emergence from anesthesia is fairly rapid. Halothane is usually administered with oxygen or with oxygen and nitrous oxide but it can also be given alone.

Halothane has the tendency to produce hypotension at the deeper levels of anesthesia because both cardiac depression and vasodilation are prominent at these levels. Respiratory rate and depth are also easily depressed, and this requires careful adjustment of anesthetic level to coincide with changes in respiration. Halothane and other halogenated anesthetics sensitize the heart to sympathomimetic amines like epinephrine and norepinephrine. Serious cardiac arrythmias including ventricular fibrillation can result.

Halothane is considered a good anesthetic for patients suffering from asthma. It is nonirritating to mucous membranes; it has no bronchoconstrictor effect and causes little increase in salivary and bronchial secretions.

Laryngospasms and laryngeal reflexes are reduced, and the masseter muscle is relaxed. General muscle relaxation is poor, and neuromuscular blocking drugs such as succinylcholine (Anectine) are usually used to produce good relaxation. Analgesia is also poor, and opiates are usually administered to prevent pain after recovery.

Approximately 20 percent of halothane is metabolized in the liver. The metabolites have been implicated in the production of liver damage which in some instances has been severe enough to cause death. Halothane is contraindicated in patients whose previous history indicates that it or other halogenated anesthetics have produced symptoms of liver disease.

Methoxyflurane (Penthrane)

Methoxyflurane is a nonflammable anesthetic. The induction period is long but can be shortened by administering IV anesthetics or nitrous oxide. Concentrations of 1 to 3% produce good anesthesia.

Methoxyflurane sensitizes the heart to sympathomimetic amines. Cardiac slowing and hypotension occur during the stage of surgical anesthesia. General anesthesia is followed by good postoperative analgesia that may last for several hours after the patient has regained consciousness. Muscle relaxation is better than with halothane and occurs during the light stages of anesthesia. However, neuromuscular blocking drugs are still used to produce a more profound relaxation. Unlike many other anesthetics, the pupils remain constricted during all stages of methoxyflurane anesthesia. Like halothane, methoxyflurane does not irritate mucous membranes or stimulate salivary and bronchial secretions. Bronchoconstriction and laryngospasms are not produced by this drug, and it is well tolerated in asthmatics. Methoxyflurane is partly metabolized in the liver to yield free fluoride ions which are toxic to the kidneys. This effect is cumulative, and patients should not receive this drug more than once in a monthly period. Renal toxicity is enhanced by the simultaneous administration of tetracyclines and other antibiotics. (See Chap. 19.) Because of this renal toxicity methoxyflurane is now limited in use to small doses for short periods of time. As with halothane, liver damage can occur. This drug is contraindicated in patients with a history of jaundice associated with the administration of a halogenated anesthetic.

Enflurane (Ethrane)

This volatile anesthetic produces a rapid induction, easy maintenance, and rapid recovery. Depression of respiration and blood pressure is similar to that of halothane. Cardiac rhythm tends to be stable, and there is only a mild sensitization of the heart to sympathomimetic amines.

Enflurane produces good analgesia and muscle relaxation. Usually, small doses of the competitive-type drugs are administered in order to produce better muscle relaxation in the lighter planes of anesthesia. Enflurane strongly potentiates the action of these drugs.

About 2 percent of patients develop signs of motor hyperactivity such as twitching of the muscles of the jaw, face, neck, or extremities. This has been demonstrated by electroencephalograph recordings to be associated with brain seizure patterns. These effects appear to be temporary.

Enflurane metabolism in the liver results in the formation of fluoride ions. However, the fluoride levels are much lower than those found with methoxyflurane, and one would expect enflurane to be much less toxic to the kidneys. Nevertheless, enflurane should be used with care in patients with renal failure or decreased urinary output. Enflurane has been used along with nitrous oxide and oxygen for outpatient anesthetic services. It has the advantage that in low doses it is cleared from the lung more rapidly than other volatile anesthetics.

INTRAVENOUS ANESTHETICS

Ultrashort-acting barbiturates (see Chap. 6) are used IV for short dental procedures. Their effects may be supplemented by inhalation anesthetics, especially for longer procedures. Induction with these agents is instantaneous and usually smooth. When combined with other agents, there is usually a reduction in postanesthetic excitement and vomiting. Recovery from anesthesia is rapid.

Thiopental Sodium (Pentothal Sodium)

Thiopental sodium produces poor muscular relaxation and poor analgesia. Respiration is easily depressed, but there is little effect on blood pressure. Coughing, bronchospasms, and laryngospasms sometimes occur. Atropine is frequently given as a premedication because it reduces secretions which predispose to laryngospasms.

Methohexital Sodium (Brevital Sodium)

Methohexital sodium has a shorter duration of action and is somewhat more potent than thiopental sodium. Otherwise the effects are similar.

ADJUNCTIVE DRUGS FOR GENERAL ANESTHESIA

In addition to the main general anesthetics various other drugs are used as adjuncts. They contribute characteristics that the main drug might lack, they improve the safety factor, or they provide maximum comfort possible for a patient about to undergo an operational procedure. Some of these drugs are sometimes used as adjuncts, whereas at other times they may serve as the main anesthestic agent. It is part of the practice of anesthesiology to combine various drugs properly to produce a balanced anesthetic state.

Preanesthetic Sedation

Drugs used for preanesthetic sedation include the sedative-hypnotics, the narcotics, and the tranquilizers. Sedative-hypnotics are used to produce sleep the night before general anesthesia is to be administered and as sedatives preceding the operation. (See Chap. 6.) If a patient has been taking a particular sedative, it is usually wise to continue with the same drug. However, tolerance may have developed, and administration of larger doses may be required. Among the barbiturates, secobarbital (Seconal) and pentobarbital (Nembutal) are among the most frequently used. A disadvantage is that occasionally a patient may become excited instead of sedated. When the barbiturates are used instead of the narcotics, there is a lower incidence of postoperative nausea and vomiting. The patient will recover more rapidly from the general anesthetic state but will experience pain earlier and will more likely experience restlessness. Chloral hydrate is frequently preferred in children and the elderly. It appears to be better tolerated and to cause a lower incidence of excitement.

Promethazine (Phenergan), droperidol (Inapsine), and hydroxyzine (Vistaril) have, in addition to their sedative effects, antiemetic and antihistaminic effects that might be advantageous under certain conditions. Respiratory depression tends to be minimal. In addition, when hydroxyzine is used along with narcotics, it potentiates the analgesic effect of these drugs. Antiemetic drugs should be prescribed if there is a history of prolonged vomiting following anesthesia. Diazepam (Valium) used orally (po) or IV is also a popular drug used for preanesthetic sedation. Its respiratory effects are minimal, but residual effects may be of long duration.

Narcotics are frequently prescribed alone or combined with nitrous oxide and thiopental sodium or with diazepam. Besides the sedative effect, the narcotics provide postoperative analgesia. Respiratory depression occurs at therapeutic doses. This may be useful in maintaining a more satisfactory rate and depth of respiration during the light planes of anesthesia with inhalation anesthetics. The rapid, shallow breathing which occurs at this time sometimes makes it difficult to take in enough anesthetic. However, respiratory depression may be great enough to delay anesthesia unless respiratory assistance is provided. Use of narcotics is associated with greater postoperative pulmonary complications. The narcotics generally have little effect on blood pressure when the patient is supine (in a horizontal position), but occasionally a profound hypotension can result. However, vascular reflexes are decreased, and postural hypotension and fainting can occur upon arising. Narcotics can cause nausea and vomiting before or after general anesthesia and should be avoided in patients with a previous anesthetic history of protracted postoperative vomiting. They should also be avoided in patients who previously responded to these drugs with symptoms of excitement, urticaria, or wheezing. Elderly patients, debilitated patients, or patients with circulatory problems should receive reduced dosage. Narcotics should be used with caution and in sharply reduced dosage in patients with liver and pulmonary disease since respiratory depression can be severe in these patients.

Anticholinergic Drugs

These drugs need not be used routinely but only when there are specific indications. Atropine and other anticholinergics are used to decrease salivary and bronchial secretions and to prevent or treat severe reflex slowing of the heart during anesthesia. The bradycardia can be due to the general anesthetic halothane, to the neuromuscular blocking drug succinylcholine, or to the operative procedure. Anticholinergic drugs are contraindicated in patients with narrow-angle glaucoma.

Neuromuscular Blocking Drugs General anesthesia must provide, in addition to unconsciousness and freedom from pain, an optimal surgical field where skeletal muscle tone has been suppressed. This can be accomplished by deep stages of anesthesia, but the amount of anesthetic needed is great and can create serious problems. The neuromuscular blocking drugs can produce good skeletal muscle relaxation during anesthesia, and operations can be performed in lighter stages of anesthesia than would be possible otherwise. Respiratory muscles are depressed, and patients frequently require assisted respiration.

The neuromuscular blocking drugs act at the junction of the motor nerve and the skeletal muscle. They combine with acetylcholine receptors on the surface of the muscle and block the effect of this neurotransmitter after it is released by the nerve. Decreased functioning results in skeletal muscle paralysis.

There are two types of neuromuscular blocking drugs. The competitive type blocks acetylcholine receptors but does not activate them, while the depolarizing drugs initially mimic the action of acetylcholine and activate muscle fibers. Following this initial effect the receptor area remains depolarized, and this prevents activity. Muscular paralysis results. The initial stimulation produces an uncoordinated contraction of muscles which may cause stiff, sore muscles in the postoperative period.

The neuromuscular block associated with depolarization is called a phase I block. If depolarizing drugs are frequently repeated or used for a prolonged period of time, the depolarization disappears yet the block persists. This is called a phase II block, and the mechanism by which it is produced is unknown at the present time.

The main neuromuscular blocking drugs presently in use include the depolarizing drug succinylcholine (Anectine) and the competitive drugs tubocurarine (Tubarine), gallamine (Flaxedil), and pancuronium (Pavulon).

Succinylcholine This depolarizing drug is administered IV in amounts of 0.5 to 1.0 mg/kg for short procedures. The duration of action is from 5 to 10 min. Muscular fasciculation occurs upon injection, and this may produce muscular pain in the postoperative period. It may be administered as an IV infusion for longer procedures. Succinylcholine has effects at cholinergic sites in the autonomic nervous system and may produce hypertension and tachycardia from stimulating autonomic ganglia, or bradycardia, salivation, and increased bronchial secretions from effects at parasympathetic sites. Succinylcholine is rapidly metabolized by serum cholinesterase which accounts for its short duration of action. Certain patients with genetically determined abnormal cholinesterase show a marked decrease in the ability to metabolize succinylcholine. The drug remains in the body for a long time, and a prolonged apnea (cessation of breathing) results. Since cholinesterase is synthesized in the liver, even moderate liver disease can result in a decreased synthesis of this enzyme. The duration of action of succinylcholine may be twice as long in these patients. The irreversible cholinesterase inhibitors used as eye drops for the treatment of glaucoma may be absorbed systemically and interfere with the metabolism and prolong the action of succinylcholine.

The apnea which results from the prolonged effect of succinylcholine does not endanger the patient if ventilation is controlled until the drug is eliminated. There are no adequate chemical antagonists to this drug. The cholinesterase inhibitors appear to intensify the phase I block and antagonize the phase II block, but there are no adequate ways to identify clinically which block is present, so these antagonists are not useful.

Tubocurarine (Tubarine) Muscle flacidity produced by this competitive blocking drug is useful for procedures that last approximately 20 min. The most common side effect is a dose-related fall in blood pressure which has been attributed to both ganglionic block and histamine release. If hypotension is already present in a patient, another blocking drug should be considered. Bronchospasms and increased bronchial and salivary secretions sometimes produced by tubocurarine have also been attributed to the release of histamine. Tubocurarine and other competitive drugs are antagonized by cholinesterase inhibitors like neostigmine, and these agents are used clinically for this purpose. Atropine is also given with it in order to abolish the parasympathetic effects (bradycardia, blurred vision, excessive salivary secretions, stimulation of the gastrointestinal and urinary tract) that are also produced by cholinesterase inhibitors. Neuromuscular block of tubocurarine as well as the other blocking drugs is enhanced by certain antibiotics and the inhalation anesthetics. The dose should be reduced when these drugs are present. The dose should also be reduced in the presence of renal failure since excretion is decreased and the drug effect is prolonged.

Gallamine (Flaxedil) This competitive blocking drug produces tachycardia and hypertension. These effects have been attributed to a parasympathetic blocking effect on the heart and to the release of norepinephrine from sympathetic nerve endings. Gallamine should not be used in patients with tachycardia or hypertension. Gallamine must not be used in the presence of kidney failure since excessive prolongation of drug response occurs.

Pancuronium (Pavulon) This drug also produces tachycardia and hypertension. It may be used in case of renal failure, but the dosage must be reduced.

ANESTHETIC PROBLEMS AND PATIENT CARE

Patients under general anesthesia have lost many of their normal protective mechanisms for survival. Cardiovascular and respiratory systems may be depressed, and the reflexes that help maintain these organs in a functional state may be obtunded. There may also be a danger of inhaling regurgitated material from the stomach.

It is the responsibility of the oral surgeon and the dental auxiliaries to maintain vital functions and care for the patient during and after this period. Care of the patient begins by first evaluating the physical and psychological status of the patient. This will help determine whether a particular person may be treated as an outpatient or will require hospitalization and what type of anesthetic and adjunctive drugs would be best under the circumstances.

In order to help with this evaluation the Society of Anesthesiologists has formulated the following classification of patients according to physical status:

Class 1. The patient has no organic or psychiatric disease. The pathological process for which the operation is to be performed is localized and does not entail systemic disturbance.

Class 2. Mild to moderate systemic disturbances caused either by the condition to be treated surgically or by other pathophysiological processes. Example: organic heart disease that is only slightly limiting, mild diabetes, essential hypertension or anemia, very old people, the extremely obese, and persons with chronic bronchitis.

Class 3. Severe systemic disturbances or disease from whatever cause even though it may not be possible to define the degree of disability with finality. Examples: severely limiting organic heart disease, severe diabetes, pulmonary insufficiency that is moderate to severe, angina pectoris, or healed myocardial infarction.

Class 4. Patients with severe systemic disorders that are already life threatening. Examples: patients with marked signs of cardiac insufficiency, persistent angina pectoris, active myocarditis, advanced degrees of pulmonary, hepatic, renal, or endocrine insufficiency.

Class 5. The patient with little chance of survival but who cannot survive without a particular operation.

E or *emergency* operation: Any patient in one of the classes listed who is operated upon as an emergency is considered to be in poorer physical condition than nonemergency patients. In order to denote this the letter E is placed after the class.

All subjects for general anesthesia should be classified. Usually a patient with poor physical status will not fare as well as a patient in good condition. No deaths should occur due to anesthesia in class 1 and 2 that can not be prevented by proper anesthesia management. Only class 1 and 2 patients should be considered for general anesthesia on an outpatient basis. Certain patients, the asthenic, the elderly, or the chronically ill, require minimal amounts of anesthesia, while robust patients require higher concentrations. Special care must be taken in the choice and administration of general anesthetics and the care of the patient when the following conditions are encountered:

1 Patients with circulatory abnormalities must be carefully supervised to make sure that they receive adequate oxygen, eliminate carbon dioxide, and maintain a safe blood pressure.

2 Patients with respiratory insufficiency are more likely to develop atelectasis (collapse of the lungs) and pneumonia. Tests of pulmonary function should be determined, infections should be treated, and bronchospasms can be counteracted with bronchodilator drugs. Intermittent positive pressure breathing should be utilized. These patients are more sensitive to the respiratory depressant effects of various drugs. For this reason, narcotics should be avoided.

3 Patients with kidney disease should not receive methoxyflurane because of the renal toxicity of this drug. Drugs like gallamine and pancuronium that are excreted by the kidney should be avoided in patients with kidney impairment.

4 Volatile anesthetics may further impair liver function in patients with liver disease. This is due to the hepatotoxicity of these drugs and their ability to reduce blood flow to the liver. Moderate disease will prolong the action of succinylcholine, while severe liver disease will interfere with the metabolism of many drugs as well as decrease the formation of prothrombin, a condition that leads to bleeding.

In addition to the physical status, the psychological status of the patient must be evaluated. The degree of apprehension and anxiety must be estimated and planned for. If preoperative anxiety is excessive, agitation and delirium are more likely to occur during the recovery period. On the other hand, excessive premedication may produce excessive cardiovascular and respiratory impairment during and after anesthesia. Usually, IV induction is preferred when strong emotional upset is present.

A medical and drug history should be taken to make sure that there are no contraindications to the planned procedure. It must also be ascertained in outpatients that a responsible adult will accompany the patient on the day of the operation. The procedure that the patient must follow before arriving at the office should be carefully explained, and the importance of following directions exactly should be emphasized: The patient should be instructed to take the medication at the proper time and to get a good night's sleep; the patient should be warned not to eat or drink during the 6 to 8 h preceding anesthesia and the reasons given.

On the day of the operation, the physical and psychological status is rechecked. The patient is questioned to make sure that all directions were followed. During and following the operation vital signs should be monitored. Emergency equipment and drugs should be available at all times, and there should be adequate recovery facilities and trained auxiliaries. The ambulatory patient must be more fit when discharged from the recovery room than the hospital patient who is returned to the hospital bed.

A patient is considered recovered enough for dismissal when vital functions are stable and few anesthetic or residual effects of the operation remain. The patient should be able to walk without dizziness or ataxia. The patient should be told of possible discomfort that may follow, given instructions and prescriptions for the control of pain, and should also be instructed to ingest only clear fluids until the stomach is settled. A phone number should be provided where the anesthetist and surgeon can be reached if necessary. It is wise to contact the patient the day after the operation to make sure that no complication is interfering with recovery.

NEUROLEPTANALGESIA

The neuroleptanalgesic state is produced by the IV administration of a major tranquilizer and a narcotic. The major tranquilizer produces a sedative effect, a state of mental and physical quieting, and an indifference to incoming stimuli. The narcotic has a sedative and analgesic effect and produces respiratory depression. A person under the influence of a narcotic tends to ignore normal physiological body signals that would usually produce a response, and when pain is felt it does not produce suffering. When the two drugs are given together, the patient appears to be in a stupor; the patient is quiet and free from pain. Minor procedures can be carried out with the cooperation of the patient. This state is not equivalent to any stages of general anesthesia and appears to be qualitatively different. The addition of nitrous oxide will produce a state in which major surgical procedures can be carried out.

The most common neuroleptic in present practice is Innovar. This is a combination of droperidol (Inapsine), a butyrophenone derivative (see Chap. 6), and fentanyl citrate (Sublimaze), a narcotic with a short duration of action. Innovar must be administered with caution since there are many disadvantages to this combination.

Innovar is always administered IV, and it takes 3 to 5 min to reach its peak effect. Attempts to administer nitrous oxide during the induction period can produce delirium, and too rapid an injection can induce chest wall spasms which interfere with respiration. This effect can be antagonized by neuromuscular blocking drugs. Hypotension and a decrease in heart rate can occur, especially during the induction period. The bradycardia can be antagonized by atropine. Respiratory depression occurs frequently and requires assisted ventilation and tracheal intubation.

Recovery from the neuroleptic state is fairly rapid, but residual effects may be present for a day or more due to the long duration of action of droperidol. When respiratory depression is still present after recovery, it is due to the effects of fentanyl citrate and may be antagonized by narcotic antagonists. Extrapyramidal symptoms consisting of tremors and spasms, and muscular rigidity can usually be controlled by antiparkinsonism drugs. Nausea and vomiting may occur following the recovery period.

Among the advantages of neuroleptanalgesia is the persistence of analgesia beyond the recovery period, the lack of toxicity to the heart, liver, and kidneys, and the ease of working with a cooperative patient.

DISSOCIATIVE ANESTHESIA

Ketamine is called a dissociative anesthetic because the patient feels unrelated to the environment during induction. This drug produces good analgesia and amnesia, but muscular relaxation is poor. There is little effect on respiration, and the blood pressure and cardiac rate are elevated. Emergence is slow. A main disadvantage of this drug is that it produces disagreeable dreams and hallucinations. These may occur during recovery and for weeks afterward. The patient must be kept quiet during recovery. Verbal, tactile, and visual stimuli must be avoided. In dentistry this drug is injected IV or intramuscularly (IM) for short outpatient procedures. It is generally reserved for children since hallucinations occur mostly in adults.

INTRAVENOUS SEDATION

Many short dental procedures do not require the stages of surgical anesthesia and the associated difficulties that occur with the use of general anesthetics. A more conservative technique involves the IV use of small amounts of depressants to produce sedation, analgesia, and amnesia. The patient remains awake and cooperative, and vital functions are minimally affected. Since analgesia is not complete, local anesthetics are also used at the same time, but there is the advantage that the patient does not mind the injections. Only a skilled, trained clinician should utilize this method since unconsciousness can easily result if care is not taken. The same precautions must be taken and the same facilities are needed for the care of the patient receiving IV sedation as was described for the ambulatory general anesthesia patient. Intravenous sedation is the most effective method of ensuring the right degree of sedation in each individual. Small amounts of drugs are given at repeated intervals until the proper result is achieved.

The most frequently used drugs for IV sedation include pentobarbital (Nembutal), diazepam (Valium), and combination of diazepam with a narcotic. (Also, see Neuroleptanalgesia and Chap. 6 for discussion of individual drugs.) Pentobarbital is administered in small increments at 1-min intervals until a happy, relaxed state is produced. At this time the patient will be talkative but speech will be slurred. The patient will have difficulty in focusing and may complain that the room is revolving. The effect will last from 2 to 4 h. Early administration of analgesics may be required since barbiturates have no analgesic effects.

Diazepam is one of the most popular IV

sedatives. Good sedation, muscle relaxation, and amnesia are produced which last approximately 1 h. The patient may have symptoms of lightheadedness, dizziness, and ataxia. Duration of action is shorter than with pentobarbital, but residual effects may sometimes be present for several days after administration. Depression of the respiratory and cardiovascular systems is less likely to occur with diazepam than with pentobarbital. Diazepam is sometimes combined with a narcotic like meperidine (Demerol) when considerable pain is present in the patient preoperatively. The combination will produce sedation, muscle relaxation, amnesia, and analgesia. Increased respiratory depression with this combination is a distinct disadvantage.

ANSWER TO CHAPTER CASE

Several deaths have been reported because tanks of nitrous oxide and oxygen were accidentally switched. Pure nitrous oxide was administered during the recovery period instead of oxygen. Lack of oxygen and CNS depression due to nitrous oxide produced respiratory failure and tissue damage which resulted in death. This type of incident should not occur since fail-safe systems are available which prevent tank mixup. In this case, the inhalation apparatus should be removed and oxygen administered from another source. Dental auxiliaries should be aware of the serious problems that can occur when equipment is damaged or improperly used and should be constantly vigilant to prevent such occurrences.

QUESTIONS

1 What is the difference between a 100% anesthetic and a 25% anesthetic?
2 What stage of general anesthesia is produced by nitrous oxide as it is usually used in dentistry? Can excitement or unconsciousness be produced?
3 What events are indicative of the various planes produced during nitrous oxide sedation and analgesia?
4 What changes occur in the pulmonary and cardiovascular systems with increasing depth of anesthesia?
5 Why should 100% nitrous oxide never be administered?

READING REFERENCES

Allen, G. D., "Nitrous Oxide-Oxygen Sedation Machines and Devices," Council on Dental Materials and Devices and Council on Dental Therapeutics, American Dental Association, *J. Am. Dent. Assoc.,* **88:**611, 1974.

Cohen, E. N., et al., "Occupational Disease among Operating Room Personnel. A National Study," *Anesthesiology,* **41:**321, 1974.

Cohen, E. N., et al., "A Survey of Anesthetic Health Hazards among Dentists," *J. Am. Dent. Assoc.,* **90:**1291, 1975.

Dripps, R. D., et al., *Introduction to Anesthesia: The Principles of Safe Practice,* W. B. Saunders, Philadelphia, 1977.

Ellis, F. R., et al., "Malignant Hyperpyrexia Induced by Nitrous Oxide and Treated with Dexamethasone," *Br. Med. J.,* **4:**270, 1974.

Langa, Harry, *Relative Analgesia in Dental Practice: Inhalation Analgesia with Nitrous Oxide.* W. B. Saunders, Philadelphia, 1968.

Reisner, L. S., and M. Lippmann, "Ventricular Arrhythmias after Epinephrine Injection in Enflurane and in Halothane Anesthesia," *Anes. Analg. (Cleveland),* **54:**468.

Trieger, N., and S. Rubenstein, "The Current Status of Halothane," *J. Oral Surg.,* **31:**595, 1973.

Walts, L. F., et al., "Critique: Occupational Disease among Operating Room Personnel," *Anesthesiology,* **42:**608, 1975.

Vitamins and Minerals

"Ms. Smith, should I buy multivitamins at the drug store or have Dr. Brown prescribe them? I think I should take large doses of vitamin D to strengthen my teeth and bones. What do you think about vitamins?"

Vitamins and minerals are important for body functions. They are found in foods, so that persons eating well-balanced diets should not need additional vitamins and minerals.

However, many patients do not eat a well-balanced diet for various reasons. Therefore, a patient may lack certain vitamins or minerals and need a therapeutic preparation. This may occur as a result of a diet deficiency during pregnancy, lactation, intestinal absorption disorders, fad diets, or periods of emotional stress when dietary intake may be inadequate. Also, vitamins and minerals may be necessary in geriatric patients, particularly those living alone, whose diets may be inadequate. A few studies have even suggested that postsurgical therapy with various vitamins and minerals may improve wound healing. However, these findings are not yet adequately documented.

Surveys have shown that vitamin and mineral intake is frequently unsatisfactory in low-income families and certain ethnic groups. Also, regardless of group status, many people have diets which are high in calcium but poor in terms of proper dietary composition.

Information on dietary supplementation of vitamins and minerals can be obtained in Table 9-1. Vitamins are either fat soluble or water soluble and are divided accordingly in Table 9-1. The allowances in this table cover individual variations among most normal persons living in the United States under average living

Table 9-1 Recommended Dietary Allowances (RDA) For Dietary Supplements*

	Units of measurement	Children 1–4 years	Children 4–10 years	Adults Male	Adults Female	Pregnancy	Lactation
Energy	Kilocalories	1300	1800–2400	2400–3000	1800–2400	2400	2600
Fat-soluble vitamins							
Vitamin A activity	Retinol	400	500–700	1000	800	1000	1200
	equiv. or IU	2000	2500–3300	5000	4000	5000	6000
Vitamin D	IU	400	400	400	400	400	400
Vitamin E activity	IU	7	10	12–15	12	15	15
Minerals							
Calcium	Milligrams	800	800	800–1200	800–1200	1200	1200
Phosphorus	Milligrams	800	800	800–1200	800–1200	1200	1200
Iodine	Micrograms	60	80–110	110–150	80–115	125	150
Iron	Milligrams	15	10	10–18	10–18	18+	18
Magnesium	Milligrams	150	200–250	350–400	300	450	450
Zinc	Milligrams	10	10	15	15	20	25
Protein	Grams	23	30–36	44–56	44–48	74–78	64–68
Water-soluble vitamins							
Ascorbic acid	Milligrams	40	40	45	45	60	80
Folic acid	Micrograms	100	200–300	400	400	800	600
Niacin	Milligrams	9	12–16	16–20	12–16	14–18	16–20
Riboflavin	Milligrams	0.8	1.1–1.2	1.5–1.8	1.1–1.4	1.4–1.7	1.6–1.9
Thiamin	Milligrams	0.7	0.9–1.2	1.2–1.5	1.0–1.2	1.3–1.5	1.3–1.5
Vitamin B_6	Milligrams	0.6	0.9–1.2	1.6–2.0	1.6–2.0	2.5	2.5
Vitamin B_{12}	Micrograms	1.0	1.5–2.0	3.0	3.0	4.0	4.0

Source: Adapted from Report of Food and Nutrition Board, National Academy of Science, National Research Council, 8th rev. ed., 1974.
* The figures presented are daily recommendations.

conditions. Many of the recommended allowances can be attained with a variety of common foods. These allowances are referred to as the recommended dietary allowances (RDA).

The RDA recommendations should not be confused with the recommendations of the Food and Drug Administration which are referred to as the U.S. recommended daily allowances (USRDA). The USRDA values represent the highest allowance for any age group and are designed for nutrition labeling. Therefore, in some cases these values will be higher than the RDA.

A knowledge of vitamins is important in dentistry since the oral cavity sometimes is the first site where vitamin deficiencies are manifested. The most common sign of vitamin disorders is soreness of the mouth and tongue.

Vitamins should be prescribed when one is fairly certain that a deficiency is present. They should not be prescribed because they are "fairly harmless" and "may make the patient feel better." Since most vitamins can be purchased without a prescription, it is necessary to be aware of the signs and symptoms of overdose.

FAT-SOLUBLE VITAMINS

The fat-soluble vitamins, A, D, E, and K, are found mainly in plants and in certain animal tissues. Since their absorption is similar to that of fat, any condition that causes malabsorption of fat may result in a deficiency of these vitamins.

These vitamins affect the permeability of cell membranes and act as oxidation-reduction agents, coenzymes, and enzyme inhibitors.

Overdosages may cause severe toxic effects since they tend to accumulate in the body and are slowly metabolized. They are stored in the liver and excreted in feces.

Vitamin A

Vitamin A, or retinol, is an unsaturated alcohol which occurs naturally in fish-liver oil, whole milk, and eggs. It is necessary for the normal development of teeth, and vitamin A deficiencies may result in enamel hypoplasia due to an impairment of odontoblastic activity. Vitamin A deficiencies may also result in eye damage, night blindness, and blindness. It may also play a role in the maintenance of normal mucosa (eyes, respiratory, gastrointestinal, and genitourinary tracts). Deficiencies have been related to keratinization of mucosal tissues, including oral mucosa.

Vitamin A deficiencies are rare in humans since the liver may store enough vitamin A to meet the body's needs. When deficiencies of vitamin A do occur, they are often associated with malabsorption problems or severe liver disease.

The recommended dietary allowance for adults is 5000 IU. Increased intake is required during pregnancy and lactation.

Overdosage of vitamin A can result in nausea, headache, lethargy, skeletal disorders, hypercalcemia, gingivitis, subcutaneous swelling, and coarse hair.

Vitamin D

Vitamin D is classified as a sterol. This vitamin exists in two forms: D_2, or ergocalciferol, and D_3, or cholecalciferol. The former is produced synthetically by the irradiation of a yeast and fungus chemical, ergosterol. The latter is naturally found in animal tissue after exposure to sunlight. Both forms have a similar effect.

Vitamin D can be found in fish-liver oil, eggs, liver, and butter. Also, common foods such as milk and bread have vitamin D added.

Vitamin D increases absorption of calcium from the intestinal tract and promotes the deposition of calcium and phosphate by specifically acting on bone cells. Its action relates to parathormone effects on calcium metabolism (see Chap. 15).

A vitamin D deficiency in children causes rickets, a disease characterized by enamel and dentin hypoplasia as well as skeletal changes. In rickets there is a lack of bone mineralization with a resultant predominance of cartilage. As a result there may be a squaring of the head, rib collapse, protrusion of the sternum, spinal curvature, and bowed legs. In the adult, a deficiency results in osteomalacia. Osteomalacia is also characterized by a lack of bone mineralization. The clinical signs differ from rickets in that deformities are a result not of decreased bone growth, but of a lack of bone mineralization in remodeled bone. Therefore, adult bones are weakened, and deformities of weight-bearing bones and pathological fractures occur.

Overdosage of vitamin D in children has resulted in hypercalcemia and ectopic calcification of soft tissues such as kidneys, blood vessels, lungs, and skin. In the adult, an overdosage has resulted in bone resorption, including loss of alveolar bone.

The recommended daily dose is 0.01 mg.

Vitamin E

This vitamin is a tocopherol which is found in vegetable oils, wheat germ, and whole grain. Although it is considered essential for humans, manifestations of dietary deficiency are nonexistent. In rats, pathologic changes in oral mucosa have been reported in deficiency states but not in humans.

Vitamin E is an antioxidant which is claimed by some to retard the aging process and may give elderly patients a feeling of vitality and well-being. However, the scientific basis for this claim is highly questionable.

It has also been used in humans for the treatment of sterility and habitual abortion, but the value of this therapy has not been adequately documented.

Excessive intake of vitamin E appears to have no harmful effects although depletion of vitamin A from liver storage may occur. Long-term dosage of large amounts (400 to 800 units) has resulted in nausea, fatigue, headache, and blurred vision in some patients. When dosage was discontinued, symptoms disappeared.

Vitamin K

This vitamin, classified as a quinone, can be found naturally or synthetized as K_1 or K_2. This vitamin is found in some leafy greens such as alfalfa, cabbage, and spinach, and in fish meal, egg yolk, soybean oil, and liver. Also, it is synthesized in the gastrointestinal tract by normally present bacteria.

A reduced vitamin K ingestion is of consequence only if its synthesis by intestinal bacteria is altered or if there is a malabsorption from the intestinal tract. Vitamin K is essential for the synthesis of prothrombin and factors VII, IX, and X (see Chap. 14). Clinically, this lack of vitamin K may lead to severe bleeding, sometimes requiring the parenteral administration of vitamin K and whole blood. Surgical procedures are contraindicated in patients with vitamin K deficiency until adequate prothrombin times have been performed. Also, vitamin K should only be given to control bleeding as a result of reduced prothrombin due to the unavailability of vitamin K.

As discussed in Chap. 14, oral anticoagulants prevent the synthesis of prothrombin by antagonism of vitamin K. Therefore, vitamin K should not be given to patients receiving these anticoagulants unless suggested by the patient's physician.

The usual causes of vitamin K deficiency include malabsorption, inadequate bacteria for synthesis, which may occur with prolonged antibiotic therapy, and hepatobiliary disease in which an inadeqate flow of bile results in inadequate absorption of vitamin K. This occurs since bile improves the solubility and absorption of fat-soluble agents.

A recommended daily allowance is not available since intestinal bacteria can synthesize vitamin K.

WATER-SOLUBLE VITAMINS

The water-soluble vitamins are vitamin C and the B complex vitamins: B_1 (thiamine), B_2 (riboflavin), B_6 (pyridoxine), niacin (nicotinic acid), pantothenic acid, biotin, B_{12} (cyanocobalamin), and folic acid.

They are widely distributed in both plants and animals. They are absorbed from the gastrointestinal tract by diffusion and active transport. They act as coenzymes, oxidation-reduction agents, and possibly facilitate the activity of mitochondria.

The water-soluble vitamins are rapidly metabolized, and excess amounts are excreted in urine. For this reason, with the exception of niacin, overdosage with these vitamins does not cause toxic effects in individuals having normal kidney function.

Vitamin B Complex

These vitamins are found in a variety of foods, including lean meats, liver, milk, whole grain, cereals, nuts, poultry, fish, and eggs.

The side effects of various members of the vitamin B group are summarized in Table 9-2. In general, deficiencies cause glossitis and a wide variety of oral mucosal changes such as angular cheilosis, stomatitis, and a sore, reddened tongue.

A number of the B vitamins are affected by

Table 9-2 The B Vitamins

Name	Deficiency state
Biotin	?
Choline	Possibly neural transmission disorders
Cyanocobalamin (B$_{12}$)	Pernicious anemia
Folic acid	Anemia, stomatitis
Inositol	?
Niacin	Pellagra
Pantothenic acid	Inadequate metabolism of carbohydrates, fats, proteins
Pyridoxine (B$_6$)	Anemia
Riboflavin (B$_2$)	Cheilosis, redness of tongue, redness and burning sensation of eyes
Thiamine (B$_1$)	Soreness of tongue and oral mucosa

other drugs and conditions, and these are listed in Table 9-3.

Biotin

Biotin is a coenzyme essential for fatty acid synthesis and other carboxylation reactions. It is normally synthesized by intestinal bacteria, and a deficiency can be induced by drugs altering gastrointestinal bacterial flora. Symptoms associated with this vitamin deficiency are rare

Table 9-3 Factors Affecting the B Vitamins

Name	Comment
Folic Acid	Deficiency can occur in patients receiving methotrexate or similar anticancer medications and phenytoin (Dilantin)
Pyridoxine	Deficiency can occur in patients receiving isoniazid or hydralazine-type drugs, oral contraceptives
Riboflavin	Urinary excretion increased by more than 1 g of oxytetracycline or chlortetracycline administered per day
Thiamine	Need increases in hyperthyroidism, pregnancy, fever, exercise

and include loss of appetite, nausea, and malaise.

Niacin

Niacin (nicotinic acid) is classified as a pyridine derivative and is converted by the body into its active form, niacinamide (nicotinamide). It is a component of two coenzymes necessary for tissue respiration and energy transfer in both glycolysis and fat metabolism.

It is present in milk, eggs, meat, yeast, and green vegetables. The body can also synthesize it from tryptophan found in animal protein. Due to increased energy needs during pregnancy and lactation, the RDA for niacin is increased.

A deficiency of niacin results in pellagra, a disorder characterized by red lesions on exposed body surfaces, stomatitis, glossitis, diarrhea, a decrease in proprioception, and mental disturbances. Deficiency states are rare in this country but may occur in individuals on diets lacking this vitamin, in malabsorption conditions, and in alcoholics. In severe deficiency, hallucinations and psychosis may occur and may be the only sign of a deficiency. Patients with pellagra are also usually deficient in iron, folic acid, vitamin B$_6$, and thiamine.

Oral signs and symptoms of pellagra include a burning sensation in the mouth, a red and swollen tongue, and in chronic cases, the appearance of a "beefy red tongue." Desquamative lesions have been reported in gingiva, including ulcerations of the interdental papilla.

Large doses of niacin cause vasodilation. However, the therapeutic value of this vasodilation is unclear since niacinamide is not used as a vasodilator and is only given in niacin deficiency.

It has also been used in schizophrenia since this condition sometimes occurs in conjunction with pellagra. However, its use for schizophrenia has not been properly documented.

Therapeutic doses of niacin may cause pruritus, flushing, headache, paresthesia, and nausea. Large doses may activate peptic ulcers, decrease glucose tolerance, and cause liver damage and hyperuricemia.

Pantothenic Acid

This vitamin is a component of coenzyme A which is necessary for the intermediate metabolism of carbohydrates, fats, and proteins. It is found in all plant and animal tissues, and deficiencies are rare. A deficiency of pantothenic acid may be seen in cases of B vitamin deficiencies as a group deficiency.

A deficiency of this vitamin may cause symptoms similar to many of the other B complex vitamins: malaise, nausea, poor muscle coordination, and mood changes.

Pyridoxine Hydrochloride (B$_6$)

Vitamin B$_6$, which includes pyridoxine, pyridoxal, and pyridoxamine, is found in whole grain, peanuts, corn, meat, poultry, and fish. Vitamin B$_6$ is important mainly in protein and amino acid metabolism. Requirements may increase with pregnancy, lactation, and age.

Deficiency of vitamin B$_6$ may result in cheilosis, glossitis, stomatitis, dermatitis, depression, convulsive seizures, peripheral nerve damage, and a tendency toward infection.

This vitamin is used to treat certain types of anemia, and to prevent peripheral nerve inflammation caused by drugs such as isoniazid, hydralazine, and penicillamine. Its use as an antinausea agent in pregnancy has not been established. It can decrease the beneficial effects of medications in patients with Parkinson's disease. Therefore, such patients should not receive vitamin B$_6$.

Riboflavin (B$_2$)

Vitamin B$_2$, a flavin of D-ribotal, acts as a coenzyme important in protein metabolism, biological oxidations, and maintenance of red blood cells. It is found in milk, meat, eggs, nuts, and green vegetables. As with the other B vitamins, increased vitamin B$_2$ is necessary during pregnancy and lactation. Also, increased amounts must be ingested by individuals requiring more energy.

Riboflavin deficiency is characterized by cheilosis, angular stomatitis, glossitis, dermatitis of the nose and scrotum, and excessive vascularization of the cornea with visual impairment. Deficiencies of this vitamin usually occur only in conjunction with other B vitamin deficiencies.

Thiamine Hydrochloride (B$_1$)

Vitamin B$_1$ is an important coenzyme for carbohydrate metabolism. It occurs in whole cereals, meats, and nuts. Requirements increase during hyperthyroidism, heavy labor, prolonged diarrhea, and liver disorders. As with some of the other B vitamins, needs increase as caloric intake increases.

Thiamine deficiency is the most common among the B vitamins. This may be partly a result of its destruction by heating foods above 100°C or washing or boiling.

Beriberi is a deficiency of B$_1$. Subjects predisposed to beriberi are alcoholics, pregnant women, and those with gastrointestinal disorders. Beriberi is characterized by peripheral nerve inflammation, muscle weakness, tachycardia, and edema. Disturbances in the gastrointestinal tract may also be present.

Patients with mild thiamine deficiencies may show symptoms similar to a deficiency of the other B vitamins as well as decreased blood pressure and body temperature.

There is some experimental evidence that thiamine and some of the other B vitamins inhibit bacterial growth in human saliva. This finding may be important to future antiplaque therapy although it is presently experimental.

Cyanocobalamin (B$_{12}$)

Vitamin B$_{12}$ is essential to the function of all cells and is a cobalt-containing compound. It occurs in all animal products, including milk.

Therefore, deficiencies are rare except in strict vegetarians.

Vitamin B_{12} is absorbed from the gastrointestinal tract with the aid of an intrinsic factor secreted by gastric mucosa and calcium. An intrinsic factor deficiency causes penicious anemia in which spinal cord degeneration may occur. Therefore, if a patient has pernicious anemia, oral forms of the drug are not useful in therapy since absorption into the body cannot occur.

Folic Acid

Folic acid, which is found in liver, leafy vegetables, and yeast, is not destroyed by heat. It is important in the metabolism of amino acids, nucleic acids, and cell mitosis.

Para-aminobenzoic acid (PABA), a component of folic acid, is antagonized by sulfonamides. This antagonism may produce a folic acid deficiency leading to anemia and symptoms of glossitis, angular cheilosis, gingivitis, weakness, weight loss, skin depigmentation, and mental irritability.

Folic acid deficiency may be seen in pregnancy, chronic alcoholism, absorption problems, and inadequate dietary intake.

Vitamin B Complex Related Agents

A number of substances are related to the vitamin B group but have no known therapeutic value and no RDAs. These include bioflavonoids, which decrease capillary permeability and fragility; choline, which is important in the synthesis of lipoproteins; inositol, which is called a lipotropic factor; and methionine, which is important in choline synthesis. Methionine must be used with caution since it may cause coma in patients with liver disease.

Vitamin C

Vitamin C, also known as ascorbic acid, is found in most foods, especially citrus fruits, tomatoes, strawberries, green peppers, raw cabbage, vegetable greens, and potatoes.

Vitamin C is important in collagen synthesis, metabolic reactions of amino acids, and synthesis of epinephrine and antiinflammatory steroids.

Scurvy, a severe deficiency of this vitamin, is characterized by a failure of connective tissues to form properly, leading to swelling and soreness of joints, capillary hemorrhage, and gingival bleeding. Gingival bleeding usually is associated with other changes throughout the body. In severe deficiency, inadequate wound healing may occur. Too often, vitamin C is incorrectly recommended for treatment of bleeding gingiva that is associated with inadequate plaque control.

Dr. Linus Pauling, a past Nobel prize winner, and others have suggested that large amounts of vitamin C may prevent the common cold. The validity of this claim is still open to considerable question.

Large doses of vitamin C are usually excreted unchanged into the urine. However, large doses cause acidification of the urine which may result in stones in the urinary tract and should be avoided in patients with a history of kidney disorders.

The recommended dietary allowance for adults is 45 mg/day with an increase to 50 to 80 mg/day during pregnancy and lactation.

MINERALS

A number of minerals are essential for normal body function. While the requirement for most minerals is extremely small, it is essential to the function of many and varied biologic systems.

Sodium and Potassium

These minerals help maintain water and electrolyte balance. Patients with edema and right heart failure are occasionally placed on sodium-restricted diets to alleviate water retention. For such patients, sodium salts of various medications should not be prescribed. The need for sodium may increase with exertion, since during heavy exercise a subject will sweat more, and the sodium level will go down due to excretion in sweat. Therefore, the subject should have an increased daily sodium intake (10 to 15 g).

Approximately 1 g of potassium and 5 g of sodium are needed daily. Increased levels of potassium can result from the administration of large doses of the potassium salts of penicillin, since 1,000,000 units of the potassium salt of penicillin contain about 10.5 percent potassium, or 65.6 mg. These increased levels can upset the body's electrolyte balance, leading to dysfunctions. Also, some drug therapies can be affected by high potassium levels. For example, a normal dose of digitalis will become a toxic dose if high potassium levels are present.

Calcium and Phosphorus

Calcium is vital for blood coagulation, formation of bone and teeth, maintenance of normal nerve conduction, maintenance of cardiac rhythm, and production of milk. Phosphorus and calcium levels in the body are interrelated so that change in the body levels of one will affect the other.

The average daily requirement of each of these minerals is 1.2 g.

Calcium and its interaction with the parathyroid glands is considered in Chap. 15 on hormones.

Fluoride

Small amounts of fluoride are present in plant and animal tissues, especially bones and teeth. Fluoride should be considered an important mineral in view of its role in the prevention of dental caries (see Chap. 10).

Iodine

This mineral helps maintain body metabolism and is necessary for the production of thyroxine and triiodothyronine. A deficiency of iodine during pregnancy may result in cretinism in the offspring and goiter in the adult.

The recommended daily amount is 1 μg/kg body weight.

Iron

Iron is necessary for the formation of normal blood cells. It is found in a variety of foods, including spinach, egg yolks, and liver.

Iron deficiency causes anemia and reddening of the oral tissues. An iron overdose may result in constipation and pigmentation of the marginal gingiva. Since iron deficiency is the most common nutritional deficiency in the United States, the dental team should watch for signs and symptoms. The daily need for iron varies with a person's stage of development. For example, normal adults and postmenopausal females need 10 mg daily. In children from birth to age 4 the requirement is 15 mg, which decreases to 10 mg between ages 5 and 9 and rises to 18 mg during adolescence.

Copper

Copper is found in liver, kidney, nuts, and raisins, and is essential to various enzyme systems. No deficiency conditions have been reported. The daily recommended amount is 2 mg.

Magnesium

This mineral is found in most foods. Deficiencies manifest as muscle tremors and uncontrolled movements, delirium, and convulsions. They are most common in patients with severe kidney and liver disease, extensive therapy with diuretics, and sustained loss of gastrointestinal secretions. Occlusal adjustments and bite registrations in magnesium-deficient patients should not be attempted in view of the patients' poor muscle activity.

The daily adult requirement is 300 mg in females and 350 mg in males but varies with the individual's stage of development. For example, infants need 40 to 70 mg daily, children 100 to 250 mg, and adolescents 300 to 400 mg.

Trace Elements

A number of chemicals are needed by the body in only trace amounts, such as zinc, manganese, molybdenum, cobalt, chromium, and selenium. These elements should not be prescribed for patients since adequate amounts are found in the normal diet and excessive amounts can be harmful to health.

DIET-DRUG INTERACTION[1]

As outlined in Chap. 19, much is known about the effect of one drug on the efficacy or metabolism of another drug. More recently, attention has been focused on the interactions between nutrients in the diet and drugs.

Absorption of nutrients depends on the presence of gastrointestinal secretions, pH, and on the enzymatic activity of absorptive cells. With the exception of vitamin B_{12}, the major bulk of nutrients is absorbed in the upper intestines by passive diffusion and active transport. The degree of lipid solubility is important only for fats, since water-soluble nutrients are absorbed and transported by the nonlipid phase of intestinal content. Some nutrients like simple sugars and amino acids display competitive inhibition.

Drugs which may cause malabsorption include:

1 Those that affect intestinal motility, such as laxatives or cathartics
2 Hypocholesterolemic (cholesterol-lowering) drugs such as cholestyramine
3 Antibiotic drugs such as neomycin
4 Anticonvulsant drugs such as diphenylhydantoin
5 Colchicine used in gout

Drug-induced impairment of nutrient absorption has been attributed to several possi-

[1] Some material taken from *Dairy Council Digest* **48**:2, 1977.

ble mechanisms. First, a drug can solubilize a nutrient as mineral oil dissolves dietary carotene which then is lost to the normal absorptive process. Second, drugs can absorb or interfere with the physiological activity of bile salts which are necessary for the absorption of fats and fat-soluble vitamins. Third, drugs can damage the intestinal mucosa or selectively block or interfere with nutrient transport mechanisms. Last, drugs can damage the pancreas, decreasing the synthesis and/or release of pancreatic enzymes with consequent maldigestion of fat, protein, and starch.

Drugs may function as antivitamins by blocking the conversion of vitamins to coenzymes, by inhibiting the synthesis of the active metabolite of a vitamin, or by promoting the retention of the inactive form of the vitamin. Structurally unrelated drugs that stimulate the activity of drug-metabolizing enzymes also can stimulate cellular breakdown, reducing body stores of fat-soluble and water-soluble vitamins. Biochemical signs and symptoms of vitamin D deficiency have been evident among children and adults on chronic anticonvulsant drug therapy.

Oral contraceptives appear to produce metabolic changes with regard to phosphorus, magnesium, calcium, vitamin A, thiamin, riboflavin, ascorbic acid, folic acid, pyridoxine, vitamin B_{12}, and vitamin E. Although these metabolic changes suggest an increased metabolic need for several nutrients, few clinical correlations have been identified.

The effects of antacids on mineral metabolism also have been reported. Small amounts of antacids containing aluminum inhibit the intestinal absorption of phosphorus and fluoride, reverse the urinary and fecal phosphorus excretion, and increase the excretion of calcium in urine and stool. If the calcium losses caused by antacid therapy continue for prolonged periods of time, it is possible that significant skeletal demineralization may occur.

There are also reports of decreased drug effectiveness with the simultaneous ingestion of certain foods. For example, tetracyclines form insoluble complexes with calcium, magnesium, iron, and aluminum salts. Food containing these salts may decrease or impair intestinal absorption of these drugs. Therefore, the dental auxiliary should emphasize the importance of strictly following label directions regarding the time when drugs may be taken in relation to meal times and foods contraindicated.

Cognizant of the constraints accompanying the use of human subjects for research purposes, Roe pointed out the need for prospective human studies to provide information on the incidence, etiology, and risk of drug-induced malnutrition. A comprehensive drug surveillance study among hospital patients may provide statistical relationships between biochemical indices of nutritional status and drug intake. Also needed are studies of the nutritional status of populations taking long-term medication (e.g., the geriatric population) or women taking oral contraceptive agents.

Public health measures (for example, nutrient supplementation of common foods to reduce risk of vitamin deficiencies among oral contraceptive users) suggested to control, minimize, or prevent drug-induced malnutrition remain controversial and have not gained widespread acceptance from the medical and scientific communities. It is imperative that the dental team be made aware of the risks of drug-nutrient interactions and support measures which will reduce the risks of drug-induced malnutrition. Among these measures are:

1 Avoidance of unnecessary prescriptions
2 Limitations of multiple drug regimens
3 Support for control of over-the-counter drug sales
4 Dissemination of information on the nutritional effects of drugs to medical, dental, and allied health personnel as well as to patients themselves

A relatively common diet-drug interaction is the combination of tyramine-containing foods and monoamine oxidase inhibitors (MAOI) which results in a sudden rise in blood pressure or the so-called hypertensive crisis. Tyramine-containing foods include aged cheddar cheese, pickled herring, Chianti wine, bananas, tinned and packaged soups, nuts, and so on.

Other factors influencing the risk of such a reaction include the interval between the taking of the drug and ingesting of the food, as well as the patient's susceptibility, which may be related to the ability to metabolize tyramine.

ANSWER TO CHAPTER CASE

In order to answer this question, one must be familiar with most of the material in this chapter. A general rule to follow is that vitamins and minerals should only be prescribed for patients in whom there is a suspected deficiency or an obvious sign of deficiency. Then, vitamins and minerals should be specifically prescribed for the deficiency state in question. Therefore, multivitamin preparations are not usually recommended unless they contain the vitamins and minerals necessary for the correction of the suspected or real deficiency state.

Large doses of vitamin D are contraindicated in the average patient since an overdosage may occur. Overdosage of vitamin D in children has resulted in hypercalcemia and ectopic calcification of soft tissues such as kidneys, lungs, blood vessels, and skin. In the adult, an overdosage has resulted in bone resorption including loss of alveolar bone. These adverse effects do not usually occur if the patient presents with a definite vitamin D deficiency as discussed in this chapter. The treatment of vitamin D deficiency requires careful monitoring of patient blood levels of this vitamin and their response to therapy so that overdosage does not occur.

QUESTIONS

1 Can nutritional supplements be of value to patients following dental surgical procedures? Discuss.

2 Which vitamins may be useful to treat disorders of oral tissues? List the disorders for which they are indicated.

3 Name five minerals and their contribution to the maintenance of normal health.

4 Name four trace elements.

5 Give three examples of diet-drug interactions.

READING REFERENCES

Cutforth, R. H., "Adult Scurvy," *Lancet,* **1958**:454–456.

Dreizen, S., "Oral Manifestations of Human Nutrition Anemias," *Arch. Environ. Health,* **5**:66–75, 1962.

March, D. C., *Handbook: Interactions of Selected Drugs with Nutritional Status in Man,* The American Dietetic Association, Chicago, 1976.

Nizel, A. E., *Nutrition in Preventive Dentistry: Science and Practice,* Saunders, Philadelphia, 1972.

Roe, D. A., *Drug-Induced Nutritional Deficiencies,* Avi, Westport, 1976.

Sebrell, W. H., Jr., "Some Clinical Aspects of Vitamin B Deficiencies," *Am. J. Med.,* **25**:673–679, 1958.

Smith, J. F., "Clinical Evaluation of Massive Buccal Vitamin A Dosage in Oral Hyperkeratosis," *Oral Surg.,* **15**:282–292, 1962.

Stanton, G., "The Vitamins and Dentistry. I. Vitamin A," *J. Oral Ther. Pharmacol.,* **1**:451–461, 1965.

Toverud, S. V., et al., "Effects of Vitamin D on Developing Bones and Teeth," *N.C. Dent. J.,* **56**:9–11, 1973.

Fluorides

Ms. Jones, will fluoride-containing vitamins prevent tooth decay in my child? My neighbor told me that such vitamins are not necessary since we have fluoridated drinking water. Is this true? How does fluoride reduce tooth decay?

Fluoride is widely distributed in varying concentrations in soil, water, and plants. Atmospheric fluorides are byproducts of the manufacture of some metal compounds and the burning of soft coal. Fluoride in water results from the leaching out of this chemical from soil and rocks, where it is the seventeenth most common element in the earth's crust.

Fluorspar (CaF_2), the most common, naturally occurring fluoride, is a component of minerals such as apatite, micos, topaz, and cryolite. When fluoride leaches out of rocks and soil into water, the fluoride compound dissociates, leading to the free fluoride ion (F^-). Surface waters tend to have a low fluoride concentration, whereas underground waters, such as springs, rivers, and wells, in intimate contact with fluoride-containing minerals may contain higher amounts.

Since fluoride is so common throughout nature, humans ingest varying amounts of this chemical from plants, animals, and beverages. Furthermore, the fluoride content of food is also dependent on the fluoride content of the water in which it is prepared.

It has been well established that fluoride prevents dental caries. There is also evidence that fluoride strengthens and hardens bone and relieves bone pain. For this reason it is being given to some patients with bone-resorbing diseases, with beneficial effects.

MECHANISM OF ACTION

The mechanism by which fluoride prevents caries is not clearly understood. It is known that the fluoride ion (F^-) can replace the hydroxyl ion (OH^-) in hydroxyapatite, the major crystalline structure of enamel. The substituted crystal, called fluorapatite, is more resistant to acids, such as those produced by plaque bacteria, than the original hydroxyapatite.

As the tooth develops and enamel is formed, ingested fluoride is incorporated into the enamel. Therefore, since enamel develops its outer layer first, more fluoride can be expected to be deposited on the outer layers as compared to the inner layers. It is this surface enamel layer containing fluoride which imparts caries resistance to a tooth. Topical fluorides also become incorporated into enamel and provide protection against acid. The incorporation of fluoride into enamel can be represented as a chemical reaction:

$$Ca_{10}(PO_4)_6(OH)_2 + F^-$$

Hydroxyapatite

$$\rightarrow Ca_{10}(PO_4)_6F_2 + 2(OH)^-$$

Fluorapatite

Since fluoride is also an antienzyme, it may inhibit enzymatic acid production by plaque bacteria. The plaque also tends to concentrate fluoride. This could increase possible antienzymatic activity. Some caries protection from this may be expected.

In areas where there is no fluoridation of the community water supply, fluoride may be added to school water. However, this is not a substitute for community water fluoridation since fluoride intake from birth is important. It is of value since a substantial number of permanent teeth will not have completed calcification by age five or six. Also, there is evidence of considerable enamel fluoride uptake after completion of calcification but before tooth eruption. Some benefit may also be derived from topical action subsequent to eruption.

In some areas, the school water supply has been fluoridated as much as 4.5 times the level usually recommended for community water levels. These studies, conducted for 12 years in fluoride-deficient areas, revealed a 40 percent reduction in DMF surfaces. Essentially, no undesirable fluorosis resulted from this procedure. However, it should be noted that ingestion occurred only during part of each day and only on school days. This level (4.5 ppm) from birth (during major formation of permanent teeth) would cause undesirable fluorosis with continued intake.

ABSORPTION, DISTRIBUTION, AND EXCRETION

Fluorides are absorbed mainly from the gastrointestinal tract and also from the lungs and skin. Fluoride diffuses across the mucosa lining the gastrointestinal tract, and the unabsorbed fluoride passes through the digestive tract and is incorporated into the feces.

Fluoride is absorbed into plasma and distributes into all body tissues. However, it is concentrated mainly in the bone, developing teeth, thyroid, aorta, and possibly kidneys. The degree of uptake by bone and teeth is related to intake and age. Growing bone and developing teeth show a greater content of fluoride than bone and teeth in mature subjects. Prolonged periods of time are required for mobilization of stored fluoride from bone.

The major route of excretion is by the kidneys, and to a lesser extent by sweat glands, lactating breasts, and the gastrointestinal tract (feces). Under conditions of excessive sweating, the fraction of total fluoride excreted by this means may approach 50 percent.

When the fluoride ion passes into the kidney, it is first filtered by the glomerulus. It then passes into the kidney tubules, and 90 percent of the amount filtered is reabsorbed and returned to plasma.

PLACENTAL TRANSFER OF FLUORIDE

Fluoride crosses the placental barrier and is found in the fetal circulation. The fetal blood levels may be equal to, greater than, or less than maternal levels.

Once it passes the placenta, the fluoride deposits in the developing bones and teeth of the fetus. The concentration of fluoride in fetal bones and teeth is directly related to maternal fluoride intake and the age of the fetus.

It has not been established if fluorides taken prenatally increase caries resistance. Most evidence suggests no significant benefit, but studies in this area are continuing. Except for the cusp tips of the permanent first molars, only deciduous teeth are mineralizing prenatally. Therefore, if prenatal exposure to fluoride imparts some caries resistance, only the deciduous teeth would be affected.

TOXIC EFFECTS

The Society of Toxicology considered the toxic effects of fluorides and has made the following comments.

From a critical review of the voluminous and steadily growing literature on the biologic effects of inorganic fluoride, no evidence has been found of an ill effect of water fluoridation at 1 ppm in temperate climates. In the United States there are over 10,000,000 people drinking naturally fluoridated water at the near optimal concentration or higher. These waters have been consumed by large numbers of people for many years. Therefore, an extraordinary and exceptional reliability is conferred on the safety of water fluoridation because nature, in a sense, has already made the demonstration in hundreds of communities where the drinking water naturally contains fluoride. Under controlled conditions as recommended by qualified public health authorities, the Society of Toxicology finds water fluoridation to be a safe measure.

Fluoride inhibits several enzyme systems and alters tissue respiration and metabolism. Its toxic effects can be classified as acute or chronic and will be discussed accordingly.

Acute fluoride poisoning first affects the gastrointestinal tract, with salivation, nausea, diarrhea, abdominal pain, and vomiting. As toxicity becomes more severe, there is paresthesia, muscle pain, hyperactive reflexes, and convulsions due to the calcium-binding effect of fluoride. Also, a sudden drop in blood pressure may occur due to direct depression of the vasomotor center and a direct depression of cardiac muscle action. Hyperpnea followed by respiratory depression has been reported and is due to initial stimulation of the respiratory center with a subsequent depression. Death results from respiratory paralysis and/or cardiac failure. The average lethal dose of sodium fluoride in adults is 5 g, and the average dose showing initial toxicity is 280 mg (4 mg/kg). Lesser amounts may cause accidental poisoning or, in small children, death.

The American Dental Association recommends that no more than 264 mg of sodium fluoride be prescribed at any one time. Since 264 mg of sodium fluoride is close to the dose showing initial toxicity, the total amount of prescribed drug would have to be ingested at one time in order for initial toxicity to occur. However, in small children, as little as 110 mg of sodium fluoride have produced acute toxic signs. For this reason, even these low amounts must be in "child-proof" containers. In evaluating the various concentrations of fluoride available, the reader should note that 2.2 mg of sodium fluoride contains 1.2 mg of sodium and 1 mg of fluoride.

The incidence of acute fluoride intoxication is remarkably low. Less than 1000 cases of acute fluoride intoxication have been reported in the world. The World Health Organization Monograph of 1970 cited only 435 cases over a period of 85 years. Of these, 303 occurred as a result of accidents. One such accident occurred in 1943 at the Oregon State Hospital, where 263 cases were reported.

TREATMENT OF ACUTE TOXICITY

The treatment of acute toxicity is as follows:

1 Start intravenous (IV) therapy with glucose in isotonic saline.
2 Flush the stomach with 0.15% calcium hydroxide solution.
3 Have calcium gluconate available for IV administration if signs of tetany appear.
4 Maintain high urine volumes with parenteral fluids.
5 Wash away vomited material, urine, and feces immediately to prevent external burns.
6 Be prepared to institute measures to support blood pressure and respiration.

Obviously, acute toxicity can be a serious problem during extensive therapy. Therefore, the dosages of fluoride supplements for home or office should not exceed the ADA recommendations. In addition, parents should be made aware of the possible overdose dangers of this drug. The article entitled "Misuse of Topically Applied Fluorides" (see Reading References) presents an example of use of a 4% solution of stannous fluoride in a careless and incorrect manner for a 3-year-old child. Stannous fluoride was incorrectly applied, and then the child drank 45 ml of the 4% solution with the result that 3 h later he died of fluoride poisoning. Death would not have resulted if the medication had been used correctly and precautions had been taken to prevent swallowing. Therefore, the hygienist must carefully control the application of topical fluorides, use them as directed, and guard against accidental ingestion in the office.

CHRONIC TOXICITY

Chronic, excessive amounts of fluoride can cause osteosclerosis and mottled teeth. The osteosclerotic phenomena may relate to osteoblastic activity. In its severest form it is a disabling disease called crippling fluorosis. The osteosclerosis may also reflect a replacement of the hydroxyapatite crystal of bone with a denser crystal called fluorapatite.

In adults, fluoride ingestion of 2 to 8 mg/day for years can increase bone density, which can be seen radiographically. Daily doses of 20 to 80 mg for 10 to 20 years have also caused skeletal deformities and crippling fluorosis. In order to receive such large doses, a person would have to drink 2 L/day of water containing 10 ppm of fluoride. Early symptoms of skeletal fluorosis have sometimes been misdiagnosed as rheumatoid arthritis or osteoarthritis.

Mottled enamel (dental fluorosis), first described over 50 years ago, results from a partial ameloblastic failure to produce enamel in a regular manner. Since mottling is a developmental defect, it does not occur when excessive fluoride intake occurs after tooth crowns have formed (after age 8).

Clinically, mild mottling consists of small, opaque, paper-white areas scattered irregularly over the tooth crown. In severe cases, deep brown to black stained areas are observed in enamel, and the coronal surface of the tooth may be rough, fissured, or pitted. The esthetic problem resulting from this condition has a strong psychological impact on the patient. Therefore, these defects should be corrected as soon as possible with either full

Table 10-1 Conversion of ppm to Milligrams*

$$1 \text{ ppm} = \frac{1 \text{ g fluoride}}{1,000,000 \text{ mL water}} = \frac{1000 \text{ mg fluoride}}{1,000,000 \text{ mL water}} = \frac{1 \text{ mg fluoride}}{1000 \text{ mL water}}$$

Note: 1 g = 1000 mg; 1000 mL = 1 L.

crowns or replacement of the involved enamel with a synthetic material.

Drinking water containing 1 ppm of fluoride results in a barely detectable mottling in 10 percent of children. However, at 1.7 ppm, 40 to 50 percent show mottling, and at 2.5 ppm concentrations, it is as high as 80 percent.

The practitioner may want to convert ppm (parts per million) to milligrams of fluoride. This calculation is presented in Table 10-1. From Table 10-1 it can be seen that 1 L of water intake per day is equivalent to ingesting 1 mg of fluoride ion per day.

Recently, it has been suggested that fluoride is carcinogenic. These claims are not based on scientific fact. However, the dental profession must be knowledgeable about fluoride's side effects, since fluoridation of water has become an emotional issue and one not always based on scientific facts.

FLUORIDE CONSUMPTION

Approximately 150,000,000 people in the world now consume optimally fluoridated water. This optimal concentration varies with the mean annual temperature. The U.S. Public Health Service has established recommended levels for fluoride concentrations in water supplies in accordance with mean annual temperatures. The values are shown in Table 10-2. The daily intake of fluoride not only comes from drinking water but also from food consumed or prepared with fluoridated water. Also, crops are frequently fertilized with phosphate fertilizers of high soluble-fluoride content, and food products including bone in animal feeds contain fluoride.

In 1974 there was an analysis of foods from 16 different cities in the United States, including cities where the water was fluoridated and others where it was not. The dietary intake of fluoride from the fluoridated drinking water cities ranged from 1.7 to 3.4 mg/day compared to 1.0 mg/day in the cities without fluoridated drinking water. Since fluoride is also found in foods, it is likely that the daily intake of fluoride is greater than that administered in water.

However, naturally fluoridated foods and water have been ingested for decades with no serious side effects. In addition, public fluoridation has been widespread in this country for approximately 10 years without serious side

Table 10-2 Temperature Ranges and Recommended Fluoride Concentrations

Annual average of maximum daily temperature	Fluoride concentrations, ppm	
	Optimum	Acceptable range
50.0–53.7	1.2	0.9–1.7
53.8–58.3	1.1	0.8–1.5
58.4–63.8	1.0	0.8–1.3
63.9–70.6	0.9	0.7–1.2
70.7–79.2	0.8	0.7–1.0
79.3–96.5	0.7	0.6–0.8

effects. The incidence of mottled enamel, one of the earliest and most sensitive signs of fluoride toxicity, has not increased significantly in the past 10 years during this public fluoridation. In view of this, there is no need for alarm about fluorides. The safety and efficacy of fluoride has definitely been established. There is no scientific evidence against water fluoridation. Communities without fluoridated water are doing a disservice to their citizens from an economic standpoint and that of dental public health.

THERAPEUTIC ASPECTS OF FLUORIDE

Fluoridated Water

The administration of fluoride in drinking water at concentrations of approximately 1 ppm significantly reduces dental caries. The anticaries benefits are similar to those due to natural fluoride in drinking water. Fluoridated drinking water produces (1) a 60 percent lower dental caries rate; (2) a 75 percent decrease in loss of 6-year molars, and (3) a 90 percent reduction in the incidence of proximal caries of the four upper anterior teeth.

Evidence suggests that greater inhibition of caries occurs when teeth receive fluoride throughout the calcification period. Therefore, maximum benefit may be expected from continued use of fluoridated drinking water. Dental professionals must make the public aware of the benefits of fluoridation in their communities. This is necessary since water fluoridation has frequently become an emotional and sometimes a political issue.

Dietary Supplements of Fluoride Tablets

Maximum benefits to both deciduous and permanent teeth may result from daily fluoride supplements from infancy until approximately 13 years of age, at which time all permanent teeth except the third molars should have erupted. Because cariostatic benefits may tend to gradually diminish after fluorides are discontinued, periodic applications of topical fluorides may then be necessary.

The use of dietary fluoride or topical applications of fluoride depends partly on the age of the child. Dietary supplements of fluoride are best for very young children, whereas topical fluoride applications are preferred for older children with permanent teeth. Younger children highly susceptible to caries may benefit from both measures.

There is a need for cooperation from the child and parents for a consistent and continuous regimen for dietary fluoride administration. Strong motivation and a clear realization of the need for careful regulation of the daily intake are required on the part of the parents.

The natural level of fluoride in drinking water where the child lives should be known before dietary fluoride is prescribed. Fluoride levels in areas with numerous and varied H_2O supplies can be accurately measured using specific ion electrodes and special meters produced for this purpose. At present, it is suggested that fluoride supplements be limited to where drinking water contains 60 percent or less of the optimal level of fluorides recommended for community water in the geographic area.

As a precaution, no large quantities of sodium fluoride should be stored in the home. It is recommended that no more than 264 mg of sodium fluoride be dispensed at any one time, which is enough for at least a 4-month period. Each package dispensed should also bear the statement: *Caution: store out of reach of children.*

Although the optimal level of fluoride in drinking water is well established, there is no established allowance for fluoride administered once a day. The tentative allowance is 1 mg/day for a child over 3 years of age and one-half this amount for a child between the ages of 2 and 3. In order to avoid the possibility of unesthetic dental fluorosis, the prescribed dietary allowance should be reduced in proportion to the fluoride levels in the drinking water. Table 10-3 illustrates empirical adjustments for varying amounts of natural fluorides in communities where the recommended optimal level of fluoride is 1 ppm. These allowances are for children over 3 years of age. The allowances should be reduced by one-half for a child between 2 and 3 years of age.

For children under 2 years of age, water containing 1 ppm fluoride from fluoride tablets or drops should be used for the child's drinking water and for the preparation of food or formula. The administration of 0.25 mg of fluoride daily for this age group appears to be a satisfactory alternative.

Sodium fluoride tablets are best for localities where the drinking water is substantially devoid of fluoride. The following prescription illustrates such use for a child of 3 years or older:

Rx: Sodium fluoride tablets 2.2 mg. Dispense 120 tablets.
Sig.: 1 tablet each day to be chewed and swished before swallowing.
Caution: Store out of reach of children.

For the child between 2 and 3 years of age, the directions for the label can be changed to specify either one-half tablet each day or 1 tablet containing 2.2 mg of sodium fluoride every other day.

One 2.2-mg tablet of sodium fluoride completely dissolved in 1 qt of drinking water may be used for infants.

Because it is difficult to follow the strict regimen required for effective administration of fluoride tablets, public health programs in which tablets have been distributed free of charge for use at home have generally been unsuccessful. However, dental caries have been prevented when fluoride tablets were administered in a school-based program. After 2 or more years of fluoride ingestion, protection against dental caries ranged from 20 to 40 percent. In the longest trial of fluoride tablets reported in the literature, there was a 36 percent reduction in dental caries after 8 years.

The use of fluoride tablets can provide both a preeruptive (endogenous) effect and a posteruptive (topical) effect. Therefore, tablets should be chewed or dissolved in the mouth and the teeth rinsed with the resultant solution before swallowing.

One advantage of fluoride tablets compared to water fluoridation is that a specific dosage of fluorides is delivered. One disadvantage is that dietary supplements of fluoride taken once a day are rapidly cleared from the body. There is reason to believe, therefore, that they might be less effective than fluoridated water, which is consumed throughout the day and thus maintains a more constant blood fluoride level.

Adding Fluoride to Salt

Fluoridated salt also prevents dental caries. Results to date indicate that fluoridated salt can be as protective as community water fluoridation.

Insufficient information exists on the consumption of salt by different age groups and ethnic groups and in different geographic areas. Salt fluoridation also has the inherent disadvantage of being difficult to adjust to varying suboptimal levels of natural fluoride occurring in water supplies.

Table 10-3 Adjustment of Prescribed Fluoride Relative to Natural Content of Drinking Water

| Water fluoride, ppm | Adjusted allowance | |
	Sodium fluoride, mg/day	Provides fluoride ion, mg/day
0.0	2.2	1.0
0.2	1.8	0.8
0.4	1.3	0.6
0.6	0.9	0.4

Fluoridation of Milk

Only a few small studies have been conducted in humans in which milk has been the vehicle for fluoride supplementation. The results of these studies, nevertheless, show a positive caries-preventive effect. More clinical data is needed, however, before the fluoridation of milk can be recommended for caries-prevention programs.

In view of the fact that fluoride complexes readily with calcium, the value and predictability of this dosage form is questionable. It should be noted that fluoride can be detected in the milk of a lactating female who has fluoride in her diet, but in doses too low to have any therapeutic or toxic effects.

Fluoride in Vitamins

Vitamin preparations containing sodium fluoride are also available as drops, tablets, and chewable tablets. This form of supplementation is useful in areas where the water supply contains less than 0.7 ppm. For children under 2 years of age the daily recommended dosage is 0.5 mg, and for those over 2 years it is 1 mg. This form of fluoride offers a way to provide fluoride to the child, if the parents are conscientious in dispensing the required amount daily, and if the child does not object to taking oral medications. In recommending vitamins with fluoride it is mandatory that the practitioner know the fluoride content of the child's water supply, as well as the fluoride content of the vitamin being recommended.

Topical Fluorides

Fluoride can be applied topically in various forms, offering the dental practitioner a number of options to choose for his or her patients. Dental professionals should be thoroughly familiar with these various dosage forms, their value, and their method of application, since they are often involved in applying these agents.

Topical agents are of questionable value in a caries-reduction program when they are used in fluoridated communities. However, when used in nonfluoridated areas, they are definitely effective. Actually, in such areas, they often are the only form of fluoride therapy available.

The dosage forms of topical fluoride currently available include dentifrices, solutions, gels, mouthwashes, and prophylaxis paste. These various forms are outlined in Table 10-4. Also, an excellent review of topical fluorides can be found in the article by Wei and Wefel (see Reading References).

Fluoride Dentifrices

The earliest fluoride dentifrices contained sodium fluoride. However, the fluoride was biologically unavailable since the calcium in the dentifrice abrasive bound the fluoride and thus inactivated it.

Although a number of dentifrices containing fluoride are on the market, the consumer must be cautioned that not all provide available fluoride since the abrasive systems in some dentifrices inactivate fluoride. Therefore, the product may contain as much fluoride as any other dentifrice but it is not available. Also, if the product has a short shelf-life, it will be ineffective if poor marketing gets it to the consumer too late.

For these reasons, only dentifrices approved by the Council on Dental Therapeutics of the American Dental Association should be recommended. These products are listed in *Accepted Dental Therapeutics,* and this book presents an excellent literature review on fluorides in various forms and accepted products.

Currently accepted dentifrices contain sodium monofluorophosphate or stannous fluoride, which reduce caries by approximately 25 percent when used daily. In some clinical studies, stannous fluoride dentifrices stained teeth, particularly in pits and fissures.

Table 10-4 Various Topical Fluoride Preparations

Drug name	Dosage form	Concentration recommended
Acidulated phosphate fluoride	Topical solution, topical gel, mouthrinse, prophylaxis paste	1.23% in 1% orthophosphoric acid 0.5% 0.02–0.04% 1.2%
Amine fluoride	Dentifrice, mouthrinse	1.6% 2.5%
Sodium fluoride	Topical solution, mouthrinse	2% 0.02–0.05% (daily) 0.2% (weekly)
Sodium monofluorophosphate	Dentifrice	0.76%
Stannous fluoride	Topical solution, mouthrinse, prophylaxis paste, dentrifice	8% 0.1% 8% 0.4%

This stain is related to the tin in this compound, which adheres to plaque. The significance of this staining and its esthetic problems have not been determined.

Dentifrices and mouthwashes containing amine fluorides (cetylamine hydrofluoride, oleylamine hydrofluoride) are currently under investigation. Initial results with these compounds are promising. The development of amine fluorides is of interest since the action of the fluoride ion is enhanced by the surface activity produced by amines. Also, the amines themselves may exert an antienzymatic effect on dental plaque.

The composition of some popular toothpastes is important for a proper understanding of this topic. *Crest* contains stannous fluoride (0.4 percent), with calcium pyrophosphate (40 percent) as an abrasive. It is marketed in a plastic container because a reaction of stannous ions at an acid pH occurs when conventional soft metal containers are used. *Colgate with MFP* contains sodium monofluorophosphate (0.76 percent), with sodium metaphosphate (42 percent) and dicalcium phosphate (5 percent) as abrasives. *Macleans Fluoride* contains sodium monofluorophosphate (0.76 percent), with calcium carbonate as an abrasive.

Further discussion of dentifrices in general can be found in Chap. 12, Prophylaxis Pastes, Dentifrices, and Mouthwashes.

Fluoride Solutions and Gels

In children, a reduction of 30 to 40 percent in dental caries is seen with: 2 percent sodium fluoride, 8 percent stannous fluoride, and acidulated phosphate-fluoride solutions and gels. No one agent appears to be superior to any other when used as directed.

Several investigators prefer the acidulated phosphate agents (APF) for the following reasons:

1 They can be applied once every 6 months on children's teeth, corresponding to the time interval for appointments in many offices.
2 They are stable when kept in plastic containers.
3 More fluoride may be taken up by enamel during a given period of time, as compared to other agents.
4 It is probable that fluoride retention lasts for 2 to 3 years following one application.

APF solutions are applied for 4 min to teeth which have been pumiced, dried, and isolated.

Solutions of sodium fluoride were the first

solutions used. Four applications of a 2% sodium fluoride solution are applied at 1-week intervals at ages 3, 7, 11, and 13. These ages represent the approximate eruption times of various tooth groups. A prophylaxis is given prior to the first of the four applications in each series. As with APF, the teeth are dried and isolated, and the solution is applied for 4 min. Advantages of sodium fluoride include a pleasant taste and stability in solution. Because of its stability it need not be mixed fresh for each day of use.

Some recent studies have suggested that the topical application of sodium fluoride once every 6 months may be as beneficial as the four-application regimen discussed above. However, the four-application regimen is recommended by the American Dental Association and has produced the most consistent therapeutic results for sodium fluoride.

Solutions of 8% stannous fluoride have been used to reduce caries. As with the other agents, the teeth are polished, dried, and isolated, and a 4-min application follows. The disadvantages of this solution are that it must be freshly prepared, some tooth discoloration (as discussed under dentifrices) has occurred, and it has an unpleasant taste which is difficult to mask.

Stannous fluoride solutions are useful in children with high caries activity since they may have both a caries-arresting property and one of caries prevention. The frequency of application varies with the caries activity of the child. For children with an average incidence of caries, it can be applied annually between ages 3 and 13.

It should be noted that when teeth are polished prior to application of any of the above, the prophylaxis paste should be carried interproximally with dental floss so that benefit will accrue to proximal surfaces. Also, following all topical fluoride applications, the patient should be told not to eat, drink, or rinse for at least 30 min. However, since fluoride uptake from topical solutions is rapid, the value of restricting food and drink for 30 min has been questioned by some investigators.

When gels are used, they are placed into a tray which is placed against the teeth so that the gel flows around all surfaces. Best results have been reported with custom-fitted trays. During the use of gels, the teeth should be kept dry during the application, which is for 4 min.

The value of topical fluorides on adults has not been established. However, some studies have suggested that the APF types may offer some caries protection. Recent reports have suggested that polishing of teeth is not necessary prior to the topical application of fluorides. These studies have stated that deplaquing of teeth with a toothbrush is adequate and offers the advantage of not removing surface fluoride from tooth structure. This concept may be valid, and future investigations in this area should be encouraged.

Fluoride Mouthwashes

Some fluoride-containing mouthwashes have been approved by the Council on Dental Therapeutics of the American Dental Association on a prescription basis. Daily rinsing with a 0.05% sodium fluoride solution has reduced caries by 40 percent and fortnightly rinsing with a 0.2% solution brought a reduction of about 20 percent. These results were seen in nonfluoridated areas. An over-the-counter mouthwash containing 0.05% sodium fluoride (Fluorigard) is currently available in the United States.

Acidulated phosphate fluoride-containing mouthrinses (0.02 and 0.04%) also reduce caries about 25 percent when used on a daily basis.

Stannous fluoride-containing preparations (0.1%) have also been reported to result in caries reduction of approximately 25 percent when used daily. Studies on fluoride-containing mouthrinses are continuing and may offer promises for the future. These products, when brought into the home, present a potential danger. Therefore, the Council on Dental Therapeutics has recommended that these rinses be packaged in individual dose containers and should not, in toto, exceed 300 mg of sodium fluoride. Dental professionals should stress the potential danger of these products to parents and children.

Prophylaxis Pastes

Prophylaxis pastes may contain fluoride as either sodium or stannous fluoride. Since a dental prophylaxis removes surface fluoride, this surface fluoride depletion can be prevented with fluoride-containing prophylaxis pastes. However, it has not been conclusively shown that use of these pastes offers any caries reduction, and therefore no definitive recommendation can be made at present. Some studies have suggested that fluoride-containing prophylaxis pastes may reduce root sensitivity.

Studies with self-administered prophylaxis pastes containing various fluorides are under consideration. The results are conflicting, and the value of this method of application is questionable.

FUTURE DIRECTIONS

Fluoride therapy is constantly changing, and new data become available daily. For example, pretreatment of teeth with aluminum causes a marked, increased uptake of fluoride by enamel. It is plausible that pretreatment of teeth with various agents such as this will be a part of tomorrow's fluoride application. More work is necessary on materials such as varnishes and plastics that may be used to "seal in" topically applied fluoride. It is also likely that new agents will be developed with different methods of application. Therefore, dental personnel should keep abreast of the fluoride literature so that the contributions of

dental scientists can be made readily available to patients.

ANSWER TO CHAPTER CASE

Vitamin preparations containing sodium fluoride are also available, as drops, tablets, and chewable tablets. This form of supplementation is useful in areas where the water supply contains less than 0.7 ppm. For children under 2 years of age the daily recommended dosage is 0.5 mg, and for those over 2 years it is 1 mg. This form of fluoride offers a way to provide fluoride to the child, if the parents are conscientious in dispensing the required amount daily, and if the child does not object to taking oral medications. In recommending vitamins with fluoride it is mandatory that the practitioner know the fluoride content of the child's water supply as well as the fluoride content in the vitamin being recommended.

QUESTIONS

1 What adverse effects have been associated with overdoses of fluoride?
2 How can dental fluorosis be treated?
3 How would you convert parts per million to milligrams per milliliter?
4 How does fluoride prevent dental caries?
5 Discuss the various ways fluoride can be administered.
6 Do all fluoride-containing dentifrices have an effect on caries reduction?
7 Compare and contrast acidulated phosphate fluoride, stannous fluoride, and sodium fluoride.

READING REFERENCES

Aasenden, R., P. F. DePaola, and F. Brudevold, "Effects of Daily Rinsing and Ingestion of Fluoride Solutions Upon Dental Caries and Enamel Fluoride," *Arch. Oral Biol.,* **17**:1705–1710, 1972.

Englander, H. R., et al., "Clinical Anticaries Effect of Repeated Sodium Fluoride Applications by Mouthpieces," *J. Am. Dent. Assoc.,* **75**:638–641, 1967.

Horwitz, H. S., "Misuse of Topically Applied Fluoride," *J. Prev. Dent.,* **7**:15–16, 1977.

Horwitz, H. S., and S. B. Heifetz, "The Current Status of Topical Fluorides in Preventive Dentistry," *J. Am. Dent. Assoc.,* **81:**166–170, 1970.

Muhler, J. C., "Stannous Fluoride Enamel Pigmentation—Evidence of Caries Arrestment," *J. Dent. Child.,* **27:**157–161, 1960.

Muhler, J. C., and A. W. Radike, "Effect of a Dentifrice Containing Stannous Fluoride on Dental Caries in Adults. II. Results at the End of Two Years of Unsupervised Use," *J. Am. Dent. Assoc.,* **55:**196–198, 1957.

Picozzi, A., and J. Smudski (eds.), *Pharmacology of Fluorides,* Cooper Video Communications, Morris Plains, N.J., 1974.

Shern, R. J., W. S. Driscoll, and D. C. Korts, "Enamel Biopsy Results of Children Receiving Fluoride Tablets," *J. Am. Dent. Assoc.,* **95:**310–314, 1977.

Wei, H. Y., and J. S. Wefel, "Topical Fluorides in Dental Practice," *J. Prev. Dent.,* **4:**25–32, 1977.

Zacherl, W. A., "Clinical Evaluation of Neutral Sodium Fluoride, Stannous Fluoride, Sodium Monofluorophosphate and Acidulated Fluoride-Phosphate Dentifrices," *J. Can. Dent. Assoc.,* **38:**35–38, 1972.

Sterilizing and Disinfecting Agents

After the patient leaves the dental chair, the chair and instrument table are wiped with a cloth impregnated with a disinfectant solution. Does this solution sterilize the area? What does it accomplish? Instruments used for cleaning the patient's teeth are placed into a "cold sterilizing solution." What does this solution really do to microorganisms?

To understand this topic, it is necessary to define some terms.

1 *Sterilization* is the complete destruction of all microbial forms, including viruses.

2 *Disinfection* refers to the destruction of infectious microorganisms only and usually does not involve the destruction of spores, tubercle bacilli, and hepatitis viruses. A disinfectant frequently is injurious to tissues and is only applied to inanimate materials such as countertops.

3 An *antiseptic* is a chemical that kills or inhibits pathogenic microorganisms and can be applied to living tissue without injury. One can think of an antiseptic as a disinfectant which can be used on living tissue.

A number of other terms are used relative to these agents, and they are presented in Table 11-1.

STERILIZATION

Sterilization is best accomplished with heat. This can be done by using steam under pressure (autoclave), a chemical plus steam under pressure, or dry heat. Sterilization can also be performed with ethylene oxide gas.

Table 11-1   Terminology of Various Agents

Bactericidal: kills bacteria

Bacteriostatic: inhibits bacterial growth

Fungicide: destroys some fungi

Germicide: destroys some bacteria but not spores of viruses

Sporicide: destroys spores

This may pose a health hazard, however, to the operator and to the patient, in that a residue of ethylene oxide is left on the instruments. Therefore, ethylene oxide will probably not be used in dental offices in the near future. Also, it is not practical for dental office use due to the amount of time required for sterilization.

No chemical agent has been shown to kill all microorganisms. This is partly due to the inability of culturing the hepatitis virus and thus demonstrating the killing effect of the chemical on this virus. However, a chemical called activated glutaraldehyde (Cidex, Sporicidin) appears to approach a level of sterilization when items are immersed in it for 10 h. After 10 h, all microorganisms tested are killed. The various sterilization methods are summarized in Table 11-2.

DISINFECTANTS

Disinfectants do *not* kill the bacillus responsible for tuberculosis, spores, or hepatitis viruses. These agents may be useful for scrubbing bracket tables, countertops, and chairs in

Table 11-2   Methods of Sterilization

Agent	Temperature required	Time	Problems and comments
Dry heat	170°C	60 min	Cleansing, packaging, and loading, critical. Sharp instruments not dulled; no rusting. Temperatures over 170°C will melt some instruments.
Gases	Ethylene oxide, 12%	4–5 h	Used in specially designed devices for sterilizing commercial products or hospital trays. Vapors are highly irritating. Both vapors and residual chemical on instruments may be carcinogenic, and use in the dental office is discouraged.
Glutaraldehyde*	Room temperature	7–10 h	Useful for items that cannot be sterilized by heat methods; highly irritating to skin when in contact; vapors may irritate eyes.
Steam and chemical under pressure (Harvey Vapor Steam Sterilizer)	127°C at 30 lb	20 min	Cleansing, packaging, and loading, critical. Sharp instruments dulled but not as extensively as steam under pressure, no rusting.
Steam under pressure (autoclave)	121°C at 15 lb pressure	15 min	Cleansing, packaging, loading, critical. Some instruments rust, and sharp ones are dulled.

* A probable sterilizing agent.

the operating area. They are also incorporated into various scrubbing solutions, which are labeled antiseptic and are of value as a scrub between treating patients.

Whenever instruments are to be sterilized or disinfected, it is mandatory that they first be thoroughly scrubbed and then washed with soap and water prior to being treated to remove any residual organic debris. With instruments such as files and reamers, a useful procedure is to first place them in an ultrasonic cleaner to remove debris. If any foreign materials, including soaps or detergents, are left on instruments prior to further treatment, the procedure may be rendered ineffective or less effective.

A number of disinfectants are commercially available and are summarized in Table 11-3.

Table 11-3 Commonly Used Disinfectants

Group	Example	Comments
Alcohols	Ethanol, isopropyl	Bactericidal in concentrations of 70% by weight and 78% by volume.
Aldehydes	Formaldehyde	Bactericidal in 40% concentration; irritating to skin and eyes.
Boiling water		Temperatures of 100°C destroy some microorganisms in 10 min. Many spores and viruses survive hours of boiling.
Chlorine	Sodium hypochlorite, 0.5%	Useful to disinfect surface areas in operating area; corrosive to surgical instruments; rapidly inactivated by organic debris.
Mercury	Merthiolate, metaphen	Minimal bacterial effect and doubtful value; may be bacteriostatic.
Oxidizing agents	Hydrogen peroxide, 3%	Minimal antibacterial properties; good as a mechanical cleaning agent due to the oxygen bubbles it releases when organic material is contacted.
Phenol	Hexachlorephene	Often used in scrubs, has some antibacterial effects; 3% solution, nonirritating to skin; not recommended for body bathing since some absorbed through skin; used as a 2% tincture; some skin irritation and allergy to it.
Povidone-iodine	Betadine	A complex of polyvinyl pyrrolidone and iodine; releases iodine slowly; less irritating than tincture of iodine; some allergy to iodine reported.
Surface-active agents	Zephiran	Bactericidal to some bacteria; easily inactivated by soaps and organic material; some gram-negative bacteria can grow in it.

Many of the disinfectants listed in Table 11-3 are useful as either presurgical scrubs or for the cleaning of chairs, bracket tables, countertops, and so on.

The majority of presurgical scrubs in use include plain soap, 70 to 90% alcohol, 3% hexachlorophene, and povidone iodine (Betadine). The scrubs reduce the bacterial count prior to a surgical procedure and are recommended for all members of the dental team prior to patient treatment.

One should remember that these agents only reduce the bacterial count temporarily. While they are sometimes applied to the oral mucosa prior to injection, their use is debatable since the same reduction in bacterial numbers is achieved by cleansing the oral mucosa with a sterile swab or sterile gauze.

COMMENTS ON FREQUENTLY USED CHEMICAL AGENTS

A number of agents are used as disinfectants, and they will be discussed in this section. One of the chemicals, glutaraldehyde, appears to be a sterilizing agent under certain conditions.

Aldehydes

Aldehydes bind to bacterial cell proteins and thus cause bacterial death. They are also effective antiviricidal agents. Two aldehydes are useful in this group: formaldehyde and glutaraldehyde.

Formaldehyde (Formalin, Formaldehyde Solution)

Formaldehyde is used in a 1 to 2% solution. Although it is antibacterial, its effect is not seen for 2 to 30 min after application. When mixed with alcohol in a solution containing 3 to 4% formaldehyde, it is an effective disinfectant with a more rapid onset of effectiveness than a 1 to 2% aqueous solution.

Formaldehyde solutions have a pungent, unpleasant odor and are irritating to skin and oral mucosa. Exposure can result in contact dermatitis of a long duration. It should not be applied to tissues and should be used only as a disinfectant on inanimate objects.

Glutaraldehyde (Cidex 7) (Sporicidin)

This chemical, in a 2% solution, is an excellent disinfectant and, when used for 7 h or more, appears to be a sterilizing agent. Commercial preparations are available, which are activated prior to use by addition of a buffer solution which raises the pH to 8.5. At this pH, glutaraldehyde is most effective against microorganisms and maintains its efficacy for 2 weeks.

When an instrument is immersed in this solution for 10 min, fungi, viruses, and bacteria, including the tuberculosis-causing microorganisms, are killed. However, spores are *not* killed unless immersion occurs over a 7–10-h period.

Contact with this solution should be avoided since it is irritating to skin and eyes. In some cases, even the vapors have resulted in eye irritation. Therefore, this agent should be carefully handled and used in well-ventilated areas. Instruments should also be removed with transfer forceps and washed with either water or alcohol prior to storage or use. In contrast to quaternary ammonium compounds, this substance's action is not affected by soaps or detergents.

When instruments are immersed in this solution for 7 h or more, it is probable that this chemical sterilizes. Since the hepatitis viruses (types A and B) cannot be cultured, sterilization is not proven. However, studies have shown this solution to be effective in killing viruses similar to those responsible for hepatitis, and therefore it is probable that a 7-h immersion does kill the hepatitis viruses.

Care should be taken when using activated glutaraldehyde on carbon steel instruments.

These instruments should not be immersed for more than 24 h since they may corrode. As a sterilizing agent, glutaraldehyde is particularly useful for substances such as rubber or plastic items, adhesive-bonded instruments such as lenses or mirrors, and dental handpieces which cannot be sterilized by dry heat or steam. However, when decontaminating the dental handpiece, it should be wiped with glutaraldehyde and the water spray be run for at least 2 min. Recent studies have shown that there is a "back suction" of the water spray, and bacteria from the patient's mouth may enter the spray system. Running the spray for at least 2 min helps reduce this bacterial count. *A word of caution:* If a handpiece or dental instrument is wiped with glutaraldehyde, the person applying it should protect his or her hands with gloves. After wiping handpieces or instruments with glutaraldehyde, a second wipe should be carried out with water or 70% alcohol to remove the agent completely. This precaution is necessary since this chemical is highly irritating to biologic tissues.

One should note that handpieces are now available which can be sterilized by steam under pressure or dry heat. In view of the speed and effectiveness of these methods of sterilization, they are preferable to glutaraldehyde.

Since glutaraldehyde may not completely enter the bore of a hypodermic needle, it should not be used for the sterilization of this instrument. In this instance, steam under pressure or dry heat is preferable. However, due to the difficulty associated with cleaning a needle's bore of all debris prior to sterilizing, disposable, presterilized needles are recommended.

Quaternary Ammonium Components

These disinfecting agents are not recommended for use on instruments or other inanimate objects but are useful as topical skin disinfectants. Therefore, they are useful as antiseptics and are nonirritating to skin and oral mucosa.

Since aluminum-containing items such as local anesthetic cartridges with aluminum caps are corroded by these chemicals, these compounds should not be used for their disinfection.

Quaternary ammonium compounds have significant drawbacks, including a marked reduction of their antibacterial activity by soap. Rust inhibitors should be added to the quaternary ammonium compounds since the water base of these solutions will rust metal instruments. The usual mixture needed to prevent rust is 4.5 g of sodium nitrate per quart of solution. Most importantly, it has also been demonstrated that these solutions harbor certain gram-negative bacteria and may introduce these into a wound as a contaminant. Another drawback of quaternary ammonium compounds is that they do not affect viruses, including those responsible for hepatitis, or bacteria, including those responsible for tuberculosis. The most common example of an agent in this category is benzalkonium chloride (Zephiran).

COMPOUNDS CONTAINING CHLORINE

Chlorine has some useful antibacterial properties. Some agents in this group are used for irrigation of root canals since they have not only antibacterial properties but also a solvent effect on organic matter such as pulp tissue. These agents act by liberating chlorine which has antibacterial properties.

Sodium Hypochlorite

A 5% concentration of sodium hypochlorite is used for the irrigation of root canals during endodontic therapy. It is strongly alkaline and, for this reason, is irritating to open wounds or areas of soft tissue infection.

Preparations containing sodium hypochlorite deteriorate quickly on standing and should be labeled at the time of preparation and replaced on a weekly basis.

A dilute solution of sodium hypochlorite (0.5%) is available as an antiseptic and can be used on mucous membranes with some antibacterial effect. The pH of this solution is usually buffered to neutrality with sodium bicarbonate.

Solutions of sodium hypochlorite are also useful as denture cleaners.

Chloramine-T

This solution contains sodium-4-toluene-sulfonchloramide and derives its name from its chemical composition. As a topical solution, concentrations of 0.1 to 0.4% are useful for application to wounds. Its action is similar to that of dilute sodium hypochlorite. Compared to sodium hypochlorite, it is more stable, less irritating, and relatively nontoxic when applied topically. In contrast to sodium hypochlorite, it lacks any solvent effect on organic matter. Its antibacterial properties are determined by an acid pH and lowering of temperature.

COMPOUNDS CONTAINING IODINE

Compounds containing iodine are used in dentistry as disinfectants, antiseptics, and disclosing agents. Since some patients are allergic to iodine, a careful history is important. Iodine is available as a 2 to 7% iodine solution, and most solutions contain iodine as 2.4 to 5% sodium iodide.

Iodine, U.S.P.

Iodine solutions may be applied to oral mucosa and also to teeth and rubber dams for antibacterial purposes. Prior to application, the surface should be dry, and following its use, any staining can be removed with alcohol.

One disadvantage of iodine solutions is that they are irritating to mucosa, resulting in a sensation of heat and itching. Blister formation has also occurred with strong solutions. Another limitation is the staining of acrylic, silicate, and porcelain restorations, which is reversible.

Povidone-Iodine (Betadine)

This is available for topical application as an aqueous solution containing 10% povidone iodine (a complex of polyvinylpyrrolidone and iodine) and for a surgical scrub as a 7.5% povidone-iodine in an aqueous base containing a nontoxic detergent.

Its antibacterial activity results from the slow liberation of iodine. As the complex dissociates, a 1 percent concentration of free iodine is available from the solution and 0.75 percent from the scrub.

It is nonirritating to mucous membranes and results in minimal discomfort to the patient. Also, it causes minimal discoloration of dental restorations.

Iodoform

Iodoform (triiodomethane) is available as a powder and ointment. It has analgesic and antibacterial properties, with minimal irritation. It can be placed in painful extraction sockets or dusted onto open wounds.

Overuse can result in absorption into the blood stream, which could be serious in a patient with a thyroid disorder.

Thymol Iodide

Thymol iodide, composed mainly of dithymol diodide, is an antiseptic available in powder and ointment form. Since it deteriorates on exposure to light and air, it should be stored in closed, light-resisting containers.

Thymol iodide powder is usually dusted onto surfaces of wounds and combined with topical anesthetics applied to soft tissue lesions. Because of its antiseptic properties, it is also used in some root canal filling materials.

COMPOUNDS CONTAINING MERCURY

Mercuric compounds have medical and dental applications. In medicine, their main use is as diuretics. Patients taking mercuric diuretics may develop localized areas of gingival inflammation, especially with poor oral hygiene. Therefore, frequent prophylaxis and meticulous oral hygiene is important.

In dentistry, mercuric compounds are sometimes used as antiseptics and disinfectants, but their bactericidal level is low and hence they are of limited value. Since inorganic mercuric compounds are highly irritating to tissues, most topical mercuric compounds contain organic mercury instead, since this form is less irritating.

Mercury is a systemic poison and should be used carefully and not excessively.

Mercocresols (Mercresin)

Mercocresols are composed of equal parts of secamyltricresol and 2-hydroxyphenyl-mercuric chloride. This compound is both antibacterial and antifungal but not sporicidal.

As a tincture it is used as an antiseptic for minor wounds and as a disinfectant on teeth and rubber dams prior to operative or endodontic procedures.

Thimerosal (Merthiolate)

Thimerosal or sodium ethyl mercurithiosalicylate is unstable on exposure to light; it should be stored in opaque or semiopaque containers. It is mainly antibacterial and has no effect on spores or the tubercle bacillus.

It is prepared in an isotonic solution for topical use and may have to be diluted in patients with excessively sensitive mucous membranes.

COMPOUNDS CONTAINING PHENOL

Phenols are hydroxylated derivatives of benzene. In general, the greater the degree of hydroxylation the greater the antibacterial and toxic properties.

Phenol, a protoplasmic poison, destroys bacteria and is mainly used as a disinfectant. It is sometimes used to cleanse cavity preparations and root canals but should not be used in deep cavities or under self-polymerizing resins. The latter point is important since phenols alter resin polymerization.

Phenol has been included in oral rinses for its potential effect as a plaque-reducing agent. However, its value for this purpose is questionable. It also has the ability to produce slight topical anesthesia.

Phenol has been used as a reference standard against which other disinfectants have been compared historically. The term phenol coefficient is the ratio of the disinfectant power of an agent as compared to the disinfectant power of phenol. The coefficient can be represented by the following ratio:

$$\frac{\text{Disinfectant power of test agent}}{\text{Disinfectant power of phenol}}$$

Phenol is usually used in low doses because high doses are highly caustic. One should note that cresols are derivatives of phenol, as is hexachlorophene.

Parachlorophenol

This phenol derivative is usually in an oil base of glycerine or camphor and is highly stable at room temperature. Parachlorophenol is used mainly as a constituent in root canal medications. When parachloraphenol is combined in a compound with at least 50 percent camphor, it is referred to as camphorated parachlorophenol.

Cresol

Cresol, a derivative of phenol, is a mixture of 2-methylphenol, 3-methylphenol, and 4-methylphenol. Cresol is 4 times more bactericidal than phenol, but its toxicity is slightly lower. It is compounded with alcohol, ether, glycerin, and soaps, but its main use is for root canal medications. However, it is irritating to periapical tissues and must be used with care.

Creosote

Creosote is a mixture of phenols which is readily soluble in alcohol. It has anodyne properties and will temporarily relieve a toothache when applied to a carious lesion. It is also used as a root canal antiseptic. Guaiacol, which is similar to creosote, is less irritating and is therefore sometimes used as a replacement for creosote.

Eugenol

Eugenol, or 2-methoxy-4-allyphenol, is highly soluble in alcohol and is the main chemical constituent of clove oil. It has both antibacterial and analgesic properties. It is used as the main liquid in many temporary cements and periodontal dressings, in toothache drops, and as an antiseptic in various root canal medications.

Hexachlorophene

This substance is included in various antiseptics in solutions of varying concentrations, with an average concentration between 1 and 3%. Its main use lies in soaps used for presurgical scrubs and for topical skin antisepsis.

An advantage over quaternary ammonium compounds lies in the fact that its activity is not affected by soaps. However, hexachlorophene does not kill all bacteria and is not effective against fungi, spores, or viruses.

Hexachlorophene is absorbed through skin and, as would be expected, especially through abraded skin. Animal studies using young monkeys have shown that these animals developed brain edema when bathed daily in 3% hexachlorophene for 90 days. For this reason, bathing in such solutions is not recommended and is contraindicated in children.

Alcohol

The main alcohols used for disinfection are ethanol and isopropanol. Although they are bactericidal, they are not sporicidal or viricidal and should not be used to disinfect dental instruments. Alcohols have maximal effect when diluted with water to 70% by weight and 78% by volume.

COMMENTS ON COMMON PHYSICAL METHODS
Heat

The most reliable sterilizing methods are heat, steam under pressure (autoclave), or dry heat.

Prior to sterilizing instruments with heat, the instruments must be thoroughly cleaned either by scrubbing or with an ultrasonic cleaner. If the latter method is used, the instruments should be rinsed prior to placing in the ultrasonic unit. Instruments used in the treatment of patients with severe infections or hepatitis should only be handled with gloves for protection.

Instruments should not be tightly packed into the sterilizer but only loosely loaded to permit sterilization. In an autoclave, instruments can be wrapped in muslin, paper, or cheesecloth; for dry heat, cotton, paper, or transparent synthetic bags can be used. The bags should not be sealed until after sterilization to permit the heated air to enter the bag. It is also important not to set dry heat sterilizers higher than 170°C since solder joints in reamers, files, some periodontal instruments, and impression trays may melt.

Superheated Salt or Glass Beads

Heated salt or glass beads at temperatures of 218 to 246°C rapidly sterilize small instruments or materials such as endodontic instruments after 10 sec. Instruments must be extremely clean before inserting them into the sterilizer. Since the salt or glass beads must be uniformly heated to 218 to 246°C, they should be preheated for 20 min prior to use. Even when this is done, it has been questioned whether the surface layer is as warm as lower levels. An excellent review of these sterilizing devices can be found in the 1962 issue of the *Journal of Dental Research* (listed at the end of this chapter).

Flaming

While passing an instrument through a flame can sterilize, this is not reliable. Sterilization is only assured if the instrument is left in the flame long enough to become red hot. However, this high temperature may destroy the temper and finish of instruments. Therefore, this method is not recommended for dental instruments.

PRESTERILIZED INSTRUMENTS AND MATERIALS

Many dental materials and instruments are available in a presterilized form. They are usually sterilized by dry heat, steam under pressure, or radiation with cobalt-60.

Presterilized gauze, absorbable points, and similar items should be labeled with the purchase date so that one is aware of their relative age. Some manufacturers also suggest maximum storage times.

Disposable needles, which are commonly employed in dental offices, come sealed in a plastic container. The outsides of these containers are not sterile, and care is necessary to prevent contaminating the needle when opening and placing the needle on the syringe. Similar care is necessary for presterilized suture material. The outer coverings for these presterilized materials should not be placed onto a sterile tray setup since this leads to contamination.

Local anesthetic solutions in cartridges or ampules are presterilized by the manufacturer. Once the metal can containing them is opened, the sterility of their outer surfaces may be compromised. Therefore, once they are removed from the can, they should be immersed in a solution of 70% alcohol for periods up to 24 h. Longer exposure to alcohol is not recommended because of possible seepage of alcohol into the anesthetic cartridge. A 10-min immersion in glutaraldehyde prior to use may serve the same purpose, but its irritating nature creates handling problems.

DISINFECTION OF AIR AND WATER TIPS

Many dental units have permanently attached air and water tips. Between patients these should be cleaned with soap and water and then wiped thoroughly with a disinfectant which has tuberculocidal properties (glutaraldehyde).

ANSWER TO CHAPTER CASE

Disinfectants do not sterilize. They destroy only infectious microorganisms and do not destroy spores, tubercle bacilli, and hepatitis virus. Sterilization refers to the complete destruction of all *microbial forms, including viruses. Most "cold sterilizing solutions" are disinfectants and do not truly sterilize. One of the few solutions which appears to result in sterilization, if objects are left in it for 7 h or more, is glutaraldehyde. Only solutions containing glutaraldehyde are currently allowed to be labeled as cold sterilizing solutions by the Environmental Protection Agency of the federal government of the United States.*

QUESTIONS

1 Differentiate the following terms: sterilizing agent, disinfecting agent, antiseptic agent.
2 Which chemical agent appears to be an effective sterilizing agent? How should it be used?
3 List the advantages and disadvantages of quaternary ammonium compounds as chairside disinfectants.
4 Discuss the use of heat as a sterilizing agent. How

does it compare to chemicals in terms of instrument sterilization?

5 What is the best way to treat countertops and handpieces between patients so that most microorganisms are eliminated?

READING REFERENCES

Calmes, R. B., and T. T. Lillich, *Disinfection and Sterilization in Dental Practice,* McGraw-Hill, New York, 1978.

Coughlin, J. W., et al., "Comparison of Dry Heat, Autoclave, and Vapor Sterilizers," *J. Tenn. Dent. Assoc.,* **47:**350–355, 1967.

Council on Dental Therapeutics Report, "Type B (Serum) Hepatitis and Dental Practice," *J. Am. Dent. Assoc.,* **92:**153–159, 1976.

Koehler, H. M., and J. J. Heffernan, "Time Temperature Relations of Dental Instruments Heated in Root Canal Instrument Sterilizers," *J. Dent. Res.,* **41:**86–90, 1962.

Miller, R. L., "Generation of Airborne Infection by High Speed Dental Equipment," *J. Am. Soc. Prev. Dent.,* **20:**14–17, 1976.

Neugeboren, N., et al., "Control of Cross-Contamination," *J. Am. Dent. Assoc.,* **85:**123–127, 1972.

Peterson, N. J., et al., "Hepatitis B Surface Antigen in Saliva, Impetiginous Lesions, and the Environment in Two Remote Alaskan Villages," *Appl. Environ. Micro.,* **32:**572–574, 1976.

Stonehill, A. A., S. Krop, and P. Borick, "Buffered Glutaraldehyde-A New Chemical Sterilizing Solution," *Am. J. Hosp. Pharm.,* **26:**458–465, 1963.

Prophylaxis Pastes, Dentifrices, and Mouthwashes

Thank you for cleaning my teeth, Ms. Brown. They look so white now that all the stain is gone! However, I hope you didn't remove too much enamel. Should I use salt or baking soda at home to keep them clean? Do you recommend any specific dentifrice?

Knowledge of the materials commonly used on patients is most important in order for patients to feel secure with their dental team. Also, this knowledge enables the therapist to perform duties more efficiently and with a sense of complete mastery of the situation.

PROPHYLAXIS PASTES

A prophylaxis paste is usually applied periodically by a trained person to remove stains and plaque and to polish the tooth surface. They contain abrasives, binders, coloring agents, flavoring agents, and sweeteners. The most common ingredient of dental prophylaxis

paste is pumice, a mixture of aluminum, sodium, and potassium silicate salts. Since it is abrasive, damage to tooth surfaces can occur if it is improperly applied. Therefore, it should not be used daily as a dentifrice or incorporated into a dentifrice. In addition to pumice, most prophylaxis pastes contain other abrasives, such as precipitated calcium carbonate. This is usually present in small amounts because it is highly abrasive. Prophylaxis pastes of low abrasiveness are preferred so that minimal tooth structure is removed when they are used. When resistant stains remain on teeth after using a mild abrasive, a stronger abrasive can be used carefully over small areas. However, it would be safer for tooth structure to use an instrument to remove resistant stain.

Various aromatic flavoring and coloring agents are also included. The most common aromatic flavoring agents used are peppermint and fruit extracts.

The abrasiveness of ingredients in prophylaxis pastes is related not only to the agent but also to the particle size. Usually, the larger the particle size the greater the abrasiveness. If a substance is too abrasive, however, it will not only remove stain but also scratch and roughen the surface. Such an irregular surface will make it more difficult to remove bacterial plaque by a daily oral hygiene regimen.

In addition to particle size, particle shape is also important. An irregular shape is more abrasive than a smooth, regular shape. Also, particles are rated in terms of hardness according to a Mohs or Knoop hardness scale. The harder a particle, the more its abrasiveness. The selection of an abrasive depends not only on its abrasiveness but also on its lack of interaction with other dentifrice components. For example, the abrasive in Crest is calcium pyrophosphate. Calcium carbonate, another common dentifrice abrasive, could not be used because it prevents release of the fluoride ion from the dentifrice.

Some pastes use glycerine as a binder and to facilitate flow. In addition, powdered magnesium oxide may also be included to facilitate flow.

To these mixtures are added nonsucrose sweetening agents such as saccharin or sorbitol, which are noncariogenic. Future mixtures may use xylitol, which imparts a sweetness equal to sucrose and is also noncariogenic.

Zirconium Silicate

This substance has irregularly shaped crystals which are easily reduced in size and become more rounded with manipulation. Therefore, while initially an abrasive, with use it becomes a polishing agent. Some studies have suggested that it is more effective in removing stain than pumice and that it leaves a smoother surface. Zirconium silicate has replaced pumice in some commercial prophylaxis pastes.

Kaolinite

This compound, a derivative of anhydrous aluminum silicate, is as effective as pumice and produces a more polished surface. When used alone, it dries on teeth and must be periodically rinsed off during stain removal. It has minimal grittiness, and patient response to it is better than to pumice.

Fluoride-Containing Prophylaxis Pastes

Since a thorough prophylaxis removes a thin layer of surface enamel, which normally has the highest fluoride concentration, fluoride-containing prophylaxis pastes have been formulated. It is thought that such a paste may replenish the fluoride removed during a prophylaxis. Fluorides have been incorporated as either sodium fluoride or stannous fluoride, ranging in concentration from 1.2 to 8%. Some formulations have included mixtures of buffers to either raise or lower the pH.

These pastes result in fluoride uptake by tooth enamel, and the loss occurring as a result of a prophylaxis with these pastes is minimal. It has not been shown that loss of surface fluoride following a prophylaxis with a nonfluoride-containing paste results in a greater susceptibility to caries. The fluoride lost from enamel as a result of this procedure may not be enough to increase susceptibility to caries. Also, there are insufficient studies to show that prophylaxis with a fluoride-containing paste results in a reduction in dental caries. Further investigations are underway. If a prophylaxis paste containing fluoride is desired, one should not add fluoride to pastes but should use commercial preparations. In this manner, there is less danger of administering high doses of fluoride as has been reported in the literature. Since children like the taste of fluoride pastes, they may enjoy swallowing them, and toxic effects may occur. An excellent case report can be found in the article by Horwitz entitled ''Misuse of Topically Applied Drugs'' (see Reading References).

Supervised self-application with either stannous fluoride pastes or acidulated phosphate fluoride pastes reduced caries by 25 to 37 percent. Other reports suggest no reduction occurred. Therefore, this therapeutic concept remains an open question and deserves further investigation.

DENTIFRICES

Approximately $600,000,000 per year is spent on dentifrices. A dentifrice is a substance used in conjunction with a toothbrush to clean surfaces of teeth. Dentifrices are available as gels, pastes, powders, and slurries. They all contain abrasives, flavoring agents, foaming agents, and, in some cases, preservatives. As a paste,

a dentifrice contains water, binders, and humectants (agents which prevent water loss on exposure to air). Examples of dentifrice components are presented in Table 12-1.

Abrasiveness

The abrasiveness of dentifrices was reported in 1970 by the American Dental Association. Table 12-2 presents an updated summary with the products listed from least to most abrasive. The degree of abrasiveness varies. A person with heavily stained teeth should use a dentifrice with a high abrasiveness, provided that the root surfaces are not exposed. When root surfaces are exposed, they abrade easily. Therefore, a low-abrasive dentifrice is recommended. Baking soda has sometimes been recommended as a dentifrice because it has low abrasiveness. Because its taste is unacceptable to most patients, they have better oral hygiene if they use a flavored dentifrice.

Manufacturers of a number of dentifrices claim they produce whiter and brighter teeth. These dentifrices usually have a strong abrasive which removes stain. Their abrasive may include calcium carbonate, silica, or anhydrous dibasic calcium carbonate. Dentifrices with high abrasiveness will not only remove stain, but also exposed cementum, dentin, and

Table 12-1   Components of Dentifrices

Component group	Examples	Comment
Abrasives	Phosphate salts, calcium and magnesium carbonates, hydrated aluminum oxides, silicates, dehydrated silica gels	Usually inorganic salts with a low solubility
Binders	Natural gums, seaweed colloids, synthetic cellulose, mineral colloids	Thickening agents
Flavoring	Sodium saccharin as a sweetener, various agents for flavoring	Average saccharin content is 0.2%
Foaming agents	Sodium lauryl sulfate, sodium-*n*-lauryl sarcosinate, soaps	Soaps not used often
Humectants	Sorbitol, glycerol, and propylene glycol	Sorbitol, glycerol have sweetening properties

Table 12-2   Abrasiveness of Some Dentifrices

Product	Abrasive index
Thermodent	24
Listerine	26
Pepsodent	26
Ammident	33
Colgate MFP	51
Ultrabrite	64
Pearl Drops	72
Crest (Mint)	81
Close-Up	87
Crest (Regular)	95
Macleans	100
Gleam II	106
Phillips	114
Aim	120
Sensodyne*	157
Iodent #2	174
Smokers Toothpaste	202

* Abrasiveness being reduced.

enamel. In addition, they can also damage the surface of some synthetic filling materials.

Some patients have used highly abrasive dentifrices for many years. Such patients usually present with areas of wear at the cementoenamel junction. They may also present with areas of enamel wear, which will appear as yellowish colored areas. This color is due to the fact that the abrasive has thinned enamel to the extent that the underlying dentin, which is yellow in color, is now more visible.

Therapeutic Value of Dentifrices

The main therapeutic value of nonfluoride-containing dentifrices is their ability to remove plaque and stain. Various chemicals, enzymes, and foaming agents have been incorporated into dentifrices, but their value as anticaries agents is questionable.

Dentifrices containing either stannous fluoride or sodium monofluorophosphate are equally effective in reducing caries in humans. However, the amount of caries reduction is not as great as that produced by fluoridated

drinking water or fluoride tablets. A good anticaries program should include inclusion of fluoride in either drinking water or tablets, in conjunction with the use of a fluoride dentifrice.

The Council on Dental Therapeutics of the American Dental Association periodically reviews the efficacy of fluoride-containing dentifrices and fluoride bioavailability. Their seal of approval is only placed on agents which are of definite therapeutic value. Therefore, only fluoride dentifrices which carry the seal of approval of this council should be recommended for your patients.

Dentifrices and Sensitive Teeth

Sometimes a patient will complain of teeth that are hypersensitive to heat and cold. These teeth usually have exposed root surfaces with a loss of cementum. Various dentifrices are recommended for the treatment of sensitivity, with minimal success.

The greatest success occurs with dentifrices containing 10 percent strontium chloride (Sensodyne), 1.4 percent formalin (Thermodent), 5 percent potassium nitrate, and some fluoride-containing dentifrices.

However, because of its high abrasive index (Table 12-2), caution should be exercised in using Sensodyne on areas of exposed cementum. When used, it should be gently applied with a soft brush. No reports can be found in the dental literature on adverse effects of Sensodyne on root surfaces. Therefore, its abrasive index apparently presents no clinical problems. The primary mechanisms postulated for these dentifrices is that they occlude dentinal tubules, preventing stimuli from the oral cavity from irritating the dental nerve via these tubules.

For maximum effect, a patient must use only one of these dentifrices for at least a month. If no benefit occurs after 1 month, a different dentifrice should be recommended or other methods employed.

Several studies suggest that sometimes root hypersensitivity may be a psychosomatic problem since relief sometimes occurs with a placebo dentifrice. Other studies, however, have shown that this hypersensitivity can also be minimized if the root surfaces are kept plaque-free.

MOUTHWASHES

Annual sales of mouthwashes are approximately $30,000,000. They flush loose debris from the mouth, provide a pleasant taste, and mask bad breath for 15 to 30 min. Some commercial mouthwashes reduce plaque; however, there is no concomitant reduction in gingivitis. This may be due to the fact that a mouthwash does not actually enter the gingival crevice. Therefore, an effect on subgingival plaque and associated gingivitis is not seen.

Some mouthwashes have a topical anesthetic effect on oral mucosa and are useful for relieving pain associated with denture sore spots, herpetic infections, and apthous ulcers (Chloraseptic, Cēpastat, Ambesol). In patients with painful lesions, these mouthwashes should be used prior to eating to improve comfort. Although this action will reduce a person's taste sensation, pain will not be associated with eating.

A number of chemicals have been placed in mouthwashes. Some commonly used mouthwashes are listed in Table 12-3. From the table one can determine the active agent in the mouthwash and its possible effect.

One of these mouthwashes contains 0.05% sodium fluoride and may be of value in reducing the incidence of caries in children living in nonfluoridated areas.

Several mouthwashes listed in Table 12-3 are being evaluated for their ability to reduce plaque and gingivitis. If the results are positive, they may be useful adjuncts to mechanical methods of oral hygiene.

Mouthwashes containing oxygenating agents such as hydrogen peroxide and sodium perborate (Amosan, Vince, Proxigel, Glyoxide) mechanically remove loose debris

Table 12-3 Commonly Used Mouthwashes

Product	Active agent	Comment
Cēpacol	Cetylpyridinium chloride	Surface active, some antibacterial properties
Fluorigard	Sodium fluoride	May prevent some dental caries
Hydrogen peroxide	1–1.5% hydrogen peroxide	Oxidizing agent, mechanical cleansing related to bubbling action
Lavoris	Zinc chloride, oil of clove	Astringent, some antibacterial properties
Listerine	Thymol, essential oils	Some antibacterial properties
Saline	0.9% saline	Soothing properties, some antibacterial
Scope	Cetylpyridinium chloride, domiphen bromide	Surface active, some antibacterial properties
Sodium perborate	Sodium perborate, varying concentrations	Oxidizing agents, highly irritating in continued use

around teeth. It has not been shown that these agents reduce plaque, but some studies suggest that oxygenating agents may reduce acute cases of gingivitis. Long-term use of these agents has occasionally been associated with the development of black hairy tongue.

Mouthwashes containing fluorides are currently on the market. These mouthwashes have been shown to be effective in the reduction of caries, particularly when used in conjunction with other forms of fluoride therapy. Further comments on this topic can be found in Chap. 10, Fluorides.

ANSWER TO CHAPTER CASE

The hygienist should review the topic of abrasiveness in this chapter in order to intelligently answer the patient's comment regarding removal of enamel. Salt should definitely not be used because it is too abrasive. Baking soda has a low abrasiveness and could be used. However, most patients object to its taste. For this reason, a dentifrice should be recommended according to the patient's needs. For example, from Table 12-2 one notes the abrasiveness of some dentifrices. If the patient presents with areas of enamel or cementum wear, a dentifrice with a low index is indicated. If the patient presents with no areas of wear and heavy staining, a dentifrice with a higher index could be recommended.

QUESTIONS

1 What are the usual ingredients of prophylaxis pastes? What is the value of each agent?
2 What are the main components of dentifrices? Give one example of each.
3 What is the therapeutic value of dentifrices?
4 What is the therapeutic value of mouthwashes?
5 Name the active agent in four commercial mouthrinses, and state its value.

READING REFERENCES

Brudevold, F., and N. W. Chilton, "Comparative Study of A Fluoride Dentifrice Containing Soluble Phosphate and a Calcium-Free Abrasive: Second Year Report," *J. Am. Dent. Assoc.,* **72:**889–894, 1966.

Ciancio, S. G., M. L. Mather, and H. L. Bunnell, "Clinical Evaluation of a Quaternary Ammonium-Containing Mouthrinse," *J. Periodontol.,* **46:**397–401, 1975.

Council on Dental Therapeutics of the American Dental Association, "Abrasivity of Current Dentifrices," *J. Am. Dent. Assoc.,* **81:**1177–1178, 1970.

Dudding, N. J., L. O. Dahl, and J. C. Muhler, "Patient Reaction to Brushing Teeth with Water, Dentifrice, or Salt and Soda," *J. Periodontol.,* **31:**386–392, 1960.

Fischman, S. L., et al., "The Inhibition of Plaque in Humans by Two Experimental Oral Rinses," *J. Periodontol.,* **44:**100–104, 1973.

Flotra, L., et al., "A Four Month Study on the Effect of Chlorhexidine Mouthwashes on Fifty Soldiers," *Scand. J. Dent. Res.,* **80:**10–16, 1972.

Hefferan, J. J., "A Laboratory Method of Assessment of Dentifrice Abrasivity," *J. Dent. Res.,* **55:**563–573, 1976.

Horwitz, H. S., "Misuse of Topically Applied Fluorides," *J. Prev. Dent.,* **7:**15–16, 1977.

Horwitz, H. S., and H. S. Lucye, "A Clinical Study of Stannous Fluoride in Prophylaxis Paste as a Solution," *J. Oral Ther. Pharmacol.,* **3:**17–25, 1966.

Muhler, J. C., "The Anticariogenic Effectiveness of a Single Application of Stannous Fluoride in Children Residing in an Optimal Communal Fluoride Area. II. Results at the End of Thirty Months," *J. Am. Dent. Assoc.,* **61:**431–438, 1960.

Vrbic, V., F. Brudevold, and H. G. McCann, "Acquisition of Fluoride by Enamel from Fluoride Pumice Pastes," *Helv. Odontol. Acta,* **11:**21–26, 1967.

Part Three

Drugs That May Alter Daily Practice

Chapter 13

Anticonvulsant Drugs

Ms. Smith, Mr. Swanson has been on anticonvulsant therapy for a month, so please have a bite block available. When you seat him, be sure not to flash the dental light in his eyes. Please take a photograph of his gingival tissues so we have a record of their topography. Also, score his plaque after disclosing. We must initiate a strict oral hygiene program for him.

Although epilepsy is not the sole cause of convulsions, it is the most common disorder treated with anticonvulsant drugs. Since approximately 1 in every 100 persons is afflicted with some form of epilepsy, epileptics will be seen in daily practice. Anticonvulsant drugs are of dental interest since some cause gingival hyperplasia and other clinical side effects.

Convulsive disorders are classified as either idiopathic, where the etiology is unknown, or symptomatic. Symptomatic convulsive disorders are associated with known cerebral pathology such as trauma, metabolic diseases, brain tumors, and brain disease. Epilepsy is classified as idiopathic.

The current International Classification of Epileptic Seizures divides central nervous system disorders into four categories:

I Partial seizures (focal seizures, local seizures)
  A Partial seizures with elementary

symptoms—usually consciousness is not lost. When motor or sensory symptoms are present, these are called Jacksonian-type seizures.

  B Partial seizures with complex symptoms (psychomotor or temporal lobe seizures). Usually consciousness is lost, characterized by initial confused behavior.

II Generalized seizures (bilateral and symmetrical)

  A Absence or petit mal seizures—brief loss of consciousness. Varies from simple blinking to violent body jerking.

  B Tonic-clonic or grand mal seizures—loss of consciousness, contraction of skeletal muscles followed by a period of depression of all body functions. Muscle contractions may last 1 to 5 min.

  C A group of seizures seen in children also fall in this category. Some involve muscle contractions in various parts of the body, and others involve autonomic manifestations. Usually a loss of consciousness is associated with these.

III Unilateral seizures. Various responses occur but they are usually unilateral; consciousness may or may not be lost for brief periods.

IV Unclassified seizures. Seizures which occur but whose cause is unknown (idiopathic).

Many patients may have more than one type of seizure, and drugs effective against one type may not help or may even mask another. Therefore, some patients are managed with more than one drug.

CONSIDERATIONS IN THE DENTAL OFFICE

Patients under medication for a convulsive disorder may still have a convulsion in the dental chair. When this occurs:

  1 A wooden bite block should be available to protect the tongue and teeth.

  2 One should not restrain patients. Instead, protect them from injury while their muscles are contracting.

  3 When the convulsion is over, emotional first aid is most important.

With some anticonvulsants, gingival hyperplasia is a side effect. This commonly occurs with phenytoin therapy and rarely with phenobarbital therapy. Hyperplasia is considered in depth later in this chapter.

Patients on anticonvulsant therapy sometimes become sedated, particularly during the early stages of therapy. Therefore, it may be particularly difficult to motivate or instruct them in proper plaque control. Because of this, plaque control instruction should be minimized during the first 2 months of anticonvulsant therapy to avoid frustration by the patient and the instructor.

Drug interactions between the anticonvulsants and drugs such as sedatives must be considered. (See Chap. 19, Drug Interactions.) Additional medication with sedatives may result in an overly sedated patient who will respond poorly to your questions and instructions.

TREATMENT WITH ANTICONVULSANTS

The dosage of a drug depends on the patient's size, age, and physical condition, response to therapy, and the potential synergistic or antagonistic effects with his or her other medications. The anticonvulsant dosages for children are proportionally larger on a weight basis than those for adults.

The therapeutic dose of an anticonvulsant is sometimes near the toxic dose. Because of this, patients are first started on small or moderate doses to see if the convulsions are controlled. If control is not achieved, the dosage can be increased until minor signs and symptoms of toxicity are manifested. If toxic signs develop before control is obtained, another drug is usually prescribed. When control cannot be achieved with a single drug, a combination of drugs may result in good control and minimal toxicity.

Most anticonvulsants modify the ability of the brain to respond to various stimuli which evoke seizures by altering normal cortical brain function. This also accounts for some side effects.

In general, drugs effective in grand mal seizures are usually not effective in petit mal seizures, and vice versa.

Barbiturates

The three most common barbiturates used to treat convulsive disorders are phenobarbital (Luminal), mephobarbital (Mebaral), and metharbital (Gemonil). Only an occasional, mild gingival hyperplasia has been reported with these drugs. Metharbital and mephobarbital, while less potent than phenobarbital, are beneficial where phenobarbital has failed.

Phenobarbital, a long-acting barbiturate, was first introduced as an anticonvulsant in 1912. It is still the most widely used anticonvulsant today. Phenobarbital is administered alone or in conjunction with phenytoin for the control of convulsions. It is sometimes the initial drug of choice because it controls multiple types of seizures. It is also relatively safe. As a sedative, a transient drowsiness is the most common adverse effect. With time, the sedative effect decreases, so the effects are primarily anticonvulsive. A pharmacologic discussion of this drug as a sedative can be found in Chap. 6.

Some children, however, exhibit an opposite effect and become hyperactive. It is thought that this excitation may indicate brain dysfunction. However, since this relationship has not been clearly established, it must be confirmed with a neurologic examination.

Barbiturates are habituating, so that chronic treatment can result in physical and psychic dependence. The abrupt cessation of therapy can lead to withdrawal symptoms, including tremors, hallucinations, convulsions, and death. Since low doses are usually given for epilepsy, however, there is usually no physical and psychic dependence. On occasion, gastrointestinal disorders are associated with use of this drug.

The barbiturates are also respiratory depressants; however, this is mainly seen with drug overdoses. In view of this, if your patient presents with breathing difficulties, a barbiturate overdosage should be suspected; the patient should be informed and his or her physician contacted. Also, in such patients, inhalation anesthetics such as nitrous oxide should not be administered. If the dental auxiliary observes any respiratory depression in the patient, it should immediately be brought to the dentist's attention. *This is another example of the need for auxiliary personnel to know the patient's history.*

When phenobarbital is administered orally (po), the onset of action is 30 to 60 min, with an effective duration of 4 to 6 h. Up to 2 weeks of therapy may be necessary before a determination can be made of the effectiveness of phenobarbital in controlling convulsions, since it sometimes takes this long for adequate distribution of this drug throughout plasma and body tissues.

The sodium salt of phenobarbital can be injected intramuscularly (IM) or intravenously (IV) for control of severe, continuous convulsions classified as status epilepticus. However, the current trend in the majority of cases is to use diazepam (Valium) for this purpose.

Primidone (Mysoline)

This drug is biochemically similar to the barbiturates and can be substituted for barbiturates in patients not responding to other drug therapy. When used for this purpose, larger doses are needed than with phenobarbital. This drug is metabolized partially to phenobarbital, which may explain some of its effects. As with the barbiturates, the undesired sedative effects diminish with continued administration. In contrast to the barbiturates, which have minimal side effects, many are associated with primidone and include anemia, dizziness, nausea, vomiting, diplopia, and nystagmus.

This drug is excreted in the milk of lactating females, and inadvertent administration to nursing infants may occur in this way. Also, patients on chronic long-term drug therapy have complained of vague gingival pains. Although the etiology of the gingival pain is not clear, an awareness is important in patient management.

HYDANTOINS

A number of drugs belong in this classification and include phenytoin or diphenylhydantoin (Dilantin), ethotoin (Peganone), and mephenytoin (Mesantoin). Lymphadenopathies simulating malignant lymphomas have been related to therapy with these drugs, particularly with the use of mephenytoin. Usually this is reversible with cessation of therapy. On occasion, liver disorders have also been related to therapy. The dental professional should watch for signs of liver damage in patients taking hydantoins, such as yellowing of the eyeballs or the fingernail bed (icterus). Gingival hyperplasia has been associated with two of the drugs in this group, i.e., phenytoin and, to a lesser extent, mephenytoin. Periodic blood studies are indicated in patients taking these medications, since anemia (megablastic type) has been associated with their use.

Phenytoin (Diphenylhydantoin, Dilantin)

This drug is the most useful drug for treatment of convulsions of the grand mal type and is used alone or in combination with phenobarbital or primidone (Mysoline). It has also been used with some success to relieve the pain of trigeminal neuralgia. This drug is thought to stabilize cell membranes and synaptic transmission by altering movement of ions across cell membranes. However, its mechanism of action has not been fully elucidated.

In contrast to barbiturates, this drug does not produce sedation in normal therapeutic doses. It is administered po and has a variable absorption, with peak plasma concentrations occurring between 3 and 12 h after ingestion. Once in plasma, most (70 to 95 percent) binds to protein, which leads to cumulative effects. The main site of metabolism is the liver.

A number of toxic effects of diphenylhydantoin have been reported, including skin eruptions, gastric distress, peripheral neuropathy, gingival hyperplasia, hirsutism, hepatitis, bone marrow depression, systemic lupus erythematosus, Stevens-Johnson syndrome, and lymphadenopathy resembling malignant lymphomas. Dental personnel should be aware of these toxicities.

Gingival Hyperplasia and Phenytoin Therapy

In children who are receiving phenytoin, the incidence of gingival hyperplasia has been reported to range from 25 to 62 percent, with a mean of 50 percent. A number of investigators have suggested that gingival hyperplasia can be prevented or at least inhibited with good oral hygiene.

Hall reported on the effects of phenytoin on gingival hyperplasia in patients studied within 10 days of the time that Dilantin therapy was instituted. No gingival hyperplasia was seen in 20 patients examined over a 120-day period. His study suggested that eliminating gingival inflammation before or immediately after the initiation of therapy would prevent gingival hyperplasia. Other investigators such as Ziskin, Baden and Zegarelli, and Aas have made similar suggestions. This effect on gingival hyperplasia is illustrated in Fig. 13-1.

The role of local irritants such as orthodontic bands was investigated by Cunat and Ciancio. They showed that gingival hyperplasia

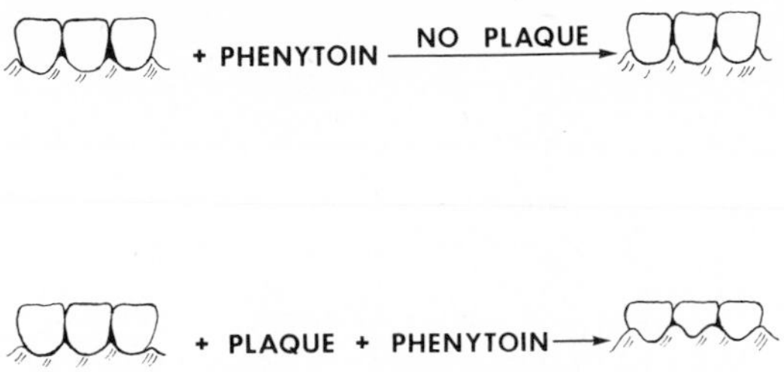

+ PHENYTOIN ——— NO PLAQUE ⟶

+ PLAQUE + PHENYTOIN ⟶

Figure 13-1 Effect of phenytoin (diphenylhydantoin, Dilantin) in producing gingival hyperplasia in the absence and presence of dental plaque.

could still be controlled in patients taking diphenylhydantoin during major tooth movement if plaque control was excellent. They also noted that the teeth of these patients were moved orthodontically at a more rapid rate than predicted.

Gingival hyperplasia is usually more severe in patients aged 15 or younger. Adults on diphenylhydantoin seldom show as high an incidence or severity of gingival hyperplasia. Gingival hyperplasia first occurs as a papillary enlargement in the interproximal area and appears to develop from this area. The gingival hyperplasia ranges from a minimum, where only the gingival papillae are enlarged, to a maximum, where the hyperplasia extends over the occlusal surfaces of the teeth and interferes with chewing. Often the hyperplasia is greater anteriorly and creates severe esthetic and psychological problems for the patient. Because of this, many patients ''hide'' their enlarged gingiva by smirking instead of smiling.

When gingival hyperplasia interferes with plaque control, or the esthetics create psychological problems, periodontal surgery is indicated. When plaque control is excellent following periodontal surgery, rate and degree of recurrence can be kept to a minimum. Thus, *success of therapy depends on patient motivation by dental professionals*.

Some success in reducing gingival hyperplasia has been reported with devices that apply pressure to gingival tissues. However, these findings have been contradictory so that the value of these devices is not clear.

The mechanism of gingival hyperplasia due to diphenylhydantoin has not been fully clarified. It appears that collagen production by fibroblasts is stimulated, with resultant clinical signs of hyperplasia. The adrenal gland may also be altered, which would influence soft-tissue metabolism.

Ethotoin (Peganone)

Ethotoin is a hydantoin derivative which is less effective than diphenylhydantoin but has the advantages of less toxicity and lack of gingival hyperplasia. Therefore, it may be an excellent alternative drug in the hyperplasia-prone patient.

Mephenytoin (Mesantoin)

Mephenytoin is as effective as diphenylhydantoin for many major convulsive disorders but is more toxic. It has a sedative effect usually absent with phenytoin but has a lower incidence of gingival hyperplasia, hirsutism, and gastric distress. However, serious side effects (more than for diphenylhydantoin) associated with its usage include skin eruptions, blood dyscrasias, hepatitis, systemic lupus erythematosus, and lymphadenopathy simulating malignant lymphomas.

Mephenytoin is generally given concurrently with other agents in the lowest dose possible, and only to patients who fail to respond to or who do not tolerate safer agents. Because of its sedative effects it is more often employed concurrently with phenytoin than with phenobarbital or primidone.

Oxazolidones

These drugs are useful in the management of petit mal. The two drugs in this category are trimethadone (Tridione) and paramethadione (Paradione). Toxic effects include drowsiness, ataxia, photophobia, visual disturbances, skin rash, alopecia, bone marrow depression, and kidney damage. Some reactions have been fatal. There is also some evidence that they may result in birth defects; therefore, their use should be avoided in pregnant women.

Succinimides

These drugs are useful in the management of petit mal. The three drugs in this category are phensuximide (Milontin), methsuximide (Celontin), and ethosuximide (Zarontin). This group of drugs is less toxic than the oxazolidones, and the major side effects associated with their use are dizziness and skin rashes. Some cases of blood dyscrasias have also been associated with their use. Currently, ethosuximide is considered the drug of choice for petit mal seizures.

Miscellaneous Anticonvulsants

Other drugs are occasionally used for the treatment of convulsions, but they are usually not as effective as those previously described. These drugs are listed in Table 13-1.

The most common side effects associated with the drugs in Table 13-1 relate to their depressive effects on the central nervous system (CNS). Patients may be drowsy, occasionally have blood dycrasias, and may complain of gastrointestinal disturbances and headaches. Behavioral changes may occur, ranging from an attitude of noncommitment to one of depression. Because of these side effects, the dental auxiliary may find that a formerly cooperative patient may no longer be a good patient. Plaque control in patients taking these

Table 13-1 Miscellaneous Anticonvulsants

Generic name	Commercial name
Acetazolamide	Diamox
Carbamazepine	Tegretol
Diazepam	Valium
Phenacemide	Phenurone

medications may be poor or lacking due to their mental outlook. Gentleness and patience are necessary for establishing patient rapport and helping the patient establish a good plaque-control program.

Two of the drugs in Table 13-1, carbamazepine and acetazolamide, have been reported to produce numbness or paresthesia in the head and neck region. Therefore, paresthesia in these patients may not be of dental origin but related to medications. Interestingly, because of the side effects of paresthesia, carbamazepine has been used to treat patients suffering from pain associated with trigeminal neuralgia.

Blood dyscrasias, or disturbances in various blood cells, have been associated with some of the anticonvulsants in a few patients. Therefore, adequate laboratory blood tests are necessary prior to the initiation of surgical therapy. If a blood dyscrasia is untreated, postoperative wound healing will be compromised, and the risk of infection will be increased.

Because dental professionals will often be the first to observe the side effects or to hear the patient's symptoms, this knowledge will be an important contribution to the successful management of these patients.

Parkinson's Disease

Although it is not a true convulsive disorder, this condition has tremors associated with it. Parkinson's disease is a disorder in which patients develop a marked rigidity coupled with slow, weak, involuntary muscle movements and increased salivation. Because these patients have difficulty with muscle control, oral hygiene procedures are difficult. It is due to a depletion of dopamine, a chemical in the CNS. This condition is treated by the administration of drugs with dopamine activity.

Parkinson's disease occurs mainly in old people but may also be seen as a side effect of therapy with drugs such as reserpine or the phenothiazines. Reserpine depletes dopamine, and the phenothiazines block dopamine receptors.

The main drug used in therapy of Parkinson's disease is levodopa. Once absorbed through the blood brain barrier, it is converted to dopamine, and gradually the concentration of dopamine in the CNS increases.

Side effects are common with levodopa, and include nausea, vomiting, postural hypotension, involuntary movements, and psychiatric disturbances. If a patient in your office is taking levodopa and develops any of these symptoms, she should be told to contact her physician, since an overdose may be present.

When levodopa does not alleviate parkinsonism, some anticholinergic drugs such as atropine and related synthetic agents are used. These drugs only reduce the tremors and decrease salivation. Since xerostomia (dry mouth) may occur in these patients, plaque control may be poor, and caries and gingivitis will be more extensive than in a normal patient.

ANSWER TO CHAPTER CASE

If a patient has been on anticonvulsant therapy for a short time, his convulsions may not be controlled. Therefore, one should be prepared for a convulsion to occur by having a wooden bite block available to protect the tongue and cheek and to protect the patient from injury during the convulsion. Following a convulsive episode, emotional support is most important.

The dental light should not be flashed into the eyes of a patient with a history of convulsions since this action could trigger a convulsion.

The dentist would like a picture of the patient's gingiva so that there will be a record to compare gingival changes which may occur because of the anticonvulsive medication. About 50 percent of patients receiving phenytoin will manifest varying degrees of gingival hyperplasia.

Strict plaque control in these patients is mandatory, since a number of studies have shown that gingival hyperplasia associated with phenytoin therapy can be minimized if strict plaque control is instituted within a few weeks of the time the patient receives the anticonvulsant drug.

QUESTIONS

1 Which anticonvulsants cause gingival hyperplasia?
2 What is the role of the dental auxiliary in minimizing the development of gingival hyperplasia associated with anticonvulsant therapy?
3 What are the most common side effects associated with anticonvulsant therapy? Can any of these side effects alter dental therapy or patient management?
4 What precautions should be taken in anticipating a convulsive episode in a patient with a history of epilepsy?

READING REFERENCES

Aas, E., "Hyperplasia Gingival Diphenylhydantoinea," *Acta Odontol. Scand.,* **21**:Suppl. 34, 1963.

Aiman, R., "The Use of Positive Pressure Mouthpiece as a New Therapy for Dilantin Gingival Hyperplasia," *Chron. Omaha Dent. Soc.,* **131**:244, 1963.

Baden, E., "Sodium Dilantin Gingival Hyperplasia and Conservative Treatment: A Case Report," *J. Dent. Med.,* **5**:46, 1950.

Ciancio, S. G., S. J. Yaffee, and C. C. Catz, "Gingival Hyperplasia and Diphenylhydantoin," *J. Periodontal.,* **43**:411, 1972.

Cunat, J. J., and S. G. Ciancio, "Diphenylhydantoin Sodium: Gingival Hyperplasia and Orthodontic Treatment," *Angle Ortho.,* **39**:182–185, 1969.

Hall, W. B., "Prevention of Dilantin Hyperplasia: A Preliminary Report," *Bull. Acad. Gen. Dent.,* 20, June 1969.

Svensmark, O., P. J. Schiller, and F. Buchthal, "5.5 Diphenylhydantoin (Dilantin) Blood Levels After Oral or Intravenous Dosage in Man," *Acta Pharmacol. Toxicol.,* **16**:331, 1960.

Ziskin, D. E., L. R. Stowe, and E. V. Zegarelli, "Dilantin Hyperplastic Gingivitis," *Am. J. Orthod.,* **27**:350, 1941.

Chapter 14

Cardiovascular Drugs

Can a patient taking a diuretic, digitalis, or an antihypertensive drug be moved abruptly in the dental chair? What are these drugs used for? What side effects should you antici- pate?

Drugs affecting cardiac and renal function are not usually administered by dentists. How- ever, there are a number of dental consid- erations of importance. Some of the drugs raise blood pressure (hypertensive agents), whereas others lower it (hypotensive agents). Others affect heart rate and the contractive force of heart muscle. Drugs affecting renal function influence the water content of the body, which can alter plasma volume. This, in turn, can alter blood pressure and cardiac ac- tivity. As patients grow older, they sometimes develop cardiovascular and renal problems. It is likely that 20 percent of the patients over 50

seen in a dental office will be taking medica- tions in this category.

DIGITALIS AND RELATED DRUGS

These drugs are cardiac glycosides and are the fourth most frequently prescribed drugs in this country. They are used in patients with con- gestive heart failure (one or both ventricles of the heart have a reduced force of contraction) and certain arrhythmias (abnormal heart rate). Some of these drugs were used in early Egypt and can be obtained from several plants as well as the skin of the common toad. Digitalis, the representative drug in this category, was described as a derivative of the foxglove plant as early as 1250 A.D. Because of its derivation, it is sometimes referred to as foxglove.

Mechanism of Action

The main action of digitalis is to increase the force of contraction of the ventricles. It thus makes the heart more efficient without increasing the heart's oxygen needs. This increased contractile force is referred to as positive ionotropism. Therapy with digitalis:

1 Increases cardiac output
2 Decreases venous pressure
3 Increases urination (diuresis) due to improved circulation through the kidney
4 Relieves edema
5 Decreases blood volume due to elimination of water

Pharmacologic Information

Early in therapy these drugs increase the elimination of water from the body. If a patient was recently started on digitalis, he may have to excuse himself from the dental chair to urinate. Therefore, such patients should be scheduled for more time.

This diuresis can be related to improved cardiac function and the resultant reduction in venous pressure which accompanies this action. Venous pressure is elevated in congestive heart failure due to a "back-up pressure" of blood in the veins, since the heart is not pumping blood into the arteries in adequate amounts. Venous pressure is reduced since the heart can pump more blood into the arteries and through the kidneys, with the result that the kidneys remove excess water from the blood more effectively. With reduced venous pressure, fluid flows from the intercellular spaces into the veins. As a result, circulation is improved and more fluid reaches the kidneys for elimination, with increased urine volume and decreased edema.

Although digitalis directly decreases the heart rate in animals, this is a minimal effect in normal humans. Digitalis does slow the conduction of impulses from the atrium to the ventricle, with the effect being a slight slowing of heart rate. However, in patients with congestive heart failure and reduced cardiac output, tachycardia (increased heart rate) may be seen as a means to improve cardiac output and thus raise pressure on the arterial side of the heart. Because cardiac output increases with digitalis, cardiac slowing is seen as a secondary effect since there is no longer a need for an increase in heart rate to try to compensate for reduced cardiac output.

Another effect of digitalis is seen in the ventricle. Here, it can increase the automaticity of the ventricles, resulting in ectopic pacemaker sites. Since large doses of epinephrine also increase ventricular automaticity, it should not be applied topically to wounds or used in retraction cords in patients taking digitalis, since a serious drug interaction may occur. However, epinephrine in local anesthetic solutions (1/100,000) is not contraindicated. The recommended dosage should not exceed 0.2 mg of epinephrine per visit.

Innervation by the vagus nerve is important to the regulation of heart rate. As vagal impulses increase, the heart slows its rate, and vice versa. Digitalis reduces the ventricular rate in atrial fibrillation by increasing impulses from the vagus nerve and by other extravagal effects. Atropine and similar drugs used to decrease salivary secretion are contraindicated since these may counteract the beneficial effects of digitalis in increasing vagal impulses (see Chap. 3).

Adverse Effects

The cardiac glycosides have a low margin of safety, and cumulative effects do occur. The early signs of toxicity are usually not serious, but serve as a warning. Therefore, dental personnel should be cognizant of these signs and symptoms so that they can advise the patient to consult with the physician regarding the dosage regimen.

These signs and symptoms include anorexia, nausea, vomiting, and sometimes diarrhea. In some patients, heart rate and rhythm may change to the extent that the patient might volunteer that he is nervous and "his heart beat doesn't feel right." Indeed, this nervousness may be a sign of overdosage.

Since these patients are more prone to vomiting, this must be considered, particularly during taking of impressions or work on posterior teeth.

Some effects of digitalis are greatly reduced by large concentrations of potassium in plasma. Therefore, dental use of large doses of drugs containing potassium should be avoided in these patients. For example, the sodium salts of antibiotics should be prescribed instead of potassium salts, when possible.

Phenobarbital also increases the metabolism of digitalis, altering its therapeutic efficacy. Therefore, dentists should avoid this sedative in patients on digitalis.

Therapeutic Usage

These drugs are used in congestive heart failure, atrial fibrillation, atrial flutter, and paroxysmal tachycardia.

A number of cardiac glycosides are available. Digoxin (Lanoxin) is the most commonly prescribed since it has a more prolonged duration of action. Other preparations include digitoxin (Crystodigin, Purodigin), lantoside (Cledilanid), deslanoside (Cedilanid-D), acetyldigitoxin (Acylanid), and quabain (G-strophanthin).

ANTIARRHYTHMIC DRUGS

A number of other drugs in addition to cardiac glycosides affect cardiac rhythm. Cardiac disease or injury may alter normal cardiac rhythm by damaging the impulse-conducting systems or by developing ectopic pacemakers and abnormal pacemaker rhythms. Drugs for normalizing these arrhythmias include: quinidine, procainamide, lidocaine, phenytoin (diphenylhydantoin), and propranolol.

Quinidine

This drug prevents or abolishes certain cardiac arrhythmias, including atrial fibrillation and flutter, paroxysmal supraventricular and ventricular tachycardia, and premature systoles. Quinidine affects cardiac rhythm by two mechanisms. First, by a direct effect on the myocardium, it decreases excitability, conduction velocity, and automaticity. Second, by an indirect effect, it reduces the influence of the vagus nerve on heart rate. Since the vagus nerve slows heart rate, this latter effect must be carefully monitored.

Adverse effects associated with this drug are common and may be serious. The early signs of an adverse response include: diarrhea, nausea and vomiting, tinnitus, vertigo, headache, and mental confusion.

Procainamide

Procainamide, a derivative of procaine, has pharmacological properties similar to procaine. Its actions on the heart are similar to those described above for quinidine.

Adverse effects associated with its usage include: anorexia, nausea, vomiting, a bitter taste, diarrhea, mental depression, and sometimes hallucinations. If patients complain of a bad oral taste, it may not be due to oral or gastrointestinal causes but rather to the side effect listed above. Some patients also develop an allergy to this drug. When this occurs, they will also be allergic to other local anesthetics derived from benzoic acid. These are the local anesthetics classified as esters (see Chap. 7).

Hypotension can occur with this drug and leads to dizziness in these patients if they are abruptly raised or lowered in the dental chair.

This phenomenon is called orthostatic hypotension. Therefore, they should be slowly moved upward following completion of dental procedures to prevent fainting due to lack of an adequate blood supply to the brain.

Lidocaine

This local anesthetic is widely used for the emergency treatment of ventricular arrhythmias associated with cardiac surgery or myocardial infarction. It has a more rapid onset of action than quinidine and procainamide and has a very short duration. Therefore, it is excellent for emergency procedures.

Since the drug is used as an injectable agent, side effects related to its use as an antiarrhythmic drug cannot be expected in the dental office. However, if the patient had an allergic reaction with lidocaine, similar allergic reactions can be expected with other chemically related local anesthetics.

Phenytoin (Diphenylhydantoin)

Although this drug is mainly used as an anticonvulsant, it is also effective for cardiac arrhythmia. Its mechanism of action is unlike that of procainamide, quinidine, or lidocaine. Phenytoin exerts its effect mainly by depressing pacemaker activity in the Purkinje fibers of the heart and by enhancing fiber conduction. Therefore, it is often used in cases of ventricular arrhythmias. Its actions are most pronounced in patients showing toxic effects of digitalis, and it is the drug of choice in the treatment of digitalis arrhythmias. Adverse effects are discussed in the chapter on anticonvulsants (see Chap. 13).

Propranolol

This drug is a beta-adrenergic blocking agent and is useful in treating a number of cardiac dysfunctions. Patients taking this drug usually receive it because they have serious cardiac arrhythmia problems. In addition to beta-blocking effects, as an antiarrhythmic agent it has a direct effect on the heart similar to quinidine.

It is principally used to control the ventricular rate in supraventricular tachycardia (atrial fibrillation, flutter, and paroxysmal tachycardia). It exerts this effect by decreasing electrical conduction through the A-V node.

It is also used in the treatment of hypertension and angina.

ANTIHYPERTENSIVE DRUGS

Cardiovascular complications such as heart failure, coronary artery disease, stroke, and kidney failure often are a result of elevated high blood pressure (hypertension). It is estimated that 20 percent of the U.S. adult population has high blood pressure. Many patients with high blood pressure are unaware of their problem. For this reason, many dental offices include hypertension screening as a health service to their patients. Effective reduction of blood pressure in males can reduce the frequency of most of the complications associated with high blood pressure. However, results of treatment in females are lacking. The reduction of blood pressure is often accomplished by diet (especially salt elimination) and drug therapy.

Hypertension is categorized according to severity as mild, moderate, or severe. This classification is based mainly on a person's diastolic blood pressure, which reflects the nature of the peripheral vasculature. Patients with mild hypertension (diastolic pressure 90 to 100 mmHg) are often controlled by diet and exercise. Those with moderate hypertension (100 to 115 mmHg) and severe hypertension (above 115 mmHg) are best controlled by a combination of drugs and diet. The drugs used in the treatment of hypertension are diuretics, inhibitors of sympathetic nervous system activity, and vasodilators. Drugs that lower elevated blood pressure are classified as antihypertensive drugs.

Prior to a discussion considering the individual drugs, some general comments are necessary. In dental patients on antihypertensive agents, the blood pressure is very responsive to positional change (orthostatic hypotension). In view of this, such patients should not be subjected to abrupt positional changes in the dental chair. The blood vessels may not constrict in time to compensate for the positional change as they do in the normal patient. Therefore, the patient may lapse into unconsciousness due to a lack of adequate blood supply to the brain.

Patients taking antihypertensive agents and also taking sedatives or sleeping pills may be even more prone to orthostatic hypotension. This results from the interaction of sedatives and antihypertensives, which enhances orthostatic hypotension.

Drugs which lower blood pressure are classified according to their mechanism of action. Those which act on the sympathetic system are classified as sympatholytic, and those which interfere with neural transmission at ganglia are called ganglionic blocking agents. Another group of drugs which act directly on smooth muscles of arterioles is classified as arteriolar muscle relaxants. Others exert their effect by a diuretic action in the kidney.

Diuretics increase the rate of urine formation by increasing the excretion of solutes and water by the kidney. Most important is their effect on the excretion of solutes, such as sodium, which influence water excretion. Diuretic therapy, therefore, removes edema-causing fluid from the body, which reduces blood volume. As blood volume decreases, blood pressure decreases. It is not clear if the decreased blood pressure results only from fluid volume changes or also from effects on vascular resistance.

The most commonly used diuretics are classified as thiazides, loop diuretics, or potassium sparing.

Thiazides

The thiazides are the main diuretics used to treat hypertension. These agents lower blood pressure by reducing the extracellular fluid volume. When used in conjunction with non-diuretic antihypertensive drugs, they prevent sodium and water retention produced by some antihypertensive agents.

Adverse effects associated with thiazides include weakness, fatigue, dizziness, and leg cramps. An awareness of these symptoms is important to the dental auxiliary in terms of the dental team's role in the overall management of a patient's health.

The thiazides increase the urinary excretion of potassium, and serum potassium levels fall during prolonged therapy. This drop in serum potassium is called hypokalemia and accounts for many of the thiazide side effects. Since potassium levels are important to the cardiac muscle's response to digitalis, patients taking digitalis may require potassium supplementation during therapy. In patients with a history of gout or renal failure, an acute attack of gout may be precipitated. Drugs included in this group are chlorthalidone, metolazone, and quinethazone.

Loop Diuretics

These drugs are identical to thiazides in pharmacological action but differ chemically. Their onset of action is more rapid, and their diuretic effect is greater than the thiazides. While they are stronger diuretics, they are not as effective antihypertensives as the thiazides. These drugs are substitutes for the thiazides when there is impaired renal function. They are not used as often as the thiazides because they have a higher incidence of side effects. Adverse effects associated with therapy include dehydration, hypotension, hypokalemia, hyperglycemia, and deafness. Drugs included in this group are classified as furosemide and ethacrynic acid.

Potassium-Sparing Diuretics

These drugs are used in conjunction with the thiazide diuretics to treat hypertension. Such combined therapy results in increased sodium excretion and decreased potassium excretion. In this manner, the hypokalemia (low blood potassium) associated with the thiazides is minimized.

One of the drugs in this group, spironolactone (Aldactone), exerts its effect by antagonizing aldosterone. Triamterene (Pyrenium), the other drug in this group, acts at the exchange sites in the kidney and promotes sodium excretion.

Adverse effects associated with these drugs include menstrual irregularities (gynecomastia). Antihypertensive drugs and their characteristics are listed in Table 14-1.

Frequently, there is sedation, postural hypotension, dry mouth, nasal stuffiness, skin rashes, and, except for the diuretics, salt and water retention with resultant edema. Certain side effects are more often associated with specific drugs, and these are listed in Table 14-2.

Dental Considerations

The use of antihypertensive agents requires special consideration, since drug interactions may occur when the drug prescribed by the dentist alters the effect of the antihypertensive drug. Potentiation and prolongation of analgesics, narcotics, barbiturates, sedatives, and tranquilizing agents may be observed, depending on the hypertensive agent involved. Because of this, the dentist may have to alter the dose of these drugs. In most cases, the drug prescribed by the dentist must be given in doses lower than usual. A safe rule is to prescribe half the usual dosage and then observe the patient's response. If a greater dose is needed, the dosage can be gradually increased, and problems related to the drug interaction will be minimized.

ANTICOAGULANTS

In order to understand the action of anticoagulants, a review of the blood-clotting

Table 14-1 Characteristics of Antihypertensive Drugs

Name				
Commercial	Trade	Mechanism of action	Daily dosage	Side effects
Clonidine	Catapres	Sympatholytic	0.4–2.0 mg	Few
Diazoxide	Hyperstat (IV)	Arteriole muscle relaxant	300 mg	Low
Hexamethonium chloride		Ganglionic blocking	125–750 mg	High
Hydralazine	Apresoline HCl	Arteriolar muscle relaxant	100–200 mg	Many
Mecamylamine HCl	Inversine	Ganglionic blocking	5 mg	High
Methyldopa	Aldomet	Action on CNS	1 g	Moderate
Monamine oxidase inhibitors	Pargyline	Sympatholytic	25–50 mg	Moderate
Nitroprusside	Sodium nitroprusside	Arteriole muscle relaxant	Variable	High
Pentolinium tartrate	Ansolysen	Ganglionic blocking	60 mg	High
Thiazides	Diuril, Esidrix, Hydrodiuric, Oretic	Diuretic	Varies with agent	Low
Veratrum alkaloids (reserpine)	Serpasil, Sandril, Reserpoid	Sympatholytic?	0.25–0.5 mg	Moderate

Table 14-2   Side Effects of Some Antihypertensive Drugs

Drug	Side effects
Clonidine	Impotence, constipation
Diazoxide	Salt and water retention, hyperglycemia, hypertrichosis
Diuretics	Feeling of weakness, blurred vision, hypokalemia
Ganglionic blocking agents	Fainting, blurred vision, constipation (side effects are so high that other drugs have replaced this group)
Hydralazine	Nausea, dizziness, headache, paresthesia, muscle cramps, kidney disorders, anemia
Methyldopa	Vertigo, lactation, extrapyramidal stimulation with possible muscle spasm, psychic depression, liver damage, anemia
Monamine oxidase inhibitors (MAOI)	Psychotic reactions, muscle cramps, strong interaction with certain foods (old cheeses, wines)
Nitroprusside	Nausea, vomiting, headache, palpitation, chest pains
Veratrum alkaloids	Nausea, vomiting, "digitalis-type" effect on the heart

system is necessary. Blood coagulation has been divided into three stages: (1) formation of thromboplastin, (2) conversion of prothrombin to thrombin, and (3) conversion of fibrinogen to fibrin. A number of tissue factors and platelet factors are necessary for the formation of thromboplastin. Vitamin K is necessary for the formation of prothrombin in the liver, thromboplastin and calcium are necessary for the conversion of prothrombin to thrombin, and thrombin and calcium are necessary for the conversion of fibrinogen to fibrin. The clotting system is presented in Fig. 14-1.

Many older patients will be taking anticoagulants. They are often prescribed following myocardial infarcts, and in patients with a history of blood clots. Different anticoagulants exert their effects at different sites in the clotting system. The main anticoagulants in use today are heparin, derivatives of bishydroxycoumarin, indanediones, and agents that alter platelet aggregation.

Heparin

Heparin inhibits the conversion of prothrombin to thrombin by complexing with certain plasma factors (IX to XII). It also has some antithrombin properties. In order for heparin to exert its anticoagulant effect, a plasma alphaglobulin, called heparin cofactor, is necessary.

Heparin must be given by the parenteral route. For this reason it has not been used as often as the oral anticoagulants. However, slow-release depository forms have been developed, and the frequency of its use is increasing.

Adverse effects associated with heparin in-

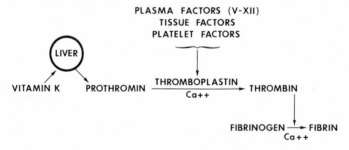

Figure 14-1   Blood coagulation system.

clude reversible thrombocytopenia, transient alopecia, increased sodium excretion, decreased potassium excretion, and osteoporosis. It is questionable whether the osteoporosis affects the maxilla and mandible.

Heparin also lowers elevated lipid levels in plasma. The significance of this lipid-clearing action is not clear at this time.

An overdose of heparin can be counteracted by the intravenous injection of protamine sulfate. Protamine sulfate is a base, and heparin is an acid. Therefore, protamine sulfate acts by chemically neutralizing the effect of heparin.

Certain clinical tests are invalid in patients receiving heparin. For example, white blood cell counts must be done within 2 h of the time the blood is withdrawn from the patient since these cells disintegrate after 2 h. Also, heparin inhibits red blood cell hemolysis. Therefore, red blood cell fragility tests are meaningless.

Coumarins

These anticoagulants are used most often. They exert their effect by decreasing the action of vitamin K on prothrombin formation. This is effected by competing with vitamin K

for an enzyme important in the synthesis of prothrombin and factors VIII, IX, and X. These drugs can be administered orally. The most common adverse effect associated with all coumarin therapy is spontaneous hemorrhage, which may first occur in the gingival tissues. This is a result of overdosage which can occur because of narrow safety range and accumulation. Accumulation occurs because coumarins are highly bound to protein and are then slowly released from their protein-binding sites. Hematuria, anorexia, nausea, and diarrhea have also been reported with their use. Also the coumarins dilate coronary arteries.

The anticoagulant effect of coumarins is overcome by a transfusion with whole blood and the simultaneous administration of vitamin K. The transfusion is necessary since vitamin K does not exert its effect for 3 to 4 h.

Indanediones

These anticoagulants differ chemically from the coumarins but have a similar mechanism of action and are also given orally.

They are not used as frequently as heparin or coumarin since they have more side effects.

Table 14-3 Commonly Used Anticoagulants

Generic name	Brand names	Route of administration
Agents altering platelet function		
Salicylic acid	Aspirin, Bayer, Anacin	PO
Phenylbutazone	Butazolidin	PO
Indomethacin		PO
Coumarin types		
Bishydroxycoumarin	Dicumarol	PO
Warfarin	Coumadin, Panwarfin	IV
Phenprocoumon	Liquomar, Marcumar	PO
Acenocoumarol	Sintron	PO
Heparin type		
Sodium heparin		IV, IM, SC
Indanediones		
Diphenadione	Dipaxin	PO
Phenindione	Danilone, Hedulon	PO
Anisindione	Miradon	PO

These include agranulocytosis, hepatitis, kidney damage, leukopenia, and massive generalized edema. These drugs also normally produce a temporary orange discoloration of urine, which is not harmful.

Platelet Function Suppression

Platelet function suppression is sometimes used for anticoagulation. Aspirin and other nonsteroid antiinflammatory drugs alter platelet function, which in turn prevents the formation of thromboplastin.

These drugs can be given orally with few side effects. Their anticoagulant effect is not as potent as the other agents, but they are being evaluated for use in patients after heart attacks.

Examples of the various anticoagulants are presented in Table 14-3. A discussion of the management of patients taking anticoagulants can be found in Chap. 17.

The anticoagulants interact with more drugs than any other drugs known. Therefore, they must be carefully prescribed when given with other drugs. The topic of drug interactions is discussed in detail in Chap. 19.

ANSWER TO CHAPTER CASE

Patients receiving a diuretic, digitalis, or an antihypertensive drug cannot be moved rapidly or abruptly in the dental chair because they are prone to orthostatic hypotension and may exhibit syncope.

Diuretics are drugs which increase the rate of urine formation by increasing the excretion of water and solutes by the kidneys. Digitalis is a drug used to increase the force of contraction of the ventricles.

Antihypertensive drugs are those which decrease blood pressure by various methods. Side effects of diuretics and digitalis are discussed under appropriate headings in this chapter and those of antihypertensive drugs are summarized in Table 14-2.

QUESTIONS

1 What conditions are treated with cardiac glycosides?
2 What are the signs and symptoms of an overdose of digitalis?
3 What is orthostatic hypotension? Why is it sometimes seen in patients taking cardiac glycosides?
4 Which drugs are useful in the treatment of cardiac arrhythmias?
5 What are the most common side effects associated with antihypertensive drug therapy?

READING REFERENCES

Aagard, G. N., "The Management of Hypertension," *J. Am. Med. Assoc.,* **224:**329–332, 1973.

Bigger, J. T., Jr., and H. C. Strauss, "Digitalis Toxicity: Drug Interactions Promoting Toxicity and the Management of Toxicity," *Semin. Drug Treat.,* **2:**147–177, 1972.

Coleman, T. G., et al., "The Role of Salt in Experimental and Human Hypertension," *Am. J. Med. Sci.,* **264:**103–110, 1972.

Moe, G. K., and A. E. Farah, "Digitalis and Allied Cardiac Glycosides," in L. S. Goodman and A. Gilman (eds.), *Pharmacological Basis of Therapeutics,* Macmillan, New York, 1975.

O'Brien, E. T., and J. Mackinnon, "Propranolol and Polythiazide in Treatment of Hypertension," *Br. Heart J.,* **34:**1042–1044, 1972.

Solomon, H. M., and W. B. Abrams, "Interactions Between Digitoxin and Other Drugs in Man," *Am. Heart J.,* **83:**277–280, 1972.

Hormones and Related Substances

"Dr. Green, since I started taking birth control pills, my gums bleed often. Are these pills causing this?"

Hormones are biologically active substances that are secreted by endocrine glands and transported by the blood to those "target" organs where they exert an effect. Endocrine glands include the hypophysis (pituitary), thyroid, parathyroids, pancreatic islets, adrenals, gonads, and the placenta. Endocrines regulate many body functions and are controlled themselves by feedback systems (Fig. 15-1).

Other substances, called autocoids, local hormones, or autopharmacologic agents, are not classified as hormones but also have strong pharmacologic properties. These include histamine, endogenous amines, angiotensin, bradykinin, kallidin, and prostaglandins. Au-

tocoids play a role in health and disease and may be important in homeostasis. Some autocoids are purified from animal glands. However, synthetic autocoids resembling the natural products have proven more useful in therapy. In this chapter, the hormones and important autocoids will be discussed with emphasis on dental problems associated with hormonal therapy and the use of hormone therapy in the correction of dental problems. Since histamine and its antagonists are discussed in another chapter, they will not be considered here.

The growth and development of the body is partially regulated by hormones. Therefore, hormonal imbalances during the growth and

163

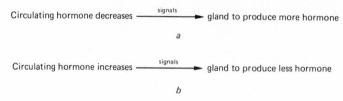

Figure 15-1 General scheme for hormonal feedback systems.

development of teeth and facial bones can lead to abnormalities. Hormonal imbalances after teeth have erupted obviously do not affect the crowns of the teeth. Instead, changes which may be diagnostic for an endocrine imbalance may be seen in the roots and periodontium.

PITUITARY HORMONES

The pituitary gland is divided into an anterior (adenohypophysis) and a posterior lobe (neurohypophysis). Secretion of pituitary hormones is influenced by hormones of the peripheral endocrine glands via a feedback system and by neurohumoral substances from the hypothalamus. The neurohumoral substances are termed releasing hormones, releasing factors, or regulatory hormones.

Anterior Pituitary

The ten hormones produced by the anterior pituitary are growth hormone, prolactin, two gonadotropins, thyrotropin, corticotropin, two lipotropins, and two melanocyte-stimulating hormones.

Corticotropin, or ACTH (adrenocorticotropic hormone), is the principal pituitary hormone and stimulates the adrenal cortex. Hypopituitarism, or decreased anterior pituitary secretion, causes a variety of symptoms, including loss of secondary sex characteristics, lowered metabolism, and even death. Failure of this gland to develop properly during embryogenesis results in dwarfism. Hypersecretion of the anterior pituitary during childhood results in gigantism.

Posterior Pituitary

The posterior pituitary, or neurohypophysis, produces oxytocin and vasopressin and also interacts with the hypothalamus. Oxytocin controls uterine contractibility and mammary gland milk ejection. Oxytocin (Syntocinon, Pitocin) has been used therapeutically to induce labor and control post-partum hemorrhage. Because oxytocin alters bone coaptation at the pubic symphysis, it may alter the attachment of tooth to bone. While orthodontists thought this activity would facilitate orthodontic tooth movement, this is not the case.

Vasopressin affects electrolyte balance and has some vasoconstrictor activity on blood vessels. Therapeutically, vasopressin (Pitressin) has been used for the treatment of diabetes insipidus (water loss due to pituitary damage).

GONADAL HORMONES

"Sex" hormones, or gonadal hormones, are secreted by the ovaries, testes, and placenta. The major female secretions are estrogens and progestins, and the major male hormones are androgens. These hormones influence the gingiva and other soft tissues and are classified in Table 15-1.

Sex hormone secretions are controlled by a feedback mechanism through gonadotropins, which are produced by the pituitary gland. As the gonads produce more hormone, the pituitary gland produces less. This hormone balance regulates menstruation and pregnancy in the female and spermatogenesis in the male.

Table 15-1 Sex Hormones

Hormone	Major gland	Minor gland(s)
Androgens	Testes	Ovary, adrenal cortex
Estrogens	Ovary	Testes, placenta
Progestins	Ovary	Testes, adrenal cortex, placenta

Estrogens

The main estrogen, estradiol, is produced by human ovaries and converted by the liver to estrone and estriol. During pregnancy, the placenta also produces large amounts of estradiol. Estrogens promote growth and development of the vagina, uterus, and fallopian tubes, breast enlargement, and pigmentation of the nipples and areolae, fat distribution, epiphyseal changes, retention of salt and water, and growth of axillary and pubic hair. They are also responsible for changes at puberty and influence the menstrual cycle. The relative concentrations of estrogen vary during pregnancy and menopause. In conjunction with progestins, they are components of birth control pills. Estrogen production by females varies daily, while daily androgen production in the male is more constant.

An increased incidence of vaginal and cervical carcinoma has been observed in children where the mother received synthetic estrogens (such as diethylstilbestrol) during the first trimester of pregnancy. Some reports have also associated carcinoma of the breast with estrogen therapy.

These hormones are readily absorbed by the gastrointestinal tract and can be given orally (po). Since they are also absorbed through skin and mucous membranes, topical application may exert a systemic response.

Progestins

Progestins play a role in the regulation of ovulation, leading to an elevation in body temperature at ovulation of approximately 1°F. The temperature declines at the onset of menstruation coincident with a decline in the progestin levels. Progestin levels, which normally change during the menstrual cycle, can actually alter the regular cycle. Because of this, they are a component of some contraceptives. Other effects of progestins are a proliferation of the mammary gland acini and maturation of the secretory lining of the uterus.

Progesterone is a naturally occurring progestin. Synthetic oral progestins with similar activity include megestrol acetate (Megace), dydrogesterone (Duphaston, Gynorest), norethindrone (Micronor, Nor-QD, Norluten), norethindrone acetate (Norlutate), and ethisterone (Duosterone).

Uses of Estrogens and Progestins

These drugs are used for oral contraception and for control of uterine bleeding, dysmenorrhea, endometriosis, relief of premenstrual tension, prevention of natural abortion, suppression of post-partum lactation, and as palliative agents in uterine carcinoma.

Oral Contraception Current oral contraceptives, which are approximately 98 percent effective, are either estrogenlike or progestinlike substances or a combination of both. Contraceptives are given daily between days 5 and 25 of the menstrual cycle on a sequential basis or as a single daily dose. This latter group has been referred to as ''minipills,'' and these contain only progesterone. Investigations are currently underway to develop a ''morning-after'' pill. At the present time, only diethylstilbestrol has been approved. Because of its possible potential to produce cancer, its use is limited to emergencies such as rape.

A combination of estrogen and progestin inhibits ovulation by suppressing gonadotropin (follicle-stimulating hormone and luteneizing hormone) production by the anterior pituitary gland. Estrogen appears to cause this suppression, while progesterone regulates and controls the bleeding in the menstrual cycle.

Progestins can control pregnancy. While they do not inhibit ovulation, they prevent implantation of the egg by altering the structure of the endometrium. By changing the consistency of uterine mucosa, progestins may also inhibit activity of sperm.

Adverse effects of these drugs include: nausea, dizziness, headache, weight gain and breast discomfort, brownish spots on the face (chloasma), gallbladder disorders, blood pressure elevation, ocular disturbances, liver damage, and gingival bleeding.

The carcinogenic activity of progestins is open to question. Some studies suggest that these drugs cause both benign and malignant tumors. Other reports indicate a decreased incidence of tumors when these drugs are used regularly.

There is also a controversy regarding the production of thrombophlebitis and thromboemboli in women taking oral contraceptives. Current evidence suggests that these individuals are more predisposed to these conditions than women not taking oral contraceptives. The incidence of thromboembolic disorders increases fourfold to tenfold with the use of combined or sequential oral contraceptives. Oral contraceptives also accelerate blood clotting and increase blood concentrations of some clotting factors.

Dental Considerations   Oral contraceptives have been suggested to adversely alter immunologic mechanisms. This would decrease immunologic defenses against plaque bacteria, leading to the initiation and/or progression of periodontal disease.

Oral contraceptives may also increase the incidence of gingival bleeding by proliferation of blood vessels in marginal gingiva, increasing clotting time, and altering the permeability of blood vessels. Some studies contradict the above activities for contraceptives, so this issue has not been completely resolved. Until it is resolved, the role of oral contraceptives

should be considered in evaluating the cause of gingival bleeding problems.

During pregnancy there may be gingival bleeding ("pregnancy gingivitis") and areas of localized hyperplasia ("pregnancy tumors") which occur after the second month of pregnancy and usually disappear after gestation. These gingival changes appear to relate to local accumulations of plaque as well as to hormonal changes during pregnancy.

During puberty, the sex hormones in males and females change sometimes with accompanying gingivitis. This "puberty gingivitis," which clinically appears as plaque-related gingivitis, may be localized or generalized. As in pregnancy gingivitis, excellent plaque control is the best therapy. Puberty gingivitis can be minimized or prevented by good oral hygiene.

Chronic desquamative gingivitis (gingivosis) is another gingival disturbance that may be hormonal in nature since it is more common in females, particularly postmenopausal females. In varying gingival locations, broad, reddened areas are seen. Some effectiveness in treatment has been reported with systemic sex hormone therapy as well as with systemic and topical steroids.

During menstruation and menopause, there are sometimes complaints of "itching gingival tissues," as well as burning and odd oral tastes. These subjective complaints may be hormonally induced by emotional and/or physiologic changes.

Osteoporosis is sometimes also seen postmenopausally, and may result from hormonal secretions associated with menopause. Whether this osteoporosis can be observed in alveolar bone is not clear. This should be considered, however, in evaluating radiographic signs of bone loss.

Androgens

These male hormones are responsible for most characteristics which distinguish the male from the female. They also have a strong anabolic effect and result in nitrogen retention in the body.

Testosterone is produced mainly by the testes and is converted to dihydrotestosterone, which is more active than the parent compound. A feedback mechanism between this gland and the anterior pituitary controls the testosterone levels similarly to that described for the estrogens.

A number of synthetic androgens are available for replacement therapy when necessary due to decreased production by the testes. They are also used for the palliative treatment of breast cancer, menstrual disorders, anemia, and suppression of lactation.

Adverse effects with systemic androgen therapy include masculinization in the female, generalized edema, liver damage, and fever. Buccal and sublingual preparations can also cause stomatitis, which may first be detected during a routine dental visit.

A male oral contraceptive is now being considered that contains androgens in combination with a progestin. Such preparations would decrease gonadotropin secretion and spermatogenesis while still maintaining secondary male traits.

ADRENAL HORMONES

The adrenal gland produces hormones from the medulla (center) and cortex (periphery). The main secretion of the adrenal medulla is epinephrine. Since this hormone is considered in the chapter on autonomic drugs, it will not be discussed at this time.

Corticosteroids, the secretions of the adrenal cortex, include glucocorticoids (antiinflammatory and catabolic effects) and mineralocorticoids (sodium retaining, potassium depleting).

Examples of glucocorticoids are cortisol, corticosterone, and hydrocortisone. They have a multitude of biologic actions, the most prominent of which are listed in Table 15-2 and briefly discussed below.

Effect on Carbohydrate, Protein, and Fat Synthesis

The glucocorticoids increase gluconeogenesis and inhibit peripheral glucose utilization. This results in a build-up of glycogen in the liver and glucose in the body which may lead to hyperglycemia (elevated blood sugar) and glycosurea (excess sugar in urine). As a result, there can be an aggravation of both insulin-dependent and noninsulin-dependent diabetes in some individuals.

Glucocorticoids also promote protein breakdown and inhibit protein synthesis, which can retard wound healing and growth in children.

Fat mobilization is also promoted by glucocorticoids with unusual focal accumulations of fat, most commonly in the back (buffalo hump).

Effect on Electrolytes

The glucocorticoids increase sodium retention and promote potassium excretion, leading

Table 15-2 Effects of Glucocorticoids

Alteration of fat distribution and catabolism of fats
Conversion of amino acids to glucose (gluconeogenesis) for storage by the liver
Enhancement of protein breakdown
Increased sodium retention and potassium excretion
Inhibition of bone growth, matrix formation, and calcification
Inhibition of proliferation and increase in collagen breakdown
Inhibition of the immune response
Inhibition of the inflammatory response
Maintenance of blood pressure and blood volume
Maintenance of excitation threshold of brain
Maintenance of muscle strength
Reduction of calcium absorption from gastrointestinal tract, and promotion of renal excretion of calcium
Reduction of lymphocytes and eosinophils
Stimulation of erythropoesis and platelet production
Thinning of gastric mucosa

sometimes to alkalosis in which body pH increases. They also play a role in the excretion of water by the kidneys, as well as in influencing the distribution of electrolytes between cells and extracellular fluid.

The glucocorticoids also favor the depletion of calcium by promoting calcium excretion and inhibiting its absorption from the intestine.

Antiinflammatory Effect

The glucocorticosteroids inhibit the inflammatory process, probably by inhibiting the migration of polymorphonuclear leukocytes, suppressing the fibroblastic reparative processes, inhibiting capillary permeability and lysosomal stabilization.

Antiallergic Effect

These steroids help counteract an allergic reaction, probably by inhibition of the host's immune response, and by their antiinflammatory action.

Effect on Blood Pressure

The corticosteroids may elevate blood pressure and result in hypertension by promoting sodium retention.

The secretion of the glucocorticoids is related to the amount of adrenocorticotropic hormone (ACTH) released by the anterior pituitary. This system is one in which there is a negative feedback; increased amounts of glucocorticoids signal the anterior pituitary to produce less ACTH. However, in severe stress, this feedback system appears to be shunted, and more ACTH is secreted to help the body meet the stress-producing situation.

Aldosterone and desoxycorticosterone are examples of mineralocorticoids. Mineralocorticoid secretions are controlled mainly by an interaction with renin-angiotensin produced by the kidney, although adequate blood levels of ACTH are needed for their secretion.

Mineralocorticoids are exceedingly potent in enhancing sodium retention and potassium excretion by the renal tubules.

Corticosteroids, which are most often used for their antiinflammatory properties, can be administered topically, orally, and parenterally. Topical application is preferred since this route has minimal systemic effects. *Systemic effects may occur since these drugs can be absorbed through skin and mucosa.* Small amounts of corticosteroids placed in the mouth and covered with an oral adhesive for 12 h can alter secretions of the adrenal cortex by being absorbed through oral mucosa.

Dental Usage

Oral lesions of chronic desquamative gingivitis and apthous ulcers have been treated with topical corticosteroids. It has also been suggested that steroids be applied to these ulcers in conjunction with an electrical current (iontoelectrophoresis), to yield more rapid relief of pain and increased rate of healing. However, with herpetic lesions this is contraindicated and can cause the spread of viral infection from the mouth to the eye.

Topical corticosteroids have also been suggested as an adjunct in pulpotomy and pulp capping. The value of this procedure is inconclusive and must be further studied.

Also, it has been suggested that various steroids can be applied to dentin both with and without an electrical current for desensitization. Studies suggest that application with an electrical current may be highly effective after only one or two applications. Using this route, no adverse pulpal effects have been reported.

The various dental uses are summarized in Table 15-3, and commonly used steroids for dental purposes are summarized in Table 15-4.

Nondental Therapeutic Uses

Corticosteroids are used in replacement therapy and for treatment of rheumatoid arthritis, osteoarthritis, rheumatic carditis, collagen diseases, allergic disorders, bronchial asthma, ocular diseases, skin diseases, chronic ulcerative colitis, some malignancies,

Table 15-3 Dental Uses of Corticosteroids

Condition	Route of administration
Apthous ulcers	Topical
Dentin hypersensitivity	Topical
Desquamative gingivitis	Topical, systemic
Oral lichen planus	Topical, systemic
Oral pemphigus	Topical, systemic
Postextraction (reduce edema)	Systemic
Pulp capping	Topical
Pulpotomy	Topical
Severe allergy	Systemic
TMJ arthritis symptoms	Systemic

liver disease, and shock. Although they are used in shock, their value is not clear.

Adverse Effects

Adverse effects occur as a result of withdrawal and overdose. Patients receiving steroids usually have a depressed adrenal cortex function, since administered steroids lead to decreased ACTH production, which in turn decreases adrenocorticoid activity (negative feedback). When the administered steroid is decreased to normal levels, the ACTH should be secreted, but the adrenal cortex may not respond and an adrenal crisis may occur. Symptoms of this withdrawal include fever, myalgia, arthralgia, hypotension, and malaise. This is similar to early signs of adrenal hypofunction (Addison's disease). Sometimes, cessation of steroid therapy does not quickly lead to normal adrenal cortex function. Therefore, immediately

Table 15-4 Steroids of Use in Dentistry

Name	Route
Dexamethasone (Decadron)	Oral, injectable, topical
Hydrocortisone (Celestone)	Oral
Hydrocortisone sodium succinate (Solu-Cortef)	Injectable
Prednisolone (Delta-Cortef, Meticortelone)	Oral, injectable, topical
Prednisone (Delta-Dome)	Oral
Triamcinolone acetonide (Kenalog)	Topical

following drug cessation, adverse effects, especially during stressful situations such as various dental procedures, can occur. In these situations, patients may need some doses of steroid prior to and following dental surgical procedures to properly protect them, since the adrenal cortex may not be able to respond to a stressful situation and an "adrenal crisis" may occur. When this occurs, 100 mg of hydrocortisone succinate (Solu-Cortef) should be administered IV and patients should be transferred to a hospital if they do not respond. All vital signs should be monitored and preparations made for cardiopulmonary resuscitation (see Chap. 18). The same principle applies to the management of patients taking steroids who are going to face a stressful situation.

Other adverse effects due to hyperfunction or overdose include fluid and electrolyte disturbance, hyperglycemia, glycosemia, osteoporosis, behavioral disturbances, visual disturbances, and increased susceptibility to infection. The patient may show signs of Cushings syndrome (moon face, abnormal fat deposits, humped back, hirsutism, and acne). It has also been shown that glucocorticoid therapy can cause peptic ulcers because of decreased protection offered by the gastric mucous barrier, which interferes with tissue repair and, in some patients, increases gastric acid and pepsinogen production. Also, therapy with glucocorticosteroids may mask the symptoms of an ulcer, and perforation and hemorrhage may occur.

Osteoporosis from steroid therapy must be considered in patients with severe alveolar bone loss. Increased susceptibility to infection may be an indication for post-surgical antibiotic coverage in these patients. This increased susceptibility to infection is not specific for any particular bacterial or fungal microorganism. It is mainly related to the fact that corticosteroids decrease the body's inflammatory and immune responses. Thus, the body's defense against infectious agents is diminished.

Use in Gingivitis

It has been suggested that topical applications of corticosteroids may decrease the severity of gingivitis. Although this may be true, this is dangerous, since only the patients' inflammatory response is reduced and their bacterial plaque is not altered. As a result, the progress of gingival infection may be accelerated.

PARATHYROID HORMONE

The parathyroid glands produce proparathyroid hormone, which is then converted to parathyroid hormone (PTH). PTH is cleaved into fragments in the bloodstream, liver, and kidneys, and possibly at the receptor site. Clinically, measurement of parathyroid hormone levels is important for the diagnosis of some clinical problems associated with calcium and bone metabolism.

Function

The main function of PTH is to maintain the concentration of the calcium ion in extracellular fluid by regulating the deposition and mobilization of calcium from bone, the absorption of calcium from the gastrointestinal tract, the excretion of calcium in urine and feces, and secretion of calcium in sweat and milk. PTH thus directly affects bone by mobilizing calcium from bone to maintain plasma calcium at about 7 mg%.

At the cellular level, PTH stimulates osteoclastic bone resorption by lengthening the life of osteoclasts. Also, it increases the rate of conversion of mesenchymal cells to osteoclasts.

In the kidney, PTH increases the renal tubular reabsorption of calcium and the excretion of phosphate. Both these effects tend to raise the extracellular calcium concentration.

It is of interest that PTH also decreases the secretion of calcium into both mother's milk and saliva. This may conserve calcium in extracellular fluid by reducing its rate of transport from extracellular fluid to milk and saliva. These various actions of PTH are summarized in Fig. 15-2.

The secretions of PTH are indirectly related to levels of ionized calcium in blood. When ionized calcium levels are high or normal, less PTH is secreted, and vice versa.

Parathyroid Disorders

Hypoparathyroidism is only one of the many causes of lowered serum calcium levels. Another condition, pseudohypoparathyroidism, is due to a lack of response to PTH in the target organs. Lowered serum calcium leads to paresthesia of the extremities, muscle spasms leading to tetany, bone loss, hair loss, brittleness of finger nails, defects in dental enamel, emotional disturbances, and even death.

Hyperparathyroidism is characterized by elevated ionized calcium plasma levels. Calcium mobilized from bone is precipitated in soft tissues, and metastatic calcification is seen in the kidneys, stomach wall, bronchi, and heart muscle. Hyperparathyroidism may cause a bone disorder known as osteitis fibrosa cystica, or Recklinghausen's disease of bone. Mild to severe skeletal changes may also be observed on radiographs. In the early stages this decalcification is associated with aches

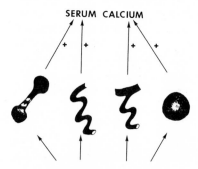

Figure 15-2 Effects of parathyroid hormone on bone, gastrointestinal tract, kidney, milk and salivary glands in the maintenance of serum calcium.

and pains in bones and joints. Since excessive amounts of calcium and phosphate are found in urine, renal calculi may occur. There is also general muscle weakness, constipation, nausea, vomiting, and anorexia. These patients have a higher incidence of peptic ulcers. For this reason, when analgesics are prescribed for these patients, drugs containing salicylic acid should be avoided because of their irritating action on the gastrointestinal tract.

Therapeutic Uses

There are no current valid therapeutic uses of parathyroid hormone. Its main use is in the diagnosis of pseudohypoparathyroidism, in which target organs do not respond to parathyroid hormone. In this test, PTH is injected; if there is no elevation in plasma calcium, the diagnosis of pseudohypoparathyroidism is established.

THYROID HORMONES

The thyroid gland produces thyroxin, triiodothyronine, and calcitonin. Thyroxin and triiodothyronine regulate growth, differentiation, and mineral and oxidative metabolism. Calcitonin regulates bone resorption.

Thyroxin and triiodothyronine are iodine-containing derivatives of thyronine which are synthesized and stored as amino acid residues of thyroglobulin. Since iodine uptake and conversion is essential to their biosynthesis, adequate dietary intake of iodine is essential for their production.

Iodine in the diet becomes incorporated into thyroglobulin in the thyroid gland. Thyroglobulin is then cleaved into thyroxine (T_4) and, to a lesser extent, triiodothyronine (T_3). Once T_4 is formed, 20 percent of it is converted to T_3.

Thyroid hormones are bound to protein in plasma. The more the hormone is complexed with (bound) protein, the less it is available in the free, active form, and vice versa. If disease or drugs alter the amount of protein binding, fluctuations in the amount of free, active hormone occur. Since there is a feedback system in which the level of free hormone regulates its production, the body can compensate for fluctuations in protein binding.

Thyroid Function—Mechanism of Control

Circulating levels of free thyroid hormone exert a negative feedback action on the control of secretion of thyrotropin by the anterior pituitary. Therefore, as the circulating levels of T_3 and T_4 increase, less thyrotropin is produced. Therefore, a balance is maintained between the secretions of these two glands. This relationship is shown in Fig. 15-3.

If less than normal amounts of thyroid hormone are produced, the anterior pituitary gland increases the production of thyrotropin. This in turn stimulates the thyroid gland to become more active, and the glandular tissue hypertrophies to compensate for the inadequate hormone production. This glandular enlargement, called common goiter, is seen in many iodine-deficient individuals. Iodine supplementation frequently corrects this condition.

There is some question as to the possible toxic effects of iodine applied topically as a medication for oral disease or as a disclosing solution, since it may be absorbed through oral

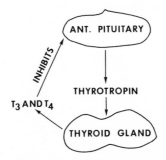

Figure 15-3 Negative feedback between the thyroid gland and the anterior pituitary.

mucosa. This could then potentially alter thyroid function.

Thyroid Disorders

Hyposecretion of thyroid hormone is referred to as myxedema, hypothyroidism, or Gull's disease. Since this leads to drowsiness and fatigue, it may be difficult to motivate plaque control. Hyposecretion in children can result in cretinism. These children are dwarfed, mentally retarded, inactive, and expressionless. Hypersecretion of thyroid hormone may result in diffuse, toxic goiter (Graves' disease, or Badedow's disease), or toxic nodular goiter, called Plummer's disease. Ophthalmopathy, protruding eyes, and anxiety may also be associated with this condition.

Agents Used to Treat Thyroid Disorders   In patients taking medication for thyroid dysfunction, the nature of the dysfunction should be determined, since such a determination may be essential in developing a plaque control program as discussed in previous paragraphs.

A number of antithyroid medications are available, and the most common ones are listed in Table 15-5. Agranulocytosis is the most serious side effect of these drugs. Therefore, prior to dental surgical procedures, a determination should be made of the possible existence of agranulocytosis since it could cause inhibition of wound healing and possibly increased susceptibility to infection. Other side effects reported with these drugs include arthalgia, paresthesia (which could manifest itself in facial areas), headache, nausea, and loss or depigmentation of hair.

Thyroid preparations for hypothyroidism are listed in Table 15-6. Adverse effects associated with these agents are rare. Overdosage will produce signs and symptoms of hyperthyroidism. Since these drugs can affect cardiac function, they must be used with caution in cardiac patients. Otherwise, they may precipitate angina, or cardiac failure.

Calcitonin

Calcitonin is produced by parafollicular cells of the thyroid gland. Its biosynthesis and secretion are regulated by the concentration of calcium in plasma. When the calcium concentration is high, the amount of calcitonin in plasma increases, and vice versa. However, its role in regulating plasma calcium is not known.

Calcitonin inhibits bone resorption by alteration of the activity of osteoclasts. Also, it enhances bone formation by stimulating osteoblastic activity and interferes with the bone resorption associated with parathyroid hormone activity; i.e., it acts in an exactly opposite manner to PTH.

Clinical Usage   Calcitonin has been used to treat a number of skeletal diseases, including Paget's disease, a bone-remodeling disorder in which bone resorption increases. In this condition, it produces symptomatic relief. It is effective as initial therapy in treating hypercalcemia, hyperparathyroidism, vitamin D overdose, and bone metastases of an osteolytic

Table 15-5   Common Antithyroid Medications

Carbimazole
Methimazole
Methylthiouracil
Propythiouracil

Table 15-6   Common Medications For Hypothyroidism

Levothyroxine
Liothyronine sodium
Thyroglobulin
Thyroid extract

nature. Therapy decreases plasma calcium and phosphate by inhibiting their resorption and increasing their deposition into bone.

Side effects associated with therapy with this drug include nausea, swelling, tenderness of extremities, and urticaria.

PANCREATIC HORMONES AND ORAL HYPOGLYCEMIC AGENTS

Insulin and glucagon are the hormones produced by the alpha and beta cells, respectively, of the pancreas. The alpha and beta cells, along with the delta cells, are sometimes called the islands of Langerhans.

Insulin

Beta cells of the pancreas produce proinsulin, which is converted to insulin and then secreted. Insulin promotes food storage and the metabolism of glucose, amino acids, and fatty acids. Insulin affects glucose metabolism by enhancing cellular uptake of glucose by cells, by promoting the conversion of glucose to glycogen, and by decreasing the conversion of proteins to glucose. Insulin also decreases fat mobilization from fat deposits and inhibits any enzymes that convert fats to fatty acids. Insulin secretion is stimulated mainly by the presence of excess glucose in blood and is altered by other hormonal and neural stimuli, including certain gastrointestinal hormones. Many hormones and autocoids affect insulin release. For this reason, insulin secretion is a complex matter involving many interrelationships.

Epinephrine and norepinephrine suppress insulin secretion. Since epinephrine and norephinephrine are released during normal exercise and during certain pathological states, these situations decrease insulin secretion and consequently may cause hyperglycemia.

In a nervous diabetic patient, with little if any insulin secretion, hyperglycemia may occur by a different route. Epinephrine and norephinephrine increase glycogenolysis in the liver with the result that glycogen is converted to glucose, the patient cannot produce enough insulin to metabolize this glucose, and hyperglycemia results.

Once insulin enters the bloodstream, the liver and kidneys are of primary importance in its metabolism and excretion. Each of these organs is capable of metabolizing 40 percent of the insulin produced per day.

Therapeutic Uses and Adverse Effects Insulin is used therapeutically for treatment of diabetes mellitus. In diabetics taking insulin, hypoglycemic reactions may result from failure to eat, unaccustomed exercise or stress, and inadvertant administration of too large a dose of insulin. Therefore, dental appointments for patients taking insulin should not interfere with meals, and stressful situations should be minimized and of short duration. Oral surgical procedures should be performed 1.5 to 2 h after the patient has eaten a normal breakfast and taken their regular antidiabetic medication. Dental therapy, especially surgery, should not be performed on uncontrolled diabetics.

The dental team should be familiar with the symptoms and treatment since such hypoglycemia reactions are not uncommon. The symptoms include sweating, weakness, hunger, tachycardia, "feeling of trembling," headache, blurred vision, mental confusion, and incoherent speech, and eventually coma, convulsions, and death. Treatment of hypoglycemia in the early stages, when the patient is awake, is with fruit juice, particularly orange juice, or soluble carbohydrates. When the patient is unconscious, treatment is by IV injection of glucose or glucagon. These items should be readily available in the dental office for emergency purposes.

Diabetes and Dental Hygiene A number of studies indicate that diabetics are prone to more severe periodontal disease. This may be because these patients accumulate plaque more readily. Part of this accumulation of plaque may be because diabetics have elevated levels of glucose in their gingival crevicular fluid. This glucose may provide an excellent nutritional base for plaque microbes.

It has also been suggested that the measurement of glucose concentration in crevicular fluid may serve as a diagnostic aid for diabetes in the future. Therefore, in the future, dental professionals may detect diabetes or monitor a diabetic's degree of control by simply collecting gingival crevicular fluid on a paper strip to be analyzed for glucose concentration.

Oral Agents Used to Treat Diabetes Mellitus These agents are classified as sulfonylureas and are summarized in Table 15-7. The sulfonylureas stimulate secretion of insulin by the beta cells in the pancreas.

Adverse Reactions The adverse effects of sulfonylureas include blood dyscrasias, cutaneous problems, gastrointestinal disturbances, and liver damage. Therefore, a thorough blood workup is important prior to surgical therapy in these patients. In view of the role of the liver in producing prothrombin, prothrombin times should be determined so that a bleeding problem can be prevented during dental surgical procedures.

In 1970, a 9-year study was completed to determine if the control of blood glucose by oral agents led to vascular disease. The results suggest that patients taking these drugs have more cardiovascular problems than diabetic

Table 15-7 Oral Drugs Used to Treat Diabetes Mellitus

Acetohexamide
Chlorpropamide
Tolbutamide

patients controlled by diet alone. Therefore, the cardiovascular system should be monitored in the dental office if a diabetic is being treated with sulfonylureas.

The same dental precautions relative to patients taking insulin should also be followed for patients taking oral hypoglycemic agents.

Glucagon

Glucagon, produced by the pancreatic alpha cells, is important in the metabolism of glucose and is actively secreted when plasma glucose concentrations decrease. Its secretion is also stimulated by a gastrointestinal hormone, epinephrine, and norephinephrine.

Glucagon causes fuel mobilization, in contrast to insulin, which promotes fuel storage. As a consequence of decreased food intake, glucagon secretion increases, insulin secretion is depressed, and fuels stored intracellularly are metabolized to meet the body's energy needs.

Another function of this hormone is the stimulation of glucose production from noncarbohydrate sources. It thus provides the glucose necessary during infection or stress.

Glucagon, in high concentrations, also increases the force of contraction of the heart.

PROSTAGLANDINS

Prostaglandins, while not actually hormones, are among the most prevalent autocoids and have been detected in most body tissues and fluids. There are six main classes, E, F, A, B, C, and D, of which the E and F groups are predominant. They are cyclic, oxygenated fatty acids and have a diversity of clinical effects. Their activities include vasodilation, increased heart rate and cardiac output, increased capillary permeability, alteration of smooth muscle contraction, inhibition of gastric secretion and increased mucous secretion in the intestine, increased renal blood flow, sedation, stimulation of pain fibers, and alteration of endocrine gland secretions. The E prostaglandins are interesting to dentistry since they exert parathyroid hormone-like effects that result in mobilization of calcium from bone in tissue culture. These compounds may thus be an etiologic factor for the alveolar bone loss seen in periodontal disease.

Mechanism of Action

While there does not appear to be a single receptor site for all prostaglandins, there are specific receptors for the various agents. Receptors may produce one effect with one class of prostaglandins, while others may have an opposite effect with a member of another class.

Mechanical, thermal, chemical, bacterial, and other traumatic effects cause prostaglandin release. Prostaglandins appear to be important factors in the inflammatory process, particularly chronic inflammation. In this respect, they may be involved in the initiation and/or progression of periodontal disease.

Value as Therapeutic Agents

Therapeutically, prostaglandins are mainly used to induce abortions, particularly in the midtrimester. Their use as a contraceptive in a "morning after" pill is also being considered.

On a limited basis, they are being used to treat bronchial asthma and ulcers. Investigations are also underway for their role as antihypertensive agents.

Antiinflammatory, nonsteroid drugs interfere with the synthesis and release of prostaglandins. The inhibitors of prostaglandins include fenamates, phenylbutazone, aspirin, and prostynoic acid. If the prostaglandins are important in the etiology of periodontal disease, future periodontal therapy may incorporate either prostaglandins or their antagonists.

KININS

Kinins are polypeptides which are distributed in a variety of body tissues. Kallidin and bradykinin, members of this group found in plasma, may play a role in dental diseases. They are formed from kininogen by proteolytic enzymes called kininogenases. The kininogenases include kallikreins, trypsin, plasmin, and components of certain snake venoms. Once formed, bradykinin and kallidin are rapidly inactivated.

The plasma kinins appear to be important in blood clotting, fibrinolysis, and complement activity. They also increase capillary permeability, cause vasodilation, edema, pain by affecting nerve endings, and contraction or relaxation of a variety of extravascular smooth muscles. These agents may mediate pulpal pain so that inhibitors may be used in the future as dental therapeutic aids.

No specific antagonists are yet available. However, salicylates and glucocorticoids which inhibit kinin-evoked responses by inhibiting the activation of kallikrein may play a role in future therapy. Also, investigations are now in progress relative to clinical antagonists of kinins.

ANSWERS TO CHAPTER CASE

Birth control pills (oral contraceptives) are classified as either estrogens or progestinlike substances, or a combination of both. If oral contraceptives produce gingival bleeding, they may do this by decreasing immunologic defense mechanisms to plaque bacteria, by altering the permeability of blood vessels, stimulating the proliferation of gingival blood vessels, and increasing clotting time. However, the role of birth control pills in producing gingival bleeding is not clear, since studies on this topic are contradictory.

QUESTIONS

1 What is a hormone? Why are they important?
2 What is a feedback system?
3 Name five hormones. What major effect does each exert on the body's systems?
4 How can hormones affect your management of a patient? Give three examples.

5 How can your knowledge of the side effects of hormonal therapy be useful in the daily practice of dentistry?

6 What are autocoids? Name two.

READING REFERENCES

Augoson, A., "Gingival Inflammation and Female Sex Hormones," *J. Periodont. Res.,* Res. Suppl. 5, 1971.

Baer, P. N., and S. D. Benjamin, *Periodontal Disease in Children and Adolescents,* J. B. Lippincott, Philadelphia, 1974.

Cohen, D. W., et. al., "Studies on Periodontal Patterns in Diabetes Mellitus," *J. Periodontol.,* Res. Suppl. 4, 1969.

El-Ashiry, G. M., "Comparative Study of the Influence of Pregnancy and Oral Contraceptives on the Gingivae," *Oral Surg.,* **30:**472–475, 1970.

Gottsegen, R., "Dental and Oral Considerations in Diabetes Mellitus," *N.Y. State J. Med.,* **62:**289, 1962.

McCarty, F. P., A. McCarty, and G. Shklar, "Chronic Desquamative Gingivitis," *Oral Surg.,* **13:**1300, 1960.

Pak, C. Y. C., "Parathyroid Hormone and Thyracalcitonin: Their Mode of Action and Regulation," *Ann. N.Y. Acad. Sci.,* **179:**450–474, 1971.

Pearlman, B. A., "An Oral Contraceptive Drug and Gingival Enlargement: The Relationship Between Local and Systemic Factors," *J. Clin. Periodontol.,* **1:**47–51, 1974.

Vaes, G., "On the Mechanism of Bone Resorption: The Action of Parathyroid Hormone on the Excretion and Synthesis of Lysosomal Enzymes and on the Extracellular Release of Acid by Bone Cells," *J. Cell Biol.,* **39:**676–697, 1968.

Chapter 16

Histamine and Antihistamines

A patient presents to your office with a cellulitis. The dentist prescribes an antibiotic. Two days later he telephones the office and complains of a rash on his chest and arms. Should this complaint be one which should be reported to the dentist? Would medication be advisable for this patient?

The commonly known antihistamines are useful mainly for the treatment of certain allergic diseases and certain allergic reactions to drugs. Many patients seen in dental offices take these drugs chronically and may show signs of drowsiness, xerostomia, and other side effects. Some of these drugs have prominent sedative effects and are sometimes used in dental offices as preoperative sedatives in anxious patients. The same precautions that are used with other central nervous system (CNS) depressants must be used with these drugs. The patient must be warned that she may become drowsy and that it would be dangerous for her to operate a motor vehicle under the circumstances. Also, if a patient is on antihistamine therapy, the administration of any other CNS depressant may produce excessive sedation.

HISTAMINE

In order to understand how antihistaminic drugs work it is important to have some concept of the location and function of histamine, the substance that these drugs antagonize.

Histamine is found in almost all tissues of the body. Although its precise function is not known, it appears to be involved in the function of the CNS, in initiating gastric secretions, and in regulation of the microcirculation after injury. In tissues undergoing rapid growth and repair, such as wound and granulation tissue, malignant growths, and fetal tissue, there is a high histamine-forming capacity which appears to play a physiological role in these processes. There is evidence that inhibition of the synthesis of histamines arrests development and delays healing. This histamine, called "free" since it is not stored, is not affected by antihistaminic drugs.

In contrast to free histamine, the mast cells and basophils contain a preformed histamine that is stored in a bound form in granules. This "bound" histamine is released during allergic reaction, and by drugs, venom, and injury. It is this histamine that is affected by the classic antihistaminic drugs (see Table 16-1).

Effects of Released Histamine

The most important actions produced by the histamine that is released from mast cells and basophils is on blood vessels. Histamine is capable of producing constriction of large veins, dilation of arterioles, and increased permeability of venules. When these vascular effects are systemic, blood pools in the small blood vessels, proteins, and fluids are lost from the circulation into the tissues, and edema and hypotension result. If these effects are severe enough, they may result in shock. When histamine is released locally, similar vascular effects will produce red or pale edematous patches of the skin and mucosa [e.g., urticaria (hives), angioedema (giant hives)].

Histamine has a stimulating action on nerve endings which produces the sensations of itch and pain. It is a powerful stimulant of gastric hydrochloric acid secretion, and it is capable of stimulating the contraction of other smooth muscles besides blood vessels.

The Role of Histamine in Allergic Reactions An allergic reaction is produced when an antigen combines with its antibody. The antigen can be a drug, pollen, or other substance that is capable of initiating the synthesis of its antibody, a protein whose active sites specifically compliment those of the antigen. The combining of antigen with antibody initiates a series of events which results in histamine release and which involves the synthesis

Table 16-1 Classification Of Antihistamines

Drugs	Dose, mg	Duration, h	Distinguishing features
Phenothiazines			
Promethazine (Phenergan)	25–50	4–6	Prominent CNS sedation
Ethanolamines			
Diphenhydramine (Benadryl)	50	4–6	Prominent CNS sedation
Ethylenediamines			
Pyrilamine (Neo-Antergan)	25–50	4–6	Gastrointestinal side effects common
Alkylamines			
Chlorpheniramine (Chlor-Trimeton)	2–4	4–6	Least CNS sedation; frequent CNS stimulation; most potent histamine antagonist
Piperazines			
Chlorcyclizine (Di-Paralene)	50	8–12	Produces genetic defects in animals

and release of other mediators of the allergic reaction, such as prostaglandins, kinins, and slow-reacting substance A (SRS-A). (All these mediators, including histamine, are classified as "autocoids," a name given to substances possessing strong pharmacologic activity that are present in many parts of the body but cannot be classified with neurotransmitters or hormones. See Chap. 15.)

Histamine is important in producing edema of the skin and mucosa such as occurs in urticaria and angioedema. It also contributes to the development of hypotension in systemic anaphylaxis. Histamine is not involved in producing bronchoconstriction in humans. Prostaglandins and SRS-A are believed to be the mediators of importance in producing this effect, while the kinins are believed important in producing the fall in blood pressure.

Histamine Liberators Certain drugs and venoms have the ability to produce the release of histamine from mast cells by a direct mechanism unrelated to the development of allergy, even though the symptoms produced are similar. While other mediators are important in the production of allergic reactions, they appear to be minimally involved in reactions produced by histamine liberators. A full-blown explosive release of histamine, referred to as a "nitritoid crisis," produces the following symptoms: A burning, itching sensation under the skin is followed by intense cutaneous warmth and redness. The blood pressure falls for a few minutes, and edematous patches appear on the skin. Nausea, colic, and vomiting occur due to stimulation of the gastrointestinal tract. The vomitus is highly acid due to excessive acid secretion. Some degree of bronchospasm also occurs.

Histamine and Injury Any injury that is sufficiently intense to damage mast cells will cause a release of histamine. This histamine is involved in the initial redness and edema of the inflammatory reaction but does not affect the delayed inflammatory response which is also characterized by increased vascular permeability and edema. Other mediators, such as kinins and prostaglandins, may also be involved in both the acute and delayed inflammatory responses. Damage to blood vessels is also a contributing factor. The classic antihistamines will block the initial vascular changes but will not affect the delayed response even when the initial response has been blocked. These drugs are not useful in reducing inflammation during injury.

Histamine Receptors

Histamine produces its effects by activating specific receptors present on the surfaces of cells. These receptors consist of two types:

1 H_1 receptors mediate contraction of bronchial muscle and intestines. They only partially mediate the effects of histamine on blood vessels. Classic antihistamines act on these receptors.

2 H_2 receptors mediate gastric secretion and cardiac acceleration. They also partially mediate the effects of histamine on blood vessels.

ANTIHISTAMINES

Antihistamines are competitive antagonists of histamine. By occupying the histamine receptors, they prevent histamine from reaching its site of action. The antihistamines do not stimulate H_1 or H_2 receptors, nor do they affect the amount of histamine released.

H_1 Receptor Antagonists

These drugs are the classic antihistamines listed in Table 16-1. In allergic reactions they are useful in counteracting the increased capillary permeability, especially of the skin and mucosa, which produces edema, as well as the itching and pain caused by histamine release.

They will only partially counteract the vas-odilation that leads to hypotension, since part of this effect is mediated by H_2 receptors and will not be blocked by H_1 antagonists. Also, other autocoids are involved in producing this effect. Since histamine is not involved in bronchoconstriction, antihistamines are ineffectual in this condition. H_1 antagonists, when given prophylactically, are useful in protecting against the effects of drugs that are histamine liberators. Here again, they can only partially counteract hypotension and will not affect the excessive gastric acid secretion, which is an H_2-mediated effect.

Other Effects Besides antihistaminic effects, these drugs produce other important actions. They frequently produce sedative effects, but occasionally they also cause excitement. Some of the antihistamines, diphenhydramine (Benadryl), promethazine (Phenergan), dimenhydrinate (Dramamine), cyclizine (Marezine), and meclizine (Antivert), are useful in the treatment of motion sickness. These same drugs have some beneficial effect in other types of vestibular disturbances that produce vertigo (dizziness). Promethazine is useful in treating nausea and vomiting from other causes. Cyclizine and meclizine belong to the piperazine group of drugs. These drugs are known to cause fetal deformities in rats and should not be administered to pregnant women.

All the antihistamines possess local anesthetic activity. Promethazine and pyrilamine (Neo-Antergan) are most potent in this regard and resemble procaine in activity. They have been used upon occasion in place of local anesthetics in patients thought to be allergic to other local anesthetic drugs. Antihistamines possess atropinelike activity. In therapeutic doses they cause a decrease in salivary and bronchial secretions.

Absorption and Biotransformation Antihistamines are rapidly absorbed from the gas-trointestinal tract and produce their effects in about half an hour. They are hydroxylated by the microsomal enzymes and may be involved in enzyme induction (see Chap. 2).

Therapeutic Uses These drugs are most effective in treating diseases of allergy involving the skin and mucosa. In seasonal rhinitis (hay fever) they reduce mucosal swelling, nasal secretions, and the itching of eyes, nose, and throat. They are more effective at the beginning of spring when the pollen count which produces this allergic condition is low. They are less effective when the pollen count is high and in perennial rhinitis. They relieve the swelling and itching of urticaria (hives), urticarial lesions in serum sickness, and angioedema (giant hives). However, antihistamines will not act rapidly enough if an attack of angioedema produces laryngeal swelling that is severe enough to prevent respiration. In this life-threatening situation, epinephrine should be used because it acts more rapidly and produces a more complete reversal of swelling. Also, in systemic anaphylaxis, epinephrine is the drug of choice, while the antihistamines are useful adjuncts but should not be used as the primary drugs. The antihistamines only partially counteract the hypotension and laryngeal swelling and have no effect on the bronchospasms that may occur during an attack. Antihistamines are ineffective in most cases of asthma and may further impair respiration because they tend to dry lung secretions. Viscus plugs form which hamper air exchange. Some of the antihistamines are useful in treating motion sickness, as well as other conditions that involve vestibular disturbances (vestibule of the inner ear).

The antihistamines promethazine and diphenhydramine, whose central nervous system depressant effects are prominent, are used most frequently as sedatives and as preoperative medication. Many antihistamines are used in over-the-counter preparations. They are included in sleeping pills for their sedative effects, but the amounts are frequently too small to produce sleep in most individuals. The antihistamines contained in cold preperations are only helpful in reducing nasal and bronchial secretions. They are not useful in reducing the swelling and congestion unless there is an allergic aspect to the cold. Antihistamines will have some protective action against blood-transfusion reactions and will help reduce symptoms when given prophylactically to patients who are about to receive drugs that are histamine liberators.

Side Effects and Toxicity In therapeutic doses these drugs produce a fair number of minor side effects which vary with the drug group and the individual. Xerostomia occurs frequently. Drowsiness is common, and patients should be cautioned about driving a car when using these drugs. Instead of sedation, excitement may occur at conventional doses. Patients may be restless, nervous, and unable to sleep at night. Occasionally a person will complain of palpatations, headache, a tight feeling in the chest, and tingling and weakness of the hands. Although these drugs have antiallergic effects, they can produce contact dermatitis when applied repeatedly to the skin.

Overdosage Increasing the dose of these drugs increases the sedative effects only to a certain point. Toxic doses cause CNS stimulation which may result in convulsions, hyperpyrexia, and death. Children, in particular, are susceptible to CNS stimulation even in therapeutic doses.

The atropinelike action of these drugs become more prominent with high doses. The mouth becomes dryer, the heart rate increases, and blurred vision, constipation, and urinary retention occur.

Contraindications The main contraindications to these drugs are due to their atropine-like action. They should be used with caution in patients suffering from asthma, narrow-angle glaucoma, pyloroduodenal obstruction, and bladder neck obstruction. In glaucoma, an abnormally high intraocular pressure causes damage to the retina. In narrow-angle glaucoma, these drugs interfere with the drainage of the fluid of the eyes, raising the intraocular pressure. Because the atropinelike action of these drugs reduces the activity of the gastrointestinal tract and the urinary bladder, they will tend to augment the effects of pyloroduodenal obstruction and bladder neck obstruction.

Drugs in the piperazine group should not be given to pregnant women because they have known teratogenic effects. It has not been determined whether the other antihistamines cause fetal deformities.

Individual Drugs Examples of the various antihistamines are listed in Table 16-1 with their distinguishing features. Also see Chap. 6 for a discussion of hydroxyzine (Atarax), an antihistamine used as a sedative.

H_2 Receptor Antagonists

These drugs, which have been recently discovered, are capable of counteracting all the effects on H_2 receptors mediated by histamine. Their ability to block the secretion of hydrochloric acid is of therapeutic importance. Cimetidine (Tagamet) is often used for this effect in the treatment of peptic ulcers.

H_2 antagonists also partially reverse the action of histamine on blood vessels. When H_1 and H_2 antagonists are used together they can completely block the effect of histamine, which produces increased vascular permeability and vasodilatation.

ANSWER TO CHAPTER CASE

This patient is probably suffering from an allergic reaction which appears to have been caused by the antibiotic prescribed. The antibiotic should be switched to one that does not exhibit cross-

sensitivity, and an antihistamine should be prescribed to relieve the rash. The patient should be carefully questioned in order to ascertain whether other drugs were being ingested at this time or whether the patient came in physical contact with irritating or allergic substances. The information must be recorded on the patient's chart.

QUESTIONS

1 What factors would influence the choice of an antihistamine?

2 What is the difference between antihistamines that act on H_1 and those that act on H_2 receptors?

3 How do antihistamines that are used for the treatment of allergic reactions produce their effects?

4 Besides antihistaminic effects, what other therapeutic effects are produced by antihistamines?

5 Why are antihistamines rarely effective in asthmatic patients?

READING REFERENCES

Chue, P. W. Y., "Management of Anaphylactic Reactions," *Oral Health,* **66:**20–22, 1976.

Davis, W. H., "Emergency Drugs and Allergy," in F. M. McCarthy (ed.), *Emergencies in Dental Practice. Prevention and Treatment,* W. B. Saunders, Philadelphia, 1972, Chap. 9.

Goth, A., "Histamine: Antihistaminic drugs," in *Medical Pharmacology,* C. V. Mosby, 8th ed., Saint Louis, 1976, pp. 180–199.

Mustard, J. F., and M. A. Packham, "Factors Influencing Platelet Function: Adhesion, Release and Aggregation," *Pharm. Rev.,* **22:**97–187, 1970.

Wyngaarden, J. B., and M. H. Seevers, "Toxic Effects of Antihistamine Drugs," *J. Am. Med. Assoc.,* **145:**277–282, 1951.

Part Four

Emergency Drugs and Adverse Effects

Chapter 17

Drugs Affecting Oral Tissue

"Can you remove these stains from my son's teeth? Since his teeth came in, they were stained and nothing seems to help. Brushing with toothpaste, salt, and soda has no effect. Why are they stained? Can anything be done about it?"

This situation sometimes occurs in clinical practice. A number of drugs can cause these and other effects on the hard and soft tissues of the mouth. Because of this, drug therapy sometimes has to be altered. Oral manifestations of drugs can be classified as shown in Table 17-1. Those drugs which affect the teeth are summarized in Table 17-2.

EXTERNAL EFFECTS OF DRUGS ON TEETH

Abrasion

Cervical abrasion of teeth frequently occurs. This appears to result from a horizontal brushing with a brush having hard bristles, applying excessive pressures during brushing, or through use of extremely abrasive dentifrices. Toothbrush abrasion is most commonly seen on the buccal surfaces of teeth, since patients spend most of their energy and time on these surfaces. A discussion of dentifrice abrasiveness can be found in Chap. 12.

The buccal cervical aspects of teeth are most commonly abraded because of the convexity of the teeth and the thinness of the enamel over the cervical portion of teeth. Once the enamel is lost through abrasion, the

Table 17-1 Classification of Oral Manifestations of Drugs

A. Drugs affecting teeth
   1. Externally
   2. Internally
B. Drugs affecting gingiva and oral mucosa
C. Drugs affecting bone
D. Drugs affecting other oral tissues

abrasion progresses more rapidly because the dentin is not as hard as enamel.

Abrasion then causes loss of tooth structure, sclerosed dentin, secondary dentin deposition, and tooth hypersensitivity to heat, cold, and acids.

Cervical abrasion differs from cervical caries in that the tooth surface in the defect is hard, smooth, and highly polished. These surface characteristics are important in reaching a diagnosis since these areas are often discolored and may appear carious.

Further abrasion is corrected through patient education as to the correct toothbrushing technique, type of toothbrush (nature of the bristle), and type of dentifrice. If there is also sensitivity to temperature extremes, "desensitization" must also be considered. Desensitization can be achieved with a therapeutic dentifrice (Chap. 12) and/or various topical desensitizing agents. Success has been reported with the topical application of zinc chloride, formaldehyde, potassium nitrate, and concentrated fluoride medications, as well

Table 17-2 Drugs Affecting Teeth

A. External effects
   1. Abrasives
   2. Acids
   3. Topical fluorides
   4. Metallic discolorants
   5. Disclosing agents
B. Internal effects
   1. Fluorides
   2. Tetracyclines

as the electrical application of medications to teeth (iontophoresis). The effectiveness of these methods is due to either a placebo action and/or the result of the sclerosis of dentin, which prevents stimulation of the pulp via the dentinal tubules. Sometimes restorations are placed in areas of abrasion to minimize pain and prevent further tooth damage.

Erosion

Erosion of teeth is defined as a loss of tooth structure by chemical action which is not a consequence of bacterial metabolism. These chemicals, which are usually acids, are drugs in the broad sense of the word. The clinical differentiation between erosion and abrasion can be difficult and sometimes is based on the subject's intake of acid foods (soda pop, lemon juice, and so on). The pattern of tooth loss also differs; erosion usually results in a shallow saucer-shaped area, while abrasion usually is wedge shaped.

Erosion is often seen along the buccal, cervical areas of maxillary teeth because the enamel is thinner and exposed to acids in foods such as carbonated beverages and lemons. Sometimes the acid is from chronic regurgitation from the stomach. This can occur in pregnant patients and patients with peptic ulcers. Erosion in these situations is usually on the lingual aspects of teeth, particularly the molars.

Other possible sources of acidity have been suggested, including salivary citrate, acid secretion of abnormal mucous glands (especially in patients with gout), and crevicular fluid due to gingival inflammation.

It is thought that erosion requires not only acid but also improper toothbrushing, as in the case of abrasion. This interaction between improper brushing and increased acidity is thought to produce the saucerlike lesion of erosion.

Areas of erosion differ from caries in the same manner as described for abrasion. Restorations can also be placed over eroded areas, but these restorations may fail due to the acidity. If this occurs, the best solution is a full-coverage crown.

Topical Fluorides

Topical fluorides alter the surface characteristics of enamel, making it more resistant to acids. This has resulted in the widespread use of fluorides as tablets, pastes, gels, and solutions, with a significant decrease in dental caries (Chap. 10).

No clinical signs of fluoride application are noted, except with stannous fluoride. Patients receiving these stannous fluorides may have a black pigmentation along the cervical margins of teeth and in occlusal crevices. Although this condition is not permanent, it is long lasting and disappears with time. It is related to the deposition of tin found in the stannous portion of the fluoride compound. As the tin is lost from enamel, the pigmentation signs disappear.

Disclosing Agents

Disclosing agents contain dyes which will stain bacterial plaque so that it can be visualized by the patient. This is important in a plaque-control program, since for most patients, "seeing is believing." A patient may claim that they "always brush" and do a good job. Application of a disclosing solution will verify or refute this claim.

Disclosing agents come as tablets, gels, and solutions. Solutions or gels are usually preferred for office use since they can be used more quickly. Tablets, on the other hand, cannot be spilled by children, are pleasant tasting, and can easily and safely be transported by the patient.

A number of dyes are used as disclosing agents including FDC Red #3, FDC Green #3, and sodium fluorescein. The fluorescein requires ultraviolet light to visualize the dye, and the patient therefore can leave the office

without residual discolored teeth or gingiva. The FDC dyes, on the other hand, stain with ordinary light, resulting in a prolonged discoloration of teeth and gingiva. Although the discoloration usually only lasts about an hour and can be removed from the teeth by brushing, patients may object to it.

In one product, FDC Red #3 and FDC Green #3 have been combined so that only plaque stains and there is no gingival staining. In some cases this may offer an advantage, but the patient still temporarily has blue-stained teeth.

A few products contain iodine. Although iodine stains plaque well, patients may object to its taste and prefer not to use it. In addition, some patients are allergic to iodine and could have a severe allergic reaction. If an iodine-containing disclosing solution is selected, it is important to ensure that the patient does not have a history of iodine allergy.

Iodine also discolors anterior restorations, but this discoloration is reversible. If the discoloration cannot be removed with water, it can be removed with 70% alcohol. However, alcohol should be left on the restorations for as short a time as possible since it may damage them. Generally, when iodine is used in a disclosing solution, the concentration is such that staining is not a problem.

Metallic Discolorations

Old amalgam restorations may cause black tooth discoloration. While this discoloration is not harmful, because of the esthetic problem, the restoration may have to be replaced.

Copper cement was once popular as a base under amalgam restorations because it was thought to have antibacterial properties which would be useful if all caries were not removed. This has been disproved, and copper cements are now rarely used. However, your patient may have old restorations with copper cement bases. Seepage of the copper ions into the adjacent tooth structure may cause a greenish

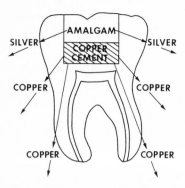

Figure 17-1 Permeability of teeth to filling materials. Copper ions pass from the copper cement through dentin and then through enamel and cementum to the periodontium. Silver ions pass from amalgam through dentin, and sometimes through enamel.

tooth discoloration. In some cases, the discoloration can extend to the roots; damage to the periodontium can result and eventually lead to extraction. Copper cements have also been shown to be damaging to pulpal tissues. Because of this, fillings with copper cement bases should be replaced to prevent such problems. See Fig. 17-1.

INTERNAL EFFECTS OF DRUGS AFFECTING TEETH

Fluoride

Systemic administration of fluoride during the time teeth are forming (birth to 7 years of age) results in the incorporation of fluoride into the tooth structure, making the teeth more resistant to caries. However, fluorides in excess of 1.8 ppm in drinking water cause mottling of teeth which appears as white spots and/or areas of brownish discoloration. The amount of discoloration depends on the fluoride concentration. Areas of discoloration represent hypocalcified areas. The cause of the brown coloration is not known, but may result from an increased porosity of the enamel surface.

Deciduous teeth are not affected to the same degree as permanent teeth. This is because deciduous teeth form partly *in utero*, where the

fluoride concentration is reduced by the selective filtration of the placenta.

Mottled enamel has to be treated for esthetic reasons, since these teeth are caries resistant. Esthetically, these teeth are best treated with full crowns. The newer ultraviolet, light-cured materials also offer some promise. Bleaching of mottled enamel, while sometimes offering limited improvement, is not adequate.

Tetracyclines

Depending on dosage and duration of administration, tetracycline antibiotics administered after the first trimester of pregnancy or to children up to age 7 can cause tooth discoloration in the infant or child. This results from the affinity of tetracyclines for calcified tissues, leading to its deposition in developing dentin and enamel and its ability to cross the placenta. Tetracyclines, therefore, should not be administered after the first trimester of pregnancy during enamel formation in the fetus. In children, tetracyclines can be safely given after age 7 when only the crowns of the third molars are still developing.

Tetracycline staining, which is an internal stain, varies from gray to yellow to green and can be differentiated from plaque which is easily removed by instruments or prophylaxis paste. Tetracycline is also fluorescent and fluoresces yellow with ultraviolet light.

Usually this problem may require treatment because of esthetics. The treatment of choice is full-coverage crowns or masking agents.

DRUGS AFFECTING THE GINGIVA AND ORAL MUCOSA

The drugs affecting gingiva and oral mucosa are summarized in Table 17-3.

Anticholinergic Drugs

Patients taking anticholinergic drugs (e.g., atropine) are usually being treated for gastrointestinal problems such as peptic ulcers. Such

**Table 17-3
Drugs Affecting
Gingiva and Oral
Mucosa**

Anticholinergics
Anticoagulants
Caustic chemicals
Heavy metals
Tranquilizers

patients may not respond as well to scaling and root planing because of the drying of the mouth (xerostomia) which is associated with this therapy. Indirectly, the xerostomia may alter the composition of bacteria in plaque to the extent that problems may occur in plaque control. This xerostomia should be anticipated in patients on drugs with anticholinergic effects.

Anticoagulants

Anticoagulants have numerous interactions with other drugs, resulting in the anticoagulant effect of the drug being either enhanced or diminished. The enhancement from drug interactions can cause spontaneous bleeding in various parts of the body, including the gingiva. Therefore, spontaneous gingival bleeding in patients on anticoagulants may not be plaque related but may be drug related. This must be carefully assessed so that a possible life-threatening situation can be prevented. If the dose of the anticoagulant is greatly diminished over a short period of time, blood clotting (thrombus formation) may occur. Although the early stages of thrombus formation are difficult to detect clinically, warning signs may include complaints of dizziness, visual disturbances, and peripheral numbness.

Tranquilizers

A number of patients are on long-term tranquilizer therapy. Clinical studies have revealed that these patients are more susceptible to monilial infections, especially if they are wearing partial dentures. Monilial infections may appear as whitish patches or broad red areas on the oral tissues, which easily bleed after rubbing the surface with gauze.

Treatment of the monilial infection includes a change in the tranquilizer (if possible) and antifungal therapy. A common drug for monilial infections is Nystatin (400,000 to 600,000 units) which is used four times a day as a rinse during the infection and for 48 h after disappearance of symptoms.

Chemical Burns

Some chemicals are highly caustic and cause whitish lesions due to tissue necrosis when in contact with oral tissue. These are termed chemical burns. One of the most common types of chemical burns occurs with aspirin. Aspirin, when improperly held next to a painful tooth instead of being swallowed, will not give relief of the toothache but creates a new source of pain—the soft tissue area now burned by the aspirin. Patients should be warned about this practice.

Metallic Pigmentations

Drugs containing mercury have been used as diuretics, and mercury and bismuth compounds were once used to treat syphilis (prior to the use of antibiotics).

Drugs containing bismuth or mercury can cause gingival inflammation even with adequate plaque control. Also, long-term use leads to black pigmentation of the marginal gingiva. Severe overdoses have been reported to cause loosening and exfoliation of teeth.

With old amalgam restorations there may be a black discoloration adjacent to the gingival margin of the restoration from a leaking out of mercury from the amalgam. Since no gingival irritation occurs and the newer amalgam formulas do not cause this, there is no cause for concern.

DRUGS AFFECTING BONE

A number of drugs which affect bone are summarized in Table 17-4.

Corticosteroids

Experimental studies in rabbits reveal that corticosteroids (cortisone) increase the incidence of cleft lip and palate. While this has not been documented in humans, corticosteroids should not be administered to pregnant females. It should be noted that these drugs are absorbed into the bloodstream when applied topically, so that topical administration may also cause changes. Long-term steroid therapy results in generalized osteoporosis. However, it has not been clarified if the osteoporosis manifests itself in alveolar bone.

Heparin

Heparin, an anticoagulant administered parenterally, is frequently given for long periods of time. Some of these patients develop generalized osteoporosis. However, as with corticosteroids, it is not known if the osteoporosis occurs in alveolar bone.

Tetracyclines

As indicated earlier in this chapter, tetracyclines are incorporated into both teeth and bone during their formation. Because alveolar bone is constantly "remodeling," tetracycline always becomes incorporated. No adverse effects, however, have been reported. On the contrary, several reports suggest that tetracyclines enhance the response to scaling and root

Table 17-4
Drugs Affecting
Bone

Corticosteroids
Heparin
Tetracyclines
Vitamin D

planing, and may aid in the formation of new bone in sites of periodontal destruction.

Since tetracyclines appear in the gingival crevicular fluid after systemic administration, it is thought they may alter the crevicular microorganisms.

Vitamin D

Vitamin D influences the absorption of calcium from the gastrointestinal tract and its subsequent deposition in bone. Vitamin D deficiency, or rickets, leads to bone loss, including alveolar bone. In infancy, rickets also results in hypoplastic enamel and retarded tooth eruption.

It should be noted that excess vitamin D levels can also cause bone loss which may be similar to that occurring with excess parathyroid hormone (see Chaps. 9 and 15).

DRUGS AFFECTING OTHER ORAL TISSUES

Acetazolamide (Diamox) is a diuretic given to patients with kidney damage and right heart failure. Occasionally, side effects of peripheral paresthesia, including paresthesia of the facial muscles, are reported. Therefore, paresthesia from this drug must be differentiated from dentally caused sources. Sometimes, a patient complains of facial numbness the day after receiving a dental injection. Needle tract infections or nerve damage as a result of the injection would be most likely. However, medication with acetazolamide could be the source of the problem, and a change to a different drug would alleviate this problem.

Phenothiazines

Phenothiazines are prescribed both as tranquilizing agents and to overcome nausea such as seen in post-partum women. As previously discussed, monilial infections (overgrowth of *Candida albicans*) can occur during chronic use of these drugs. This may result from reduced salivary flow and the resultant change in the oral microflora. Another side effect with phenothiazines is muscular spasms of the face and neck as a result of the stimulation of the central nervous system (extrapyramidal tracts). These patients may complain of not being able to open their mouths for long periods of time. Such spasms must be differentiated from those associated with occlusal trauma. Occlusal adjustment, which is usually of benefit in occlusal trauma, is ineffective in phenothiazine-induced spasms. Treatment of these drug-induced spasms is cessation of drug therapy and substitution of another drug.

ANSWER TO CHAPTER CASE

Since the stain cannot be removed, it is probably due to the fact that the child received a tetracycline while his teeth were calcifying (prior to age 8) or his mother received a tetracycline after the first trimester of pregnancy. Since tetracyclines have an affinity for calcified tissues, they deposit in developing dentin and enamel. Tetracycline staining varies from gray to yellow to green and can be differentiated from plaque stain, which is easily removed by instruments or prophylaxis paste.

QUESTIONS

1 Classify the oral manifestations of drugs.
2 Compare and contrast erosion and abrasion of teeth.
3 Which drugs can cause tooth discoloration?
4 Name five drug groups which can adversely affect gingiva and oral mucosa, and give an example of each.
5 Name four drugs which can adversely affect bone.
6 Why might an occlusal adjustment be contraindicated in a patient taking phenothiazine drugs?

READING REFERENCES

American Dental Association, *Accepted Dental Therapeutics,* 37th ed., Chicago, 1977, pp. 3–18.
Arnim, S. S., "The Use of Disclosing Agents for Measuring Tooth Cleanliness," *J. Periodontol.,* **34:**277, 1963.
Cohen, D. W., et. al., "A Comparison of Bacterial Plaque Disclosants in Periodontal Disease," *J. Periodontol.,* **43:**333–338, 1972.
Ogle, R. E., and S. G. Ciancio, "The Effect of Anticholinergic Agents on the Periodontium," *J. Periodontol.,* **42:**280–282, 1971.
Scopp, I. W., et. al., "Dryness of the Mouth with the Use of Tranquilizers; Chlorpromazine," *J. Am. Dent. Assoc.,* **71:**66, 1965.
Shira, R. B., R. J. Hall, and L. H. Guernsey, "Minor Oral Surgery During Prolonged Anticoagulant Therapy," *J. Oral Surg. Anes. Hosp. Dent. Serv.,* **20:**93–99, 1962.

Drugs Useful in Dental Office Emergencies

"Ms. Jones, bring me some epinephrine, spirits of ammonia, and oxygen immediately!
Mr. Gray has fainted, and I may need emergency supplies! Hurry!"

A number of emergency situations may occur in the dental office. Although they are uncommon, they can be life threatening. Therefore, there must be early recognition of the problem and an immediate, correct response. Dental professionals must be knowledgeable so that when an emergency arises, the entire office staff is immediately prepared.

PREPARATION FOR EMERGENCIES

Prevention is best in terms of emergencies. This consists of:

1 Knowing if there are any adverse factors in the patient's medical history.

2 Knowing how to monitor vital signs of a patient.

3 Reminding patients to take their normal medication the day of their appointment. Patients with a history of angina pectoris should have their medication at chairside in case the stress of the dental appointment provokes an angina attack.

4 Scheduling appointments so as not to interfere with medicated patients' eating habits.

5 Being aware of signs and symptoms of allergic reactions, and knowing how to respond to them. These signs and symptoms include angioneurotic edema (angioedema), purpura, urticaria, or anaphylaxis, which may be fatal.

6 Having working emergency equipment

and biologically active supplies. Equipment should be checked periodically, and drugs should be replaced upon expiration. Be thoroughly familiar with emergency drug use, dosage, and route of administration.

7 Having telephone numbers of physicians, hospitals, and ambulance services readily available for quick medical assistance.

8 Having all dental personnel familiar with resuscitative techniques.

BASIC STEPS FOR ALL EMERGENCIES

1 Place the patient flat on his or her back on a firm surface with head tipped back. In case of a coronary stroke, congestive cardiac failure, or high blood pressure problem, a semisitting position is preferred if the patient is still conscious.

2 Monitor vital signs.

3 Be sure the airway is clear.

4 Administer oxygen (except in cases of hyperventilation), preferably with positive pressure, or give mouth-to-mouth resuscitation.

5 Be prepared to support circulatory arrest.

6 Do not hesitate in obtaining help from other personnel.

BASIC STEPS FOR CARDIOPULMONARY RESUSCITATION

Cardiopulmonary arrest is a sudden and unexpected cessation of effective respiration and circulation. In the dental office it may occur as a systemic reaction following general anesthesia or as a reaction to administration of drugs such as local anesthetics or antibiotics. It may also occur in a patient experiencing a heart attack in the dental office.

Immediate recognition of respiratory and circulatory arrest is important, since irreversible biologic changes may occur after 4 min.

Respiratory arrest is characterized by the absence of chest or abdominal movements. Circulatory arrest is characterized by an absence of a pulse and heartbeat. If the subject's pupils are dilated, one can assume that circulatory arrest has been present for at least 1 min.

Appropriate training in the techniques of cardiopulmonary resuscitation (CPR) should be undertaken by dental personnel, and short courses on this subject are available throughout the United States. Necessary techniques include mouth-to-mouth resuscitation, oxygen administration, external cardiac massage, and the use of appropriate drugs.

Steps in Cardiopulmonary Resuscitation

1 Place patient in horizontal position on a hard surface, call physician and ambulance.

2 Clear the airway, support respiration.

3 Institute closed cardiac massage if neither pulse nor heartbeat is detectable.

4 After 5 to 10 min of CPR, administer 1 mL of $\frac{1}{1000}$ epinephrine into a convenient vein or the undersurface of the tongue (if no pulse).

5 If possible, an intravenous (IV) infusion should be established, and 50 mL of sodium bicarbonate (3.75 g per 50 mL) injected to counter pH changes in the body. Within a few minutes after cardiac arrest, metabolic acidosis occurs, and sodium bicarbonate prevents it from reaching a critical stage.

The administration of other drugs depends on the interpretation of electrocardiographic information. These various drugs are discussed elsewhere in the text. (See Chaps. 3 and 14.) It is important that drug therapy does not interrupt the procedures being used to support circulation and respiration. Drugs are useful but not imperative, and repeated doses may be needed at 5-min intervals until the patient begins to respond with a carotid femoral pulse, constriction of dilated pupils, occasional gasping respiration, purposeful body movements, and improved skin color.

The major points to keep in mind in CPR are:

1 Be sure the oropharynx is clear at all times.

2 Maintain an open airway by lifting the neck and tilting the head backward.

3 For mouth-to-mouth breathing, pinch the nose closed.

4 For mouth-to-nose breathing, keep the subject's mouth tightly closed.

5 While the dentist conducts cardiac compression, the assistant should support breathing so that the chest expands once every 5 sec.

6 If the stomach fills with air, compress the abdomen.

7 For cardiac massage, place pressure on the lower end of the sternum to avoid fracturing the sternum or ribs. Pressure should be enough to depress the sternum $1\frac{1}{2}$ to 2 in for adults and $\frac{1}{2}$ to $1\frac{1}{2}$ in for children.

8 The rate of cardiac compression is 60/min for adults and 100/min for children.

MANAGEMENT OF FAINTING

Fainting, or syncope, is usually caused by an inadequate blood supply to the brain. The patient frequently will state that he feels faint or weak. At the same time, there may be sudden perspiration, or discoloration of the skin of the extremities. This is treated by increasing the blood supply to the upper portion of the body. Tight clothing should be loosened, the patient positioned horizontally or with the head lower than the feet, and aromatic spirits of ammonia should be administered. Oxygen should be given if the patient does not respond. All vital signs must be monitored and the cause of the syncope determined. Syncope can be caused by cardiac or respiratory problems, hypotension, cerebral vascular accident, hyperventilation, anaphylaxis, or anxiety. In the dental chair the usual cause of syncope is anxiety, but other factors must be considered.

Hyperventilation

Hyperventilation is one of the most frequent causes of syncope, "lightheadedness" or "faintness." It is usually a sign of acute anx-

iety. It may also result from a fall in blood pressure. Hyperventilation can also reduce carbon dioxide (CO_2) levels, which lowers serum carbonic acid, and tetany may result from this.

Hyperventilation is best controlled by having the patient breathe slowly or by breathing into a paper bag to increase CO_2 levels in inspired air. This then results in more CO_2 passing into the bloodstream. Increased levels of CO_2 in blood signals the respiratory center in the central nervous system to slow down the breathing rate.

Phenylephrine and Ephedrine   These agents produce vasoconstriction without much effect on the heart. Phenylephrine is the more potent. They are useful for syncope due to circulatory depression. A diagnosis of circulatory depression is necessary for use of these agents since they are ineffective for other causes of *unconsciousness*. These drugs are discussed in Chap. 3.

INSULIN REACTION

An insulin reaction, or hypoglycemia, can result from excess insulin, reduced food intake, or excessive exercise. It is usually very rapid in onset. It contrasts with diabetic coma which is due to hyperglycemia and is very slow in onset. However, if a patient is unconscious, differentiation between the two is difficult without a blood analysis. If sugar is given to a patient in diabetic coma, no further adverse effects will occur. Therefore, in the unconscious diabetic, sugar therapy is indicated as outlined below.

If a diabetic has an insulin reaction in the dental chair, give the patient a glass of orange juice or 2 sugar cubes. If the patient loses consciousness, monitor vital signs, prepare for CPR, and arrange for immediate transfer to a hospital. Administer 1 unit (1 mg) of glucagon parenterally which can cause an increase in blood glucose by converting liver glycogen to glucose. Glucagon is a polypeptide which is produced commercially from pancreatic extracts. Usually, one injection of glucagon will awaken the patient so that oral sugar can be given (see Chap. 15).

MANAGEMENT OF ANGINA

Patients with a history of angina should be advised to bring their antianginal medication with them to the dental office since stressful situations sometimes result in an angina attack. Angina is due to an inadequate supply of blood to the heart muscle and is treated with drugs which dilate the cardiac vasculature. Such agents include nitroglycerin in tablets of 0.3 to 0.6 mg, and amylnitrite as an inhalant. The vasodilation produced by these agents may be so great that the patient may temporarily faint due to lack of adequate blood supply to the brain.

MANAGEMENT OF CHEST PAIN OTHER THAN ANGINA

A dental patient with persistent nonangina chest pain may be having a myocardial infarct. Seat the patient upright, administer oxygen, and make arrangements for immediate transfer to a hospital. Be prepared to initiate CPR. Do not inject epinephrine or other drugs.

CENTRAL NERVOUS SYSTEM STIMULATION

This usually is seen as excitement tremors, or convulsions. It is most often related to epilepsy or inadvertant IV administration of a local anesthetic.

After following the basic steps outlined for all emergencies, continue to administer oxygen. Place a firm pad between the teeth to prevent tongue biting. Do not physically restrain the patient, but guard against injury. If the convulsions persist and are severe, medical assistance is indicated. Following the convulsion, emotional support is mandatory.

Most convulsions related to local anesthesia are short-lived and result in no serious after effects if proper oxygenation is carried out. If convulsions persist for more than 3 min, they should be treated by IV injection of diazepam (Valium). Since most convulsions are followed by depression, care must be given when injecting a depressant like Valium, which may result in more depression and possibly serious side effects.

RESPIRATORY DEPRESSION

During respiratory depression, breathing may become difficult and the patient may state it is "hard to breathe." If these signs and symptoms occur, a number of aids to breathing can be used, including mouth-to-mouth breathing or use of a breathing bag and mask.

A breathing problem with choking and skin and mucous membrane discoloration may indicate an obstruction in the respiratory pathway. The patient should be turned laterally in the chair with her head downward. Then the mandible should be pulled upward and forward to overcome the obstruction.

An alternate method of removing an obstruction is to stand behind the patient, encircle him in your arms, make a fist with thumb side against his upper abdominal area below the sternum, and press inward and upward in a quick motion. The upward force may "pop" the obstruction out. In using this method, however, care should be taken not to fracture the rib cage.

If the obstruction cannot be removed, a tracheotomy at the level of the cricothyroid membrane may be necessary, and all personnel should know this technique. Once the incision is made, maintenance of the opening is essential.

In most respiratory problems drugs are not indicated initially. However, if the respiratory difficulty is due to a severe asthmatic attack (bronchospasm), 0.25 to 0.5 mg of $\frac{1}{1000}$ epinephrine should be injected IM and the area thoroughly massaged to favor passage of the drug into the bloodstream. Also, prompt relief is sometimes obtained by the inhalation of 0.1 mg of isoproterenol which relaxes the bronchi (Chap. 3). In patients with cardiovascular disease these drugs should be used at minimal concentrations with extreme caution since a cardiac crisis can result.

Respiratory depression may also be due to an overdosage of narcotics. When this occurs, the drug of choice is naloxone (Narcan), 0.2 mg IV (Chap. 5). The onset of action of this drug is 2 min after an IV injection. If the depression is not reversed with one dose, additional doses can be given since they will not increase the depression present. It precipitates withdrawal symptoms in individuals dependent on morphinelike drugs and must be administered cautiously and in small doses. It has no effect on respiratory depression caused by other classes of drugs except that caused by propoxyphene (Darvon), which is chemically related to the narcotic methadone.

MANAGEMENT OF CIRCULATORY DEPRESSION

During circulatory depression, the blood pressure drops, the pulse is rapid and weak, and the skin color is pale. After following the basic steps, and determining that the pulse is weak and blood pressure has dropped, establish an IV infusion and slowly inject 1 to 2 mL of $\frac{1}{2500}$ phenylephrine. If a vein cannot be entered, inject 2 mL of the same drug under the tongue or intramuscularly (IM). If it is injected IM, vigorously massage the injection site to stimulate circulation and improve the drug uptake into the bloodstream. Following this, if the pupils dilate and do not respond to light, employ closed-chest cardiac massage. Also, at all times during these procedures, respiration must be monitored and maintained.

MANAGEMENT OF LOCAL ANESTHETIC TOXIC REACTIONS

A toxic reaction to local anesthetics may result from overdosage, inadvertant IV injection, rapid absorption, or allergic hypersensitivity. Treatment for allergic reactions should follow that described below for allergy. If the reaction is due to an excess of intravascular local anesthetic, effects on the central nervous system (CNS) and/or the cardiovascular system may be seen.

With CNS-mediated responses patients initially appear restless, excited, and confused. Sometimes there are tremors and convulsions. This excitation stage may be followed by a depressive phase with unconsciousness, respiratory depression, hypotension, bradycardia, and sometimes cardiac arrest.

These reactions are treated as follows:

1 Clear airway.
2 Support respiration, and administer oxygen.
3 If the reaction worsens, and convulsions occur for more than 1 min administer diazepam (Valium) IV, 10 to 15 mg (Chap. 6). Most convulsions terminate within 1 min, and no drug therapy is needed. Since convulsions are usually followed by depression, premature injection of Valium could result in further depression and should be avoided unless necessary.
4 Monitor all vital signs, and be prepared to institute CPR.

MANAGEMENT OF ALLERGIC REACTIONS

Patients with a history of allergies and/or adverse drug reactions may be expected to be more prone to allergic reactions.

The initial drug of choice for most allergic reactions occurring in the dental office is epinephrine. It can be administered by one of three routes, depending on the severity of the reaction. Usually 0.3 to 0.5 mL of a $\frac{1}{1000}$ solution is used regardless of the route. For mild symptoms such as itching or rash, a subcutaneous (SC) injection is adequate. If the reaction is more severe, an IM injection is preferred. If the reaction is one of shock, the drug should be slowly injected IV.

If a patient develops a delayed allergic reaction after leaving the office, it will manifest as itching, a skin rash, or mild angioneurotic edema. In this case, diphenhydramine hydrochloride (Benadryl) can be prescribed in a dose of 50 mg given orally (po) every 4 h until symptoms are gone. If the reaction is severe and prolonged, the patient should be referred to an allergist.

In all allergic reactions, the circulatory and respiratory systems must be monitored for involvement and proper measures taken for support, if necessary.

Anaphylactoid Reactions

Anaphylactoid reactions are acute allergic reactions which are sudden, severe, and may be life threatening. These reactions include acute urticaria, angioneurotic edema, anaphylactic shock, bronchoconstriction, and laryngoedema. When they are characterized by bronchoconstriction and massive depression of the respiratory and circulatory systems, they must be treated immediately. Even with immediate attention, some reactions are fatal.

The management of these reactions is as follows:

1 Monitor vital signs, and determine the nature of the reaction.
2 Inject 0.5 mL $\frac{1}{1000}$ epinephrine IM or into the ventral surface of the tongue, or establish an IV infusion and inject 0.3 to 0.5 mL of $\frac{1}{1000}$ epinephrine slowly.
3 Support respiration, if necessary, by mouth-to-mouth breathing or with a bag and mask unit.
4 Closed-chest cardiac massage may be necessary to support the circulatory system and should be considered.
5 Consider an IV injection of Benadryl (50 mg) and the use of IV steroids to support respiration and combat the reactions on a sustained basis. Either 100 mg of hydrocortisone sodium succinate (Solu-Cortef) or 8 mg of dexamethasone (Decadron) can be given IV.

Pharmacology of Drugs Used in Allergic Reactions

The pharmacology of drugs used in these reactions is discussed in Chap. 3 for epinephrine, Chap. 16 for Benadryl, and Chap. 15 for steroids. A summary follows.

1 *Epinephrine* is a strong vasoconstrictor which also directly stimulates the heart. In anaphylaxis it acts as a physiological antagonist to the various chemicals released from body sources that produce bronchoconstriction and vasodilation.
2 *Diphenhydramine* (*Benadryl*) is an antihistamine which counteracts the action of histamine, a mediator of allergy. The action of diphenhydramine is slow, so that it is only used for treatment of delayed reactions. The usual dose is 50 mg, 4 times per day.
3 *Corticosteroids* support circulation and provide prolonged activity. They are secondary drugs of choice. The most commonly used steroids for allergic reactions are hydrocortisone sodium succinate (Solu-Cortef, 100 mg) and dexamethasone (Decadron, 8 mg) (see Chap. 15).
4 *Infusion solutions*. Whenever an infusion solution is needed for an IV injection, a sterile solution of isotonic saline or sodium bicarbonate (3.75 g per 50 mL) is appropriate. Other solutions may be used after the initial emergency is managed.

MANAGEMENT OF HEMORRHAGE

To properly understand the various agents useful in the control of bleeding, a knowledge of the clotting process is important. This is reviewed in Fig. 14-1. (See Chap. 14.)

Prothrombin production by the liver requires vitamin K. After formation, the prothrombin enters the bloodstream and tissue fluids. At sites of tissue injury, the prothrombin is converted to thrombin with the aid of calcium and thromboplastin (thromboplastin is formed with the aid of platelet and plasma factors). The thrombin then converts fibrinogen to fibrin, which causes clotting. Figure 14-1 clearly reveals the role of the liver in the clotting process. (See Chap. 14.)

Oral anticoagulants prevent coagulation by exerting effects on the liver site, while heparin exerts its effect outside the liver mainly on thrombin. Also, salicylates and certain other anti-inflammatory drugs exert an anticoagulant effect in the body by altering platelet adhesiveness. A discussion of anticoagulants can be found in Chap. 14.

USEFUL LOCAL HEMOSTATIC AGENTS

A number of agents are available for the local control of bleeding. They are useful following various dental surgical procedures.

Epinephrine, USP

Epinephrine, also known as adrenaline (in (Great Britain) has been discussed in Chap. 3. It's vasoconstrictor properties sometimes make it useful for local hemostasis. It is available in a $\frac{1}{1000}$ solution.

Since epinephrine stimulates the heart and can be absorbed from topical sites, it should not be used in patients with cardiac problems. This absorption occurs whether the epinephrine is applied as a solution or as an impregnated retraction cord.

The effect of epinephrine is temporary unless a clot has been formed. Its use is limited to capillary bleeding since its major effect is on small blood vessels. If a clot has not formed, the initial vasoconstriction may be followed by vasodilation, leading to more bleeding.

Thrombin, USP

Thrombin, prepared from bovine or human plasma, is commercially available as a powder or liquid. It is only active in bleeding areas free of clotted blood.

When used, the powder is sprinkled directly on the bleeding site or onto gauze which is then applied. It is most useful in cases of venous bleeding rather than capillary bleeding, which is better treated with epinephrine. It should not be injected, since injection can result in massive thrombosis and death.

Absorbable Gelatin Sponge, USP (Gelfoam)

Gelfoam, available as a powder or as a porous gelatin substance, is particularly useful for hemorrhaging tooth sockets. When placed in a socket it is absorbed within a few weeks. Prior to insertion, the socket should be thoroughly debrided. The Gelfoam is then placed and sutured into position. Gelfoam can be moistened with thrombin solution or sterile saline prior to placement.

Oxidized Cellulose, USP (Oxycel)

This artificial clot (cellulosic acid) consists of surgical gauze treated with nitrogen dioxide and cut to the necessary size. When wet, it becomes sticky and adheres to tissue surfaces. It should only be used to control bleeding and not as a dressing to cover tissue wounds since it retards epithelialization and prevents proper wound healing. It is most often used to control bleeding from the socket of an extracted tooth.

Oxidized Regenerated Cellulose (Surgicel)

This is a modification of Oxycel which does not retard epithelialization and is easier to work with. Because of this it is more useful as a surface dressing than Oxycel. However, as with Oxycel, it should not be placed deep in sockets since wound healing may be impaired. Also, it should not be placed in a socket for more than 2 days since it retards bone regeneration. Its main use is to control bleeding from capillaries, veins, and small arteries in both tooth sockets and surgical wounds. Its hemostatic effect is greatest when applied dry. It is resorbed only in small amounts from the site of application. Therefore, after 1 to 2 days

Table 18-1 Drugs Useful in Emergencies

Drug name	Route of administration	Emergency used for
Amylnitrite	Inhalation	Angina pectoris
Dexamethasone (Decadron, 8 mg)	IV	Anaphylaxis
Diazepam (Valium)	IV	Convulsions over 3 min, usually due to local anesthetic emergencies
Diphenhydramine (25–50 mg 4 times/day)	po	Delayed or mild allergic reaction
Ephedrine (25–50 mg)	IV	Certain cases of cardio-vascular collapse or depression
Epinephrine (1/1000) 0.3–0.5 mL 0.5 mL		Immediate allergic reactions, asthmatic reactions Anaphylactic reaction
Glucagon (1 mg)	IV	Insulin shock
Hydrocortisone sodium succinate (Solu-Cortef, 100 mg)	IV	Anaphylaxis
Isoproterenol (0.2 mg; Medihaler, Isuprel)	Inhalation	Asthmatic attack
Local hemostatic	Topical	Local control of bleeding
Naloxone (Narcan; 0.2 mg)	IV, IM	Respiratory depression related to narcotic overdosage
Nitroglycerin	Sublingual	Angina pectoris
Oxygen	Inhalation	Fainting, cardiac problems, allergy, angina pectoris, convulsions
Phenylephrine (2 mg)	IV	Certain cases of cardiovascular collapse or depression
Spirits of ammonia	Inhalation	Fainting

of hemostasis, it should be removed from the bleeding site.

Astringents

Astringents are agents which condense the surface of edematous tissue. A concentrated form of astringent, sometimes called a styptic, aids in sealing off bleeding areas caused by broken capillaries.

Astringents and styptics act by precipitating blood proteins, causing a mechanical obstruction to hemorrhage from injured blood vessels. Since large amounts of these agents cause tissue irritation, only small amounts should be applied to prevent further tissue damage with increased bleeding.

Aluminum Chloride Solutions of 5 to 10% have been used, and these produce some hemostasis. Concentrations stronger than this have resulted in tissue destruction and are not recommended.

Other Examples of Astringents

Ferric Sulfate Solution, NF (Monsel's Solution) This solution is a styptic form of astringent which is applied with cotton pellets. The value of iron-containing solutions is questionable in terms of their local hemostatic properties. It is more effective if applied under pressure and may also be left over an area for up to 24 h. However, salts of iron (ferric) may produce a black stain on teeth and are objectionable to some patients.

Tannic Acid, NF This agent, as a 0.5 to 1% solution, is usually applied on gauze and placed on the bleeding site with pressure. Since tea bags contain tannic acid, as a home remedy a patient can bite down on a tea bag to control bleeding. This is particularly useful if a patient cannot reach a member of the dental team and has a postoperative bleeding problem.

A number of valuable studies have been published on the subject of local hemostatics and are listed in the Reading References of this chapter. A summary of useful emergency drugs can be found in Table 18-1.

Gingival Retraction Cords

When taking impressions it is useful to expose the gingival margins. This is sometimes accomplished by placing gingival retraction cords into the gingival crevice for several minutes to mechanically retract the gingiva away from the tooth. Often these cords are impregnated with local hemostatics such as epinephrine or aluminum chloride.

Because of the high epinephrine concentration in epinephrine-soaked cords, they are a potential hazard in patients with a history of cardiovascular disease.

Epinephrine is available chemically in two forms: racemic and levo rotatory. Although most cords use the racemic form of epinephrine, which is far less potent than the levo rotatory form, systemic responses must still be considered. Where there is a history of cardiovascular problems, retraction cords are available which contain nonepinephrine agents. These appear to be just as effective as epine-

Table 18-2 Agents for Gingival Retraction

Commercial name	Active agent	Comment
Adrenosem	Carbazochrome salicylate	May decrease capillary permeability
Epinephrine	Racemic epinephrine	Consider cardiovascular complications
Hemodent	Aluminum chloride	Acts as an astringent

phrine. In Table 18-2 some retraction solutions commercially available are listed.

ANSWER TO CHAPTER CASE

A patient may faint for a number of reasons and the reader should review these. All vital signs must be monitored and the cause of the syncope determined. Syncope can be caused by cardiac or respiratory problems, hypotension, cerebral vascular accident, hyperventilation, anaphylaxis, or anxiety. In the dental chair the usual cause of syncope is anxiety.

When syncope occurs, loosen tight clothing, position the patient horizontally or with the head lower than the feet, and administer aromatic spirits of ammonia. Oxygen should then be given if the patient does not respond. Monitor the patient's pulse.

The various uses of epinephrine as an emergency drug should be reviewed so that one is familiar with it as a first-line emergency drug.

QUESTIONS

1 What basic steps should be taken in all emergencies?
2 What is the most common emergency situation in the dental office? How is it managed?
3 List the drugs most commonly used in emergency situations, and state the conditions they are used to treat.
4 Name five local hemostatics, and briefly comment on each.
5 Can gingival retraction cords affect a patient systemically? Discuss.

READING REFERENCES

Ciancio, S. G., and S. P. Hazen, "Local Hemostatic Agents Following Gingivectomy," *J. Periodontol.*, **38**:518–520, 1967.

Kelly, J. F., and R. Patterson, "Anaphylaxis," *J. Am. Med. Assoc.*, **277**:1431–1436, 1974.

Leake, D., and D. Deykin, "The Diagnosis and Treatment of Bleeding Tenderness—A Brief Review," *Oral Surg.*, **32**:852–864, 1971.

McCarthy, F. M., *Emergencies in the Dental Practice*, W. B. Saunders, Philadelphia, 1972.

Nichols, W. A., and D. E. Cutright, "Intralingual Injection Site for Emergency Stimulant Drugs," *Oral Surg.*, **32**:677–684, 1971.

Pogue, W. L., and J. D. Harrison, "Absorption of Epinephrine during Tissue Retraction," *J. Prosthet. Dent.*, **18**:242–247, 1967.

Ramaden, F. A., M. El-Sadeek, and E. S. Hassanein, "Histopathologic Response of Gingival Tissues to Hemodent and Aluminum Chloride Solutions as Tissue Displacement Materials," *Egypt. Dent. J.*, **19**:35–48, 1973.

Sadove, M. S., et al., "Classification and Management of Reactions to Local Anesthetic Agents," *J. Am. Med. Assoc.*, **148**:17–22, 1952.

Woycheshin, F. F., "An Evaluation of the Drugs Used For Gingival Retraction," *J. Prosthet. Dent.*, **14**:769–776, 1964.

Drug Interactions

A treatment plan for a patient calls for a large restoration which could produce pain. This patient has a history of cardiac disease and is taking the oral anticoagulant, warfarin. The dentist wishes to prescribe an analgesic in case it is needed. What precautions would be indicated? Should the patient's physician be consulted? Which analgesic should definitely not be used?

Drug interactions are important to dentistry since many people receiving dental treatment are receiving medication from other sources. Dental personnel should be aware that medications prescribed by the dentist or administered in the dental office may interact with other drugs to produce adverse effects in the patient.

Strictly speaking, a drug interaction is defined as the effect that one drug produces upon another drug. Additive effects (see Chap. 1) are not true drug interactions but will be included in this chapter because they are clinically important. When drugs interact, either an enhancement or an antagonism of one or more of the actions of the interacting drugs is produced. It is unlikely that any new pharmacological action would occur.

Drug interactions can be clinically beneficial or adverse, and the significance can vary depending on dosage, the condition of the patient, and other factors. An example of a beneficial interaction is the production of the enhanced analgesic effect that occurs when codeine and aspirin are administered together.

However, when aspirin is administered with oral anticoagulants, an adverse response, bleeding, can be the result. The systemic effects of vasoconstrictors can be potentiated by drugs like guanethidine, giving rise to cardiac arrhythmias and hypertension. However, the usual small amounts administered with local anesthetics in dentistry do not appear to produce this effect. In this situation, a clinically insignificant interaction can become adverse if excessive amounts of vasoconstrictors are injected or if an accidental intravenous (IV) injection is made. Generally, only adverse drug interactions will be considered in this chapter, since ignorance in this area may lead to serious or lethal reactions.

TYPES OF INTERACTION

Drugs may interact because: (1) in vitro chemical incompatibilities may exist; (2) additive effects may be produced due to drug activity involving the same or different structures of the body; (3) one drug can influence the absorption, distribution, biotransformation, or excretion of another drug; and (4) one drug can influence the activity of another drug at receptor sites.

In Vitro Incompatibilities

A drug may inactivate another drug when mixed before administration. For instance, a vitamin B mixture with vitamin C will inactivate tetracyclines.

Drugs in solution may precipitate out when mixed with certain other drugs because of poor solubility of one drug or because one drug may not be soluble at the pH of the other solution. There is less of a problem when a large amount of precipitate occurs because this will usually be observed, but a fine deposit may be dangerous since it is likely to go undetected. These microcrystals, when injected, may lodge in blood vessels of vital organs and produce thrombi or infarcts.

Additive Effects

Simultaneous administration of drugs whose pharmacologic effects are additive may produce responses equivalent to overdosage, if these characteristics are not taken into consideration. A prime example of this is the ability of many drugs to produce central nervous system (CNS) depression. The general anesthetics, the sedative-hypotics, the tranquilizers, alcohol, the antihistamines, the narcotics, and the tricyclic antidepressants all have this additive effect. Dosages of each of the drugs should be decreased when these drugs are administered together.

Absorption

Absorption of a drug from the gastrointestinal tract can be increased or decreased by another drug which alters the pH of gastrointestinal fluids, enzyme activity, or intestinal mobility. Absorption can also be decreased when one drug binds another drug. Antacids containing divalent or trivalent cations bind to tetracyclines and prevent their absorption. Acids in fruit juice hydrolyze penicillin G. Therapeutic effectiveness of these antibiotics is decreased in this manner because less drug is available for absorption.

Distribution

Drug interactions affect the distribution of a drug to its active site mainly because one drug can interfere with the plasma and tissue binding of another drug. Since protein binding serves as a drug storage depot, the drug that has been displaced is now free and available for the production of a pharmacological response. Since more drug is available, the response is greater. This enhanced effect tends to be temporary because the increase in blood level of released drug eventually returns toward the initial level even though the dosage of both drugs remains the same. This occurs because a higher blood level of free drug is metabolized more rapidly.

However, when the blood level of free drug is initially increased, toxic effects can occur. This is especially true if the amount of bound drug is proportionally much greater than the amount of free drug, so that, when even a small amount is displaced, the level of free drug is increased by a large percentage. For instance, approximately 97 percent of the oral anticoagulant warfarin is bound to plasma protein, while 3 percent of the drug remains in an active, free form. Only 3 percent of warfarin needs to be displaced in order to double the amount of pharmacologically active free drug. This effect is particularly important with oral anticoagulants since the safety range between therapeutic and toxic blood levels is narrow, and overdosage can be life threatening. Long-acting sulfonamides, and various antiinflammatory drugs, including aspirin, produce this effect.

Enzyme Inhibition and Induction

Certain drugs increase or decrease the metabolism of other drugs. Phenobarbital increases the synthesis of liver microsomal enzymes and as a result increases the rate of biotransformation of other drugs (see Chap. 2). Drugs whose effects are decreased in this manner include oral anticoagulants, phenytoin (Dilantin), tricyclic antidepressants, corticosteroids, oral contraceptives, and other barbiturates. On the other hand, monoamine oxidase inhibitors inhibit the metabolism of narcotics, barbiturates, and tricyclic antidepressants.

Excretion

Excretion of weak acids will be enhanced by drugs that raise the pH of the urine and will be decreased when the urinary pH is on the acid side. For example, phenobarbital and aspirin are excreted more rapidly when sodium bicarbonate is administered. The opposite is true of weak bases. Excretion of weak bases such as narcotic analgesics is enhanced by an acid urine and inhibited by an alkaline urine.

Elimination of acids and bases which are actively secreted into the urine by the renal tubules may be blocked by drugs that utilize the same mechanism. For instance, the cationic secretory pathway utilized by penicillin can be blocked by probenecid, thus decreasing the elimination of penicillin.

Receptors

Besides the blocking of carrier mechanisms described above, drug interactions occur at other receptor sites. For example, atropine blocks the parasympathetic effects of cholinesterase inhibitors and cholinergic drugs. Sympathetic blocking drugs antagonize the effects of epinephrine, while narcotic effects are completely reversed by the narcotic antagonists.

PROBLEMS OF INTERACTION
Multiple Sources

Problems of interaction are compounded because people acquire and consume drugs from many sources. A patient may be taking drugs prescribed by a dentist and several physicians. Each drug may contain two to four active ingredients, as well as other chemicals which improve taste, texture, and solubility. Other substances added to this list include alcohol, over-the-counter drugs, preparations obtained from friends, and, for some individuals, drugs of uncertain composition purchased on the street.

It is estimated that adverse drug reactions increase disproportionately with an increasing number of drugs consumed. In one study conducted at the University of Florida in a group of 700 patients, the average patient had used over five different drug preparations in the 30 days preceding their hospital visit. In another study, hospitalized patients averaged over eight drugs each. In addition to the number of drugs consumed, each drug may have many effects. For instance, chlorpromazine alone can produce 12 different pharmacological re-responses. *Taking a careful medical and drug history is an important step in preventing adverse drug reactions.* This is a critical role for the dental professional, and all efforts should be made to ensure that a complete drug history is recorded on the patient's chart.

Genetic Predisposition and Disease States

Differences in individuals exist because of genetically inherited traits or alterations due to disease. These factors may produce drug interactions of greater intensity than would occur in normal individuals. Any condition that would affect the pharmacological activity of a drug would also influence the intensity of drug interactions.

Genetic predispositions are known only in a few cases. For instance, isoniazid, by inhibiting the metabolism of phenytoin (Dilantin), increases the toxicity of the latter. Some patients who are slow metabolizers of isoniazid will experience much more severe toxicity.

Impaired renal function may increase the toxicity of drugs by increasing their retention. Large concentrations are more likely to cause interactions. Loss of serum albumin due to kidney disease may lead to toxicity for drugs that normally would bind to plasma protein. The presence of liver disease in patients taking drugs that cause liver toxicity will greatly enhance drug interactions involving this response. Severe liver disease will also result in decreased metabolism of many drugs. This will enhance the toxicity of many drugs involved in interactions.

Other Factors

Whether an interaction has important clinical significance may depend on dosage, the timing and mode of administration, the safe dose range, the risk factor, and the seriousness of the interaction.

Drug dosage is usually an important factor that determines whether an interaction takes place. Serious effects are more likely to occur when high doses of either or both drugs are administered (e.g., additive effects of drugs that produce renal toxicity, ototoxicity, or potassium deficit). If necessary drugs that produce interactions may be given to a patient when the doses are reduced and the patient is monitored for the expected adverse reaction.

In certain situations the *timing or mode of administration* of drugs may be responsible for an interaction that would not occur otherwise. Frequently, an effect produced because a drug reduces the absorption of another drug can be avoided if the two drugs are carefully spaced (e.g., reduction in absorption of tetracyclines caused by antacids). Neomycin reduces the absorption of penicillins when both drugs are given orally (po). This interaction can be avoided by parenteral administration of penicillin.

Whether two potentially interacting drugs are given together may depend on whether beneficial effects outweigh the *risk factor*. The use of aspirin as an analgesic in dentistry in patients on oral anticoagulant therapy represents an unacceptable risk, since a possible hemorrhage can occur which can be life threatening. However, these two drugs are being used together experimentally under carefully controlled conditions to decrease the coagulability of blood. In the second condition, beneficial effects which may occur under careful supervision may outweigh the risk.

The interaction of oral anticoagulants with aspirin also provides examples for the importance of the *safe dose range* and the *seriousness of the interaction.* The fact that this drug combination is potentially lethal increases the magnitude of clinical significance. This is compounded by the fact that the safety dose range of oral anticoagulants is narrow. Each patient must be maintained within a narrow dose range that is individually determined and monitored. Any interaction that increases the effectiveness of these drugs can be dangerous.

For this reason, any new drug that is added to the regimen of a person on oral anticoagulant therapy calls for consultation with a physician and careful monitoring of the patient, even if the significance of the interaction is not established.

INTERACTIONS OF DRUGS IMPORTANT TO DENTISTRY
Vasoconstrictors

Vasoconstrictors interact with antidepressants, antihypertensive drugs, general anesthestics, and cardiac glycosides. In some instances the drug interaction may be severe. However, in dentistry, when vasoconstrictors are used in local anesthetics in small amounts and with great care to prevent an intravascular injection, their use is generally not contraindicated. However, they should not be used as hemostatic or gingival retraction agents, and great caution should be taken if they are used as emergency drugs.

It should also be kept in mind that many of these drugs are present in medications used as nasal decongestants, bronchodilators, and over-the-counter cold remedies. Tyramine,

Table 19-1   Interactions of Vasoconstrictors

Drugs administered by dentist	Other ingested drugs	Type of inter-action*	Adverse effect	Clinical signifi-cance	Recom-mendations
Epinephrine; levarterenol (Levophed); levonordefrin (Neo-Cobefrin)	Monoamine oxidase inhibitors (MAOI) Pargyline (Eutonyl); tranylcypromine (Parnate)	1	Enhanced cardiovascular effects	Interaction unlikely to be severe	Use minimal amounts with caution in local anesthetics; avoid other uses
Phenylephrine (Neo-Synephrine); also foods with tyramine; phenylpropanol-amine in cold remedies		2	Hypertensive crisis	Potentially dangerous	Avoid use
Epinephrine; levarterenol; levonordefrin; phenylephrine	Antihypertensives Guanethidine (Ismelin)	3	Hypertension, tachycardia, cardiac arrhythmias	Potentially dangerous	Use minimal amounts with caution in local anesthetics; avoid other uses
	Reserpine (Serpasil); methyldopa (Aldomet)	3	Enhanced cardiovascular effects	Interaction unlikely to be severe	Use minimal amounts with caution in local anesthetics; avoid other uses
	General anesthetics Cyclopropane; halothane (Fluothane); methoxyflurane (Penthrane); enflurane (Ethrane)	4	Cardiac arrhythmias	Potentially dangerous	Use minimal amounts with caution in local anesthetics; avoid other uses

Table 19-1 *(Continued)*

Drugs administered by dentist	Other ingested drugs	Type of inter-action*	Adverse effect	Clinical significance	Recommendations
	Cardiac glycosides (digitalis)	5	Cardiac arrhythmias	Significance not established	Use minimal amounts with caution in local anesthetics; avoid other uses
	Tricyclic antidepressants Imipramine (Tofranil); desipramine (Norpramin); amitriptyline (Elavil); protriptyline (Vivactil)	6	Increase in blood pressure; greatest pressor response with norepinephrine; cardiac arrythmias greatest with epinephrine	Potentially dangerous	Use minimal amounts with caution in local anesthetics; avoid other uses

* The numbers below indicate the type of interaction.

1   MAOI prevent metabolism of "direct-acting" amines like epinephrine, levarterenol, and levonordefrin by MAO. Since these vasoconstrictors are also inactivated by another enzyme, catechol-*O*-methyltransferase (COMT), only slight drug enhancement is produced. This may be due to increased sensitivity of adrenergic sites.

2   Phenylephrine has both "direct" and "indirect" effects. It acts indirectly on sympathetic nerves to release norepinephrine. MAOI decrease metabolism of phenylephrine and increase the amount of norepinephrine present in the nerve. Increased release of norepinephrine by phenylephrine produces hypertension.

3   The antihypertensive drugs produce increased sensitivity of adrenergic sites. This effect is much greater with guanethidine.

4   Cause not established. Patients receiving this combination should be free of hypoxia, acidosis, and cardiac conduction defects.

5   Both groups of drugs increase ectopic myocardial pacemaker activity. Additive effect.

6   Not established. May be due to tricyclics preventing the uptake of the vasoconstrictors by adrenergic nerves.

found in various foods such as beer, old cheese, pickled herring, and chicken liver may produce a hypertensive crisis when consumed by patients being medicated with monoamine oxidase inhibitors.

A patient's history should be checked to see whether he is taking any of the combinations mentioned above, since there should be awareness that a possible hazard could exist because of injection of vasoconstrictors and the stress of dental procedures. The interactions of vasoconstrictors are summarized in Table 19-1.

Local Anesthetics

Few drug interactions involve local anesthetics as they are used in dentistry. Cholinesterase inhibitors, by inactivating the enzyme (cholinesterase) that metabolizes procaine and other ester-type anesthetics, may increase the toxicity of the latter. Serious reactions can occur in patients with hereditary abnormal plasma cholinesterase. Succinylcholine, a neuromuscular blocking drug that is used by anesthesiologists to produce muscle relaxation in oral surgery, is also metabolized by cholinesterase. Patients with abnormal cholinesterase will exhibit the same type of reaction, with a resultant prolonged increase in respiratory depression produced by succinylcholine. Lidocaine can increase the cardiac depressant effects of cardiac antiarrhythmic drugs, but again the amounts used in dentistry do not usually present a problem. The interactions of local anesthetics are summarized in Table 19-2.

Table 19-2 Interactions of Local Anesthetics

Drugs administered by dentist	Other ingested drugs	Type of interaction	Adverse effect	Clinical significance	Recommendation
Procaine (Novocaine); tetracaine (Pontocaine); propoxycaine (Ravocaine)	Cholinesterase inhibitors, especially echothiophate iodide (Echodide)	Decreased metabolism of ester-type local anesthetics	Increased toxicity of local anesthetics	Not established; patients with abnormal plasma cholinesterases have developed serious reactions	Use amide-type local anesthetic
	Sulfonamides, especially when used for the treatment of toxoplasmosis	The metabolite of local anesthetics, para-aminobenzoic acid, competes with sulfonamides for incorporation into folic acid synthesized by microorganisms	Infections in area of local anesthetic infiltration	Interactions appear to be infrequent	Use amide-type local anesthetic
Procaine (Novocaine); lidocaine (Xylocaine)	Succinylcholine	Displacement of succinylcholine from plasma-protein binding sites	Enhanced response to succinylcholine	Insignificant for amounts used in dentistry	Avoid excessive amounts of local anesthetics and IV injections
Lidocaine (Xylocaine)	Antiarrhythmic drugs	Additive effect	Cardiac depressant effect	Probably none in dentistry	Avoid excessive amounts of local anesthetics and IV injections

Sedative-Hypnotics and Minor Tranquilizers

Drugs in this category have additive CNS depressant effects, as described above. In addition, the barbiturates, glutethimide, meprobamate, and ethchlorvynol increase the metabolism of other drugs and decrease their effectiveness. These effects are described above. In situations where these drugs have been administered together over a period of time, withdrawal of the CNS depressants has resulted in an increased blood level (decreased metabolism) of the other drugs, with resultant increased toxicity. The interactions of these drugs are summarized in Table 19-3.

Analgesics

The ability of aspirin to produce gastrointestinal bleeding and to decrease platelet adhesiveness may produce hemorrhagic episodes in persons receiving oral anticoagulants. The ability of aspirin to raise the blood level of oral anticoagulants by displacement from plasma-protein binding sites contributes to the possibility that bleeding will occur. Aspirin is also capable of decreasing the formation of prothrombin, but this effect is small and unlikely to be of clinical significance. Although it is unlikely that an occasional analgesic dose will produce harm, it is best to avoid aspirin al-

Table 19-3   Interactions of Sedative-Hypnotic-Antianxiety Drugs

Drugs administered by dentist	Other ingested drugs	Type of interaction	Adverse effect	Clinical significance	Recommendation
Sedative-hypnotic-anti-anxiety drugs	Sedative-hypnotics; general anesthetics; narcotics; alcohol; antihistamines; tricyclic antidepressants; tranquilizers; propoxyphene (Darvon)	Additive effect	CNS depression	Dependent on dose: can be dangerous	Reduce dosage
	Antihypertensives	Additive effect	Hypotensive effect	Possibility of fainting	Patient should rise slowly from dental chair
Barbiturates	Oral anticoagulants	Enzyme induction; increased metabolism of oral anticoagulants	Decreased activity of oral anticoagulants	Loss of therapeutic control	Avoid barbiturates, do not withdraw barbiturates if patient is receiving both drugs since hemorrhage may occur
	Corticosteroids	Enzyme induction; increased metabolism of oral anticoagulants	Decreased activity of corticosteroids	Loss of therapeutic control	Avoid barbiturates, prednisone dependent asthmatic patients have suffered increased asthmatic attacks after ingesting barbiturates
	Alcohol (acute use)	Additive effect; inhibition of barbiturate metabolism	Enhanced CNS depression	Increased toxicity; potentially dangerous	Avoid use
	Alcohol (chronic use)	Increased metabolism of barbiturates; tissue tolerance	Development of tolerance	Decreased effectiveness of barbiturates	Larger doses of barbiturates needed
	Barbiturates phenytoin (Dilantin); doxycycline (Vibramycin);	Enzyme induction; increased metabolism of drugs in	Decreased activity of drugs in second column	Loss of therapeutic control potentially serious	Avoid barbiturates

Table 19-3   Interactions of Sedative-Hypnotic-Antianxiety Drugs (Continued)

Drugs administered by dentist	Other ingested drugs	Type of interaction	Adverse effect	Clinical signifi-cance	Recom-mendation
	tricyclic antidepressants Imipramine (Tofranil); amitriptyline (Elavil)	second column			
	MAOI	Metabolism of barbiturates decreased	Increased CNS depression	Respiratory depression can be severe	Avoid barbiturates
Chloral hydrate	Oral anticoagulants	Competition for protein binding	Increased effects of oral anticoagulants; danger of hemorrhage	Potentially dangerous, although a transient effect; will not occur with long-term therapy	Avoid chloral hydrate, or physician should monitor patient
Glutethimide (Doriden); meprobamate (Miltown); ethchlorvynol (Placidyl)	Oral anticoagulants	Enzyme induction; increased metabolism of oral anticoagulants	Decreased activity of oral anticoagulants	Serious loss of therapeutic control, especially with glutethimide; unlikely with meprobamate	Avoid CNS depressants; do not withdraw depressants if patient is receiving both types of drugs since hemorrhage may occur
Chlordiazepoxide (Librium)	Antacids	Delayed absorption	Delayed onset and effectiveness when administered together	Loss of therapeutic control	Avoid administering together
	Phenytoin (Dilantin)	Inhibition of phenytoin metabolism	Increased phenytoin toxicity	Not established	Avoid use or watch for toxicity
Diazepam (Valium)	Levodopa for Parkinson's disease	Not established	Symptoms of disease increases	Loss of therapeutic control	Avoid diazepam
Hydroxyzine	(see narcotics)				

together. [Platelet adhesiveness decreases at single doses as low as 300 mg (1 tablet); chronic use of aspirin at > 3 g/day or 2 tablets every 3 to 4 h can produce displacement from plasma proteins; decrease in prothrombin usually occurs at high doses of 6 g/day, but effects with 2 g have been reported.] Sodium salicylate is less likely to produce gastrointestinal bleeding and does not affect platelets to any great extent; therefore, bleeding episodes are much less likely to occur than with aspirin. Nevertheless, it is best not to use salicylates but to substitute other analgesics.

Acetaminophen (Tylenol) also produces hypoprothrombinemia in higher than analgesic doses or with prolonged use, but this response appears to be small. The usual analgesic doses administered over a short period of time are unlikely to have an effect.

Meperidine (Demerol) can produce severe toxic effects when administered to a patient receiving monoamine oxidase inhibitors.

Hyperpyrexia, hypertension, and excitement can occur in some patients, while severe respiratory depression, hypotension, and coma will be present in others. Enhanced respiratory depression and hypotension can occur when other narcotics are used but are unlikely to be severe.

Narcotics also have an additive effect with CNS depressants, and dosage should be reduced when these two groups of drugs are administered together. The FDA is presently requiring all manufacturers of propoxyphene (Darvon) to include warnings in package inserts about possible serious reactions when propoxyphene is taken with CNS depressants. Many of these reactions have occurred because of serious abuse of this drug. Propoxyphene should not be given with antiparkinsonism drugs because the combination produces CNS stimulation. The drug interactions of importance in analgesic therapy are summarized in Table 19-4.

Table 19-4 Analgesics

Drugs administered by dentist	Other drugs patient is receiving	Type of interaction	Adverse effect	Clinical significance	Recommendation
Salicylates	Heparin; Oral anticoagulants	1*	Possibility of hemorrhage, especially of gastrointestinal mucosa	Interaction likely to occur with aspirin; unlikely with small doses of sodium salicylate	Best to avoid use of salicylates, especially aspirin
	Probenecid (also other uricosuric agents used in the treatment of gout)	Ability to excrete uric acid is inhibited	Decreased effectiveness of probenecid	Loss of therapeutic control especially with prolonged use or large doses	Avoid use; small doses used occasionally do not have an adverse effect; substitute with acetaminophen

Table 19-4 Analgesics (*Continued*)

Drugs administered by dentist	Other drugs patient is receiving	Type of interaction	Adverse effect	Clinical significance	Recommendation
	Sulfinpyrazone (Anturane)	Ability to excrete uric acid is inhibited	Decreased effectiveness of sulfinpyrazone	Loss of therapeutic control	Do not use aspirin even in small doses
	Methotrexate	Decreased elimination and displacement from plasma protein of methotrexate	Increased blood level and toxicity of methotrexate; destruction of bone marrow and blood cells; liver toxicity	Danger of severe toxic effects	Avoid salicylates
	Corticosteroids	Decreased blood levels of salicylates; possible additive gastrointestinal effects	Gastrointestinal ulceration and bleeding; salicylate toxicity	Not contraindicated; must watch for toxic effects	Best to avoid use; continuous use of both drugs may result in salicylate toxicity if corticosteroid is withdrawn or reduced
	Sulfonylureas	Not established; possible additive or potentiating effect	Increased hypoglycemic effect	Loss of therapeutic control of diabetic is potentially serious	Avoid use of moderate to large doses of salicylates: usual analgesic doses cause no problems
	Other antidiabetic drugs	Not established; possible additive or potentiating effect	Possible increased hypoglycemic effects	Not established	Same as above
	Alcohol	Additive	Increased gastrointestinal bleeding	May be serious	Avoid use
	Ascorbic acid	Increased reabsorption of salicylate by kidneys	Increased toxicity of salicylates	Seen with large doses	Avoid large doses of both

Table 19-4 · Analgesics (Continued)

Drugs administered by dentist	Other drugs patient is receiving	Type of interaction	Adverse effect	Clinical significance	Recom-mendation
	Nonsteroid antiinflam-matory drugs: ibuprofen (Motrin); fenoprofen (Nalpon); naproxen (Naprosyn); tolmetin (Tolectin); indomethacin (Indocin); phenylbutazone (Butazolidine); oxyphenbutazone (Tandearil)	Possibility of additive gas-trointestinal effect; animal studies indi-cate that aspirin de-creases blood levels of drugs in second column	Possible gas-trointestinal ulceration and bleed-ing; de-creased ef-fects of drugs in second column	Not estab-lished	Use with caution
Other nonsteroid antiinflammatory drugs	Oral anticoagulants	Additive ul-cerogenic ef-fect and de-creased platelet ad-hesiveness; phenylbuta-zone dis-places oral anticoagu-lants from plasma pro-tein	Possibility of hemorrhage, especially gastrointesti-nal	Severe inter-action ex-pected with phenylbuta-zone; gastro-intestinal bleeding possible with indomethacin and ibu-profen	Never use phenylbuta-zone; best not to use in-domethacin and ibu-profen; use others with caution
	Corticosteroids	Additive ul-cerogenic effect	Possible gas-trointestinal ulceration and bleed-ing	Known to occur with indomethacin	Best to avoid use of indo-methacin; use others with caution
Indomethacin	Probenecid	Probenecid blocks renal tubular se-cretion of in-domethacin	Increased tox-icity of indo-methacin	Severity of response not established	Best to avoid use or reduce dosage of indomethacin
Acetaminophen (Tylenol)	Oral anticoagulants	Enhances hy-poprothrom-bin effect of oral anti-coagulants	Possible hemorrhage	Probably not significant in usual anal-gesic doses for several days	Avoid use for prolonged periods; avoid moder-ate to large doses
Narcotic analgesics	Monoamine oxidase inhibitors (MAOI)	Not estab-lished; partly due to inhibi-tion of me-	Hypotension and coma; also fever, hypertension,	Severe reac-tions with merperdine; not as severe	Do not use meperidine; use others with caution

Table 19-4 Analgesics (*Continued*)

Drugs administered by dentist	Other drugs patient is receiving	Type of interaction	Adverse effect	Clinical significance	Recom-mendation
		tabolism of narcotics	and excite-ment with meperidine	with other narcotics	
	Hydroxyzine	Not estab-lished; partly additive ef-fect	Enhanced sedative and respiratory depression	Not contrain-dicated	Reduce dose of narcotics
	Phenothiazine tranquilizers	Not estab-lished; partly additive ef-fect	Enhanced sedative and respiratory depression	More severe with meperi-dine; not con-traindicated	Reduce dose of narcotics; use caution with meperi-dine
	Tricyclic antidepressants	Not estab-lished; partly additive ef-fect	Enhanced sedative and respiratory depression	More severe with meperi-dine; not con-traindicated	Reduce dose of narcotics; use caution with meperi-dine
Para-aminobenzoic acid (contained in some proprietary analgesic mix-tures)	Sulfonamides	(See sulfonamides)			
Propoxyphene (Darvon)	Antiparkinsonism drugs	Not estab-lished	CNS stimula-tion; anxiety, mental con-fusion, tremors	Significant side effects	Avoid use
	CNS depressants	Additive effects	Excessive CNS depression	Coma and death have occurred from abuse of this com-bination	Use with care

* Aspirin prolongs bleeding time by decreasing platelet adhesiveness and also may produce gastrointestinal (G.I.) bleeding at usual analgesic doses. Large doses of salicylates decrease prothrombin and displace o.a. from plasma protein.

Antibacterial Drugs

Various drugs can decrease the therapeutic effectiveness of penicillins. Bacteriostatic drugs, such as chloramphenicol, tetracyclines, and erythromycin, that suppress protein synthesis will tend to abolish the bactericidal action of drugs like penicillin that inhibit cell synthesis. Since some sulfonamides will decrease the absorption of oxacillin, these drugs should not be administered together. On the other hand, aspirin and certain other antiinflammatory drugs will inhibit the excretion and prolong the life of penicillins. Cephalosporins and tetracyclines should be avoided in persons receiving certain drugs that can cause renal toxicity because of an additive effect. Broad-spectrum antibiotics enhance the effect of oral anticoagulants by decreasing the intestinal flora that produces vitamin K (vitamin K is an effective antagonist of the oral anticoagulants). This interaction is usually considered clinically significant if a vitamin K deficiency coexists in the diet. The interactions of various antibacterial drugs are summarized in Table 19-5.

Corticosteroids

Corticosteroids should be used with caution when treating patients on other antiinflamma-tory drugs like salicylates and indomethacin, since all these drugs are capable of producing gastrointestinal ulceration as well as bleeding. In addition, corticosteroids may reduce blood levels of salicylates. This interaction should be kept in mind when both drugs are used chronically, since withdrawal of the corticosteroid may result in an increase in blood levels and toxicity of the salicylates.

The ability of corticosteroids to produce hyperglycemia antagonizes the hypoglycemic effects of antidiabetic drugs. The two groups of drugs may be used together only if a patient's glucose blood level is monitored and an increase in dosage of antidiabetic drug is made by the physician when needed. Corticosteroids are also able to decrease potassium

Table 19-5 Interactions of Antibacterial Drugs

Drugs administered by dentist	Other ingested drugs	Type of interaction	Adverse effect	Clinical significance	Recom-mendation
Penicillins	Chloramphenicol; tetracyclines; erythromycin	Antagonism of penicillin effect	Loss of anti-bacterial ac-tivity	Most likely to occur when barely sufficient amounts of drugs are used	Best to avoid combination therapy
	Oral anticoagulants	Decrease in gas-trointestinal flora that pro-duces vitamin K; rare	Hemorrhage	Likely to be sig-nificant in pres-ence of vitamin K deficient diet only	Check pro-thrombin time
	Aspirin; phenylbutazone; probenecid	Inhibit excre-tions of peni-cillin; penicillin displaced from plasma-protein binding sites	None expected	Increases effec-tiveness of peni-cillin; may be beneficial	No precaution necessary
	Indomethacin; sulfonamides	Inhibit excre-tion of peni-cillin	None expected	Increases effec-tiveness of peni-cillin; may be beneficial	No precaution necessary
	Neomycin	Oral neomycin interferes with penicillin V ab-sorption	Loss of anti-bacterial ac-tivity	Significant when administered to-gether by oral route	Administer penicillin parenterally

Table 19-5   Interactions of Antibacterial Drugs (*Continued*)

Drugs administered by dentist	Other ingested drugs	Type of interaction	Adverse effect	Clinical significance	Recommendation
Oxacillin	Sulfamethoxy-pyridazine; sulfaethidole	Decreased absorption of oxacillin	Decreased effectiveness of oxacillin	Significant when given in high doses	Avoid combined oral therapy
Cephalosporins	Gentamicin; colistin; furosemide; ethacrynic acid	Additive effect	Enhanced renal toxicity	Potentially dangerous; most serious effects with furosemide and ethacrynic acid	Avoid combined therapy
Chloramphenicol	(See penicillins)				
	Folic acid; iron preparations; vitamin B_{12}	Not established	Delayed response to folic acid, iron, and vitamin B_{12} when deficiencies exist	Not established; potentially dangerous	Use other drug, or monitor patient
	Oral anticoagulants	Metabolism of oral anticoagulants inhibited; possible decrease in production of prothrombin	Possible hemorrhage	Potentially dangerous	Avoid use, or check prothrombin time
Lincomycin	Kaopectate; antacids; activated charcoal; milk	Decreased absorption of lincomycin; effect not as great with milk	Decreased effectiveness of lincomycin	Significant when given together	Give drugs in second column 2 h before or 3–4 h after lincomycin
Sulfonamides	Oral anticoagulants	Decrease in gastrointestinal flora that produces vitamin K	Hemorrhage	Likely to be significant in presence of vitamin K deficient diet only	Check prothrombin time
	Para-aminobenzoic acid (PABA)	See procaine	Antibacterial activity of sulfonamides antagonized	Spread of infection potentially serious	Avoid use
	Methotrexate	Methotrexate is displaced from plasma protein	Increased toxicity	Toxic effects dangerous	Avoid combined therapy

Table 19-5 Interactions of Antibacterial Drugs (*Continued*)

Drugs administered by dentist	Other ingested drugs	Type of interaction	Adverse effect	Clinical significance	Recom- mendation
	(See penicillin)				
Sulfaphenazole (Sulfabid)	Tolbutamide (Orinase)	Tolbutamide is displaced from plasma protein and metabolism is inhibited	Increased hypoglycemic effect	Loss of thera- peutic control can be danger- ous	Avoid com- bined therapy, or physician should ad- just doses
Other sulfonamides	Other sulfanylureas	(May be similar to above)			
Tetracyclines	Antacids; milk; iron preparations	Impaired ab- sorption of tetracyclines	Decreased ef- fectiveness of tetracyclines	Important when given together	Allow 1.5 h between ad- ministration of tetracy- clines and other prep- arations
	(See interactions of barbiturates with doxycycline)				
	Carbamazepine (Tegretol)	Enzyme induc- tion; decreased blood level of doxycycline	Loss of anti- bacterial activity	Spread of infec- tion can occur in patients treated with doxycycline	Avoid com- bined use
	Diuretics	Both groups of drugs elevate blood urea ni- trogen levels	Possible renal impairment	Most likely to be significant in patients with renal malfunc- tion	Best to avoid use of tetra- cyclines
	Methoxyflurane	Possible additive effect; both drugs produce nephrotoxicity	Enhanced nephrotoxi- city	Deaths have occurred	Do not give tetracycline to patients who will be or have re- cently been exposed to methoxy- flurane anesthesia
	Oral anticoagulants	Decrease in gas- trointestinal flora that pro- duces vitamin K	Hemorrhage	Likely to be sig- nificant in pre- sence of vitamin K deficient diet only	Check pro- thrombin time

Table 19-5   Interactions of Antibacterial Drugs (Continued)

Drugs administered by dentist	Other ingested drugs	Type of interaction	Adverse effect	Clinical significance	Recommendation
	Sodium bicarbonate	Decreased dissolution of tetracyclines	Loss of antibacterial activity	Significant if administered together	Do not administer simultaneously
Erythromycin	(See penicillins)				
Aminoglycosides	Ethacrynic acid	Additive effect: both drugs produce ototoxicity	Enhanced ototoxicity	Potentially serious	Do not use
	Methoxyflurane	Additive effect; both drugs produce nephrotoxicity	Enhanced nephrotoxicity	Potentially serious; toxicity occurs at low dose	Do not give to patients who will be or have recently been exposed to methoxyflurane
Neomycin	Digoxin	Decreased gastrointestinal absorption of digoxin	Decreased effectiveness of digoxin may lead to cardiac failure	Significant when administered simultaneously	Best not to use, space drug administration; monitor patients
	Penicillins	Oral neomycin interferes with penicillin V absorption	Loss of antibacterial activity	Significant when administered together by oral route	Administer penicillin parenterally
Amphotericin B (Fungizone)	Digitalis; compounds	Additive effect; both drugs produce loss of potassium	Increased toxicity of glycosides; cardiac arrhythmia	Potentially dangerous	Best not to use, or monitor patients for potassium deficit

levels in the body. When given to patients on antidiuretic drugs that also produce potassium loss, significant potassium depletion can occur, especially in patients whose potassium intake in the diet is inadequate. It is probable that this interaction will also occur with other drugs, such as amphotericin B and the digitalis compounds that produce potassium loss. The

interactions of corticosteroids are summarized in Table 19-6.

Vitamins

Interactions can also occur when vitamins are administered along with certain drugs. The most significant interaction involves the combined use of pyridoxine (vitamin B_6) and the

Table 19-6   Interactions of Anticholinergic Drugs

Drugs administered by dentist	Other ingested drugs	Type of interaction	Adverse effect	Clinical significance	Recommendation
Atropine; scopolamine; banthine; probanthine	Antihistamines; anticholinergic-antiparkinson drugs; glutethimide; meperidine; isoniazid; tricyclic antidepressant	Additive anticholinergic side effects expected; additive CNS depression with scopolamine	Dry mouth, urinary retention, constipation, and so on	Side effects expected to be mild in manner that anticholinergics are used in dentistry	Not contraindicated; combination of more than two drugs may have more serious consequences—use caution in old people subject to atonic ileus, glaucoma, or urinary retention
	Phenothiazines	Additive effect; delayed emptying and increased metabolism in gastrointestinal tract of phenothiazines	Enhanced anticholinergics and CNS depressant effect; repeated use of anticholinergics will lead to decreased effectiveness of phenothiazines	Anticholinergic effects same as above; sedative effects unlikely with occasional doses of anticholinergics	Watch for increased sedation due to phenothiazines; also anticholinergic effects same as above

antiparkinsonism drug levodopa. To be effective, levodopa has to reach the CNS without being metabolized. Vitamin B_6 increases the metabolism of this drug and therefore decreases the amount that reaches the CNS. The drug level becomes inadequate to control the disease. However, if the vitamin is essential, it may be administered with carbidopa, a drug which blocks the metabolism of levodopa and reverses this interaction.

The effect of folic acid, cyanocobalamin (vitamin B_{12}), and iron on red blood cells may be interfered with by chloramphenicol. Although the mechanism is not established, it may be due to interference with erythrocyte maturation by chloramphenicol.

The ability of ascorbic acid (vitamin C) to acidify the urine decreases the ionization of salicylates, resulting in increased reabsorption by the renal tubules. Higher salicylate blood levels may produce toxic effects. This interaction could also be expected with other drugs that are weak acids. See Table 19-7 for a summary of drug interactions with vitamins.

Anticholinergic Drugs

Anticholinergic drugs used in dentistry to decrease salivation will have an additive effect with many other drugs that have anticholinergic side effects. Usually the side effects are mild and consist of symptoms such as dry mouth, constipation, palpitations, and difficulty in urination. However, this combination can precipitate adynamic ileus, urinary retention, and acute glaucoma in older people that are susceptible to these conditions. The problems may be more serious when several of these drugs are used in medicine for long-term

Table 19-7   Interactions of Vitamins

Drugs administered by dentist	Other ingested drugs	Type of interaction	Adverse effect	Clinical significance	Recommendation
Pyridoxine (vitamin B$_6$)	Levodopa	Increased metabolism of levodopa; decreased effectiveness	Effect of levodopa for control of Parkinson's disease is reversed	Expected to occur	Do not use, or consult with physician
Folic acid	Phenytoin (Dilantin)	Increased metabolism of phenytoin; anticonvulsant effect may be partly due to depletion of folic acid	Increase in convulsion frequency	Some patients may be significantly affected; most will not be	Do not use, or consult with physician
Folic acid, vitamin B$_{12}$, iron		(See chloramphenicol) (See tetracyclines)			
Ascorbic acid		(See salicylates)			

therapy. There are several reports in the literature where excessive dry mouth was produced by a combination of three drugs with anticholinergic effects. Nasal bleeding, acute dryness of the mouth (xerostomia), fissures of the tongue, and cracked lips occurred when diphenhydramine, methaqualone, and thioridazine were combined. Loss of dentition due to prolonged xerostomia was reported in a patient taking diphenhydramine, trihexyphenidyl, and imipramine. Xerostomia due to drugs can frequently be treated with the cholinergic drug pilocarpine.

The anticholinergic drugs also have additive anticholinergic effects when given with the phenothiazine tranquilizers. In addition, long-term therapy with both groups of drugs can result in increased blood levels of phenothiazines. It is unlikely that an occasional use of an anticholinergic will produce this reaction, but one should watch for an increased sedative effect due to the increased blood levels of phenothiazines (see Table 19-6).

ANSWER TO CHAPTER CASE

No drug should be administered to patients on oral anticoagulants without consultation with the patient's physician. Aspirin or analgesic mixtures containing salicylates are contraindicated in these patients since bleeding can result. If the physician agrees, acetaminophen (Tylenol) mixtures with propoxyphene (Darvon) or codeine can be administered for a period of several days or acetaminophen can be prescribed alone for this period of time. Since large doses and prolonged use of acetaminophen have been reported to lower prothrombin levels, it would be wise to administer the lowest dose possible. Analgesic mixtures would be preferred since the amount of acetaminophen in each dose is usually one-half (325 mg) the amount administered when the drug is used alone (usually 650 mg). Darvon, pentazocine (Talwin), or codeine can also be used alone without anticipating any ill effects.

Table 19-8   Interactions of Corticosteroids

Other ingested drugs	Type of interaction	Adverse effect	Clinical significance	Recommendation
(See salicylates)				
(See other steroid antiinflammatory drugs)				
(See barbiturates)				
(See amphotericin B)				
Oral anti-coagulants	Complex; production of hypercoagulability of blood and gastrointestinal ulceration by corticosteroids	Possible gastrointestinal bleeding; possible decreased effectiveness of oral anticoagulants	Interaction not predictable	Do not use, or consult physician; dosage of oral anticoagulants might need adjustment at beginning and end of corticosteroid therapy
Antidiabetic drugs	Hyperglycemic effect of corticosteroids antagonizes hypoglycemic effect of antidiabetic drugs	Loss of control of diabetes	Drugs may be used together if interactions are kept in mind	Do not use, or consult physician; increase in anticonvulsant drug dose may be needed
Phenytoin (Dilantin)	Enhanced metabolism of corticosteroids due to enzyme induction	Decreased effectiveness of corticosteroids	Magnitude and significance of response not established	Monitor patient; dose adjustment of corticosteroids may be needed
Estrogen	(Same as above)			
Diuretics Chlorthalidone; furosemide; ethacrynic acid; thiazides	Additive effect; potassium (K^+) loss occurs with both groups of drugs	K^+ deficit may lead to cardiac arrhythmias	Most likely to occur in patients with inadequate K^+ intake	Do not use, or monitor K^+ balance

QUESTIONS

1 How do enzyme inhibition and induction and tissue protein binding of one drug influence the activity of another drug?

2 If phenobarbital and oral anticoagulants were administered together over a period of time, would withdrawal of phenobarbital produce adverse effects?

3 In what manner can one drug interfere with the absorption of another drug from the gastrointestinal tract?

4 What drug interactions occur with salicylates?

5 How do guanethidine and the tricyclic antidepressants influence the systemic effects of vasoconstrictors in local anesthetic solutions?

READING REFERENCES

Bourgault, P. C., and N. M. Ross (eds.), "Drug Interactions," The Third Symposium of the Pharmacology, Therapeutics, and Toxicology Group, IADR, March 25, 1976.

Greenblatt, D. J., and R. I. Shader, *Benzodiazepines in Clinical Practice,* Raven, New York, 1974.

Gysling, E., and S. Heisler, "A Practical Classification of Untoward Drug Effects," *J. Can. Med. Assoc.,* **113:**32–34, 1975.

Hansten, P. D., *Drug Interactions,* Lea & Febiger, Philadelphia, 1975.

Karch, F. E., and L. Lasagna, "Adverse Drug Reactions, A Critical Review," *J. Am. Med. Assoc.,* **234:**1236–1241, 1975.

Lennoila, M., and S. Hakkinen, "Effects of Diazepam and Codeine, Alone and in Combination with Alcohol, on Simulated Driving," *Clin. Pharmacol. Ther.,* **15:**368, 1974.

Part Five

Applied Pharmacology

Chapter 20

The Role of the Dental Professional in the Pharmacologic Management of Oral Disorders

"Ms. Brown, please place some topical anesthetic on the palatal aspect of the maxillary right second molar and allow it to remain approximately one minute. Then have the patient rinse her mouth out thoroughly. Be careful that the anesthetic does not flow into the throat."

Sometimes the dental professional applies medications without knowing their mode of action, side effects, or efficacy. The objective of this chapter is to highlight the most common types of therapy performed. Details not discussed in this section can be found in the chapter dealing with the specific drug. For example, fluorides will not be discussed here since they are thoroughly presented in Chap. 10.

ORAL SOFT TISSUE LESIONS

Some oral soft tissue lesions may not be treated or cured with drugs, but the patient can be made more comfortable with palliative measures. Examples are acute necrotizing ulcerative gingivitis, aphthous ulcers, herpetic lesions, and chemical burns. These lesions generally become asymptomatic within 4 to 7 days after onset, with complete remission within 10 days. During this time the patient can be made more comfortable by several palliative measures.

Topical Anesthetics

These can be applied prior to dental procedures to provide some comfort to patients during oral manipulations. The operator must exercise some caution during application to prevent contamination of his own hands and possible subsequent development of an allergy. After application, the patient should rinse the mouth thoroughly to remove excess drug.

The effects of topical anesthetics on patients must also be considered since they are absorbed through the oral mucosa into the bloodstream. As little as a 30-min topical application can significantly elevate blood levels of the local anesthetic. Therefore, local anesthetics should only be applied to necessary areas. (See Chap. 7.)

Caution must be employed during applications to the palate, to prevent trickling of the agent down the throat. In some patients this can initiate a laryngospasm if the material reaches the larynx.

Before use of a topical anesthetic, a possible history of allergy must be considered. If there is a history of allergic reaction to local anesthetic injections, it is probable a similar response would occur to topical application.

Mouthrinses

Mouthrinses may also ameliorate painful symptoms of oral lesions. Most mouthwashes produce topical anesthesia even though they do not actually contain a local anesthetic. Topical anesthesia can result from the surface action of phenol (Chlorseptic, Cēpastat) or cetylpyridinium chloride (Cēpacol). Dilute 1 to 2% solutions of hydrogen peroxide and saline rinses (1 tablespoon of salt in one-half glass of warm water) have also been reported to produce temporary relief.

Some mouthrinses contain oxygenating agents which may also bring relief although they probably do not cure lesions. The oxygenating agents contain either carbamide peroxide (Glyoxide, Proxigel) sodium perborate (Amosan, Vince), or a 3% solution of hydrogen peroxide. Long-term therapy with these agents can on rare occasion cause black hairy tongue, which is due to an overgrowth of

the filiform papillae. If this occurs, it is cured by a vigorous brushing of the tongue for several days and discontinuance of the causative drug.

Oxygenating agents release bubbles of oxygen upon contacting organic material, leading to mechanical debridement. In addition to mechanical debridement, it has been postulated that the increased oxygen reduces tissue inflammation and accelerates wound healing. This is controversial and has not been experimentally verified. While these agents might be expected to be plaque inhibitors due to their ability to modify the metabolism of anaerobic bacteria, this has not been demonstrated. It should also be noted that organic matter decomposes most oxygenating agents. For this reason their antibacterial effect is short-lived.

Surface Protectants

A number of topical agents protect the surface of ulcerative lesions from local trauma, permitting normal healing. These include sodium carboxymethylcellulose (Orabase), compound benzoin tincture, and denture adhesives.

MANAGEMENT OF DRY SOCKET

Dry socket, or alveolar osteitis, is a painful postextraction complication. Usually, systemic medications are not useful, and the best treatment is local application of a medicated dressing. Before placing a dressing the socket must be thoroughly debrided. Then, the dres-

Table 20-1 Drugs Commonly Used in "Dry Socket" Dressings

Drug	Purpose
Benzocaine	Anesthetic
Chlorobutanol	Anesthetic
Eugenol	Antiseptic, analgesic
Glycerin	Vehicle
Guaicol	Antiseptic, analgesic
Iodine	Antiseptic
Peruvian balsam	Analgesic, vehicle

sing must be gently placed to minimize aggravation of the pain and still contact the exposed bone. The dressing may require daily changing until symptoms are absent. Some of the most commonly used drugs incorporated in these dressings are listed in Table 20-1. Usually an analgesic is combined with an antiseptic.

MANAGEMENT OF ORAL DISEASES

Lichen Planus

Lichen planus is a chronic, recurring condition which cannot be cured and is not life threatening. However, it can be controlled and the patient can be made comfortable. Lacelike white patches and sometimes localized ulcerations on gingiva and oral mucosa are characteristic. Sometimes skin lesions may be present which require treatment by a dermatologist.

The symptoms of lichen planus can be relieved by topical application of steroids. To minimize unwanted absorption through the skin of fingers, the patient should be instructed to apply the steroid with a cotton applicator. Also, to minimize absorption through oral mucosa, the agent should only be applied to the site of the lesion. The reader is referred to Chap. 15 for a more detailed discussion of steroids.

Pemphigus

Pemphigus is a chronic disease which can be life threatening. It is characterized by vesicles or bullae on skin and oral mucosa and is managed by systemic therapy. On occasion the dental team is called on regarding the management of oral lesions. As in the case of lichen planus, topical steroids are the drugs of choice.

Erythema Multiforme

This chronic non-life-threatening disease is characterized by a symmetrical skin rash, oral vesicles, and sometimes bullae which usually become ulcerated. Management is mainly systemic, but sometimes topical steroids are useful.

Warning: Topical steroids should not be applied indiscriminately to all lesions since application to oral herpetic lesions may aid the spread of the herpes virus to the eye, with severe complications. Herpetic lesions are often difficult to diagnose, varying in appearance from ulcers to small vesicles.

Acute Necrotizing Ulcerative Gingivitis

Acute necrotizing ulcerative gingivitis (ANUG) is characterized by necrosis and ulceration of the gingiva which may be localized or generalized. The interproximal papillae may be destroyed or "punched out," a grayish white membrane may cover the tissue, and halitosis may be present. Extreme pain is noted in the early stages of this disease. Etiology has been related to lack of oral hygiene, emotional stress, and increased numbers of oral bacteria such as spirochetes and fusiform bacteria. The condition does not appear to be transmissible in humans. Also, animal transmittability has not been noted in various studies.

The best treatment is irrigation of the periodontal tissues and gentle local debridement. On occasion, when pain is severe, a topical anesthetic may be applied prior to debridement. The patient can also be advised to use a mouthwash (discussed in Chap. 12) which has a topical anesthetic effect. Use of such a mouthwash may facilitate the patient's home-care program.

The patient should be seen daily for 3 days after the initial visit. At these appointments, oral hygiene should be evaluated and reinforced, followed by scaling and root planing. The patient should not be discharged until plaque control is excellent and the acute phase has subsided. Following this, peridontal surgery must be considered to correct residual abnormal gingival architecture in the form of craters.

Antibiotics are not necessary except where there is systemic involvement in the form of severely elevated temperature or spread of the infection into the pharynx.

Hypersensitive Dentin

The dental professional may apply topical agents to teeth hypersensitive to various stimuli because of exposed dentin. Appropriate therapy requires the identification of the etiology of the hypersensitivity. Causes of hypersensitivity are listed in Table 20-2.

For hypersensitivity due to exposed dentin (Table 20-3), topical agents should be applied as follows:

1 Isolate the tooth from saliva, and keep the area dry.
2 Burnish the medication onto the tooth surface with a nonmetal instrument (metal may evoke a painful response in the patient).
3 If pain occurs, rinse the agent away, reisolate the tooth, and reapply.
4 Leave the agent on the tooth for 5 min.

Application of Topical Antiseptics

The dental professional sometimes applies a topical antiseptic such as iodine or mercurial products (antiseptics are discussed in Chap. 7). In applying these agents, three points are most important:

1 Be sure the patient is not allergic to the agent.
2 Since these agents may have a bad taste, apply them only to the area indicated.

Table 20-2   Causes of Tooth Hypersensitivity

Exposed dentin
Fractured tooth
Malocclusion
New caries
Recurrent caries

Table 20-3   Agents Useful in Treating Hypersensitive Dentin

Home use
Sensodyne dentrifrice
Thermodent dentifrice
5% potassium nitrate
Acidulated monofluorophosphate dentifrice
2% paraformaldehyde paste

Office use
40% solution of zinc chloride followed by 20% solution of potassium ferrocyamide
33⅓% sodium fluoride mixed equally with kaolin and glycerin
0.7–0.9% sodium silicofluoride
8.9% stannous fluoride paste

3 Small amounts should be used to minimize absorption through the mucosa.

Management of Teething

Teething occurs during the eruption of primary teeth. In some children, no problems are encountered, while in others, there is severe tenderness and pain. If the pain prevents the child from sleeping, a local anesthetic can be topically applied to the mucous membrane over the erupting tooth, with a cotton-tipped applicator. However, remember that topically applied anesthetics can be systemically absorbed, and large amounts in the infant could result in serious complication. In addition, care should be taken to not permit the anesthetic to flow into the pharynx. An excellent review of teething has been written by Seward and is included in this chapter's references. Symptoms of teething, even in a teething child, may actually relate to a medical condition. If medical symptoms persist (elevated temperature, coughing, crying, and so on), the child should be seen by a physician to rule out any systemic medical problem.

Halitosis

Halitosis is defined as unpleasant breath. It can be caused by local factors, systemic factors, or a combination of both. Almost 80 to 90 percent of mouth odors, however, are caused by local factors within the oral cavity. Halitosis is particularly related to caries, gingivitis, and periodontitis.

The causes of halitosis are listed in Table 20-4. Oral malodors occur because of the action of various microorganisms on proteinaceous substances such as exfoliated oral epithelium, salivary proteins, food debris, and blood.

Saliva from individuals free of dental disease produces malodor less rapidly than saliva from patients with dental disease. The most objectionable odors occur after prolonged periods of decreased salivary flow and abstinence from food and liquids.

While microorganisms are essential to odor production, no single microorganism has been implicated as the primary cause of oral malodor. In fact, most oral microorganisms have a marked odor-producing potential. These bacteria produce products which are degraded to a number of compounds, including sulfides and mucoproteins, which have been implicated in the production of odor. It appears that oral malodor results from methyl mercaptan and hydrogen sulfide in mouth air as a result of these degradative processes. Although ammonia is also produced, it does not contribute to the production of malodor. It has

been suggested that ammonia may improve the odor of mouth air.

Control of halitosis is directed at its etiology. If systemic factors are responsible, they must be corrected. However, commercial mouthwashes (Cēpacol, Scope, Lavoris) may mask the patient's breath temporarily (30 min). If local factors are responsible, institution of a thorough program of oral hygiene to include tongue brushing and elimination of gross cavities will result in control. An excellent review of halitosis can be found in the article by Tonzetich.

ANSWER TO CHAPTER CASE

Topical anesthetics are useful adjuncts to dental therapy. However, both the dentist and assistant should avoid contact with topical agents by having the patient rinse the mouth thoroughly following use of topical anesthetics. This rinsing minimizes the exposure to the dentist and the staff when they then initiate dental therapy.

When a topical anesthetic is applied in the posterior region of the oral cavity, care must be taken to prevent trickling of the agent into the throat since contact with the larynx can initiate a laryngospasm or difficulty in swallowing.

QUESTIONS

1 What three drug groups could be used topically to relieve pain associated with various oral lesions? What precautions should be taken during their use?

2 Name two diseases of the oral mucosa which are sometimes treated with topical corticosteroids. What dangers are associated with topical steroid therapy?

3 What precautions should be taken in applying topical anesthetics?

4 What are the causes of halitosis? How can halitosis be treated?

5 Discuss the proper management of a patient with acute necrotizing ulcerative gingivitis.

6 How would you apply an agent to hypersensitive dentin?

Table 20-4 Possible Causes of Halitosis

Systemic factors	Local factors
Bronchitis	Caries
Diabetes	Dental plaque
Gastrointestinal problems	Fistulas
Lung disorders	Gingivitis
Odor-producing foods and alcohol	Periodontitis
Pharyngitis	Ulcerative lesions
Postnasal drip	
Sinus infections	
Smoking	
Tonsil infections	

READING REFERENCES

Adriani, J., and D. Campbell, "Fatalaties Following Topical Application of Local Anesthetics to Mucous Membranes," *J. Am. Med. Assoc.,* **162:**1527–1530, 1956.

Dayton, R. E., T. J. DeMarco, and D. Swedlow, "Treatment of Hypersensitive Root Surfaces with Dental Adhesives," *J. Periodontol.,* **45:**873–878, 1974.

Gangarosa, L. P., and N. H. Park, "Practical Considerations in Iontophoresis of Fluoride for Desensitizing Dentin," *J. Prosthet. Dent.,* **39:**173–178, 1978.

Massler, M., "Desensitization of Cervical Cementum and Dentin By Sodium Silicofluoride," *J. Dent. Res.,* **34:**761–762, 1955.

Schluger, S., R. A. Yuodels, and R. C. Page, *Periodontal Disease,* Lea and Febiger, Philadelphia, 1977, pp. 240–250.

Seward, M. G., "The Treatment of Teething in Infants," *Br. Dent. J.,* **132:**33–36, 1972.

Spouge, J. D., *Oral Pathology,* C. V. Mosby, St. Louis, 1973, pp. 406–414, 1973.

Tonzetich, J., "Production and Origin of Malodor: A Review of Mechanisms and Methods of Analysis," *J. Periodontol.,* **48:**1–20, 1977.

Case Reports

The clinical cases presented in this chapter summarize material throughout this book. These are actual cases from the authors' experiences. An important point to remember is that whenever dental therapy may alter medical therapy, a consultation with the patient's physician is indicated. Also, when a medical problem is suspected, the patient should be referred to a physician for final diagnosis and treatment.

PROBLEMS

1 Nitrous oxide analgesia is planned for an apprehensive dental patient. Prior to administration of the nitrous oxide, the patient indicates that his physician has placed him on an antibiotic for a minor upper respiratory infection. Will this influence the use of nitrous oxide?
Answer: The main contraindication to nitrous oxide administration is upper respiratory infections. Administration of nitrous oxide should be delayed until the patient is asymptomatic.

2 A dentist decides to use a barbiturate for a nervous patient who requested a sedative prior to his next dental appointment. The patient's medical history, however, reveals that he has a chronic renal disorder. Which barbiturate groups might be prescribed? Why?
Answer: The best choices are short-acting or intermediate-acting barbiturates since they are metabolized mainly by the liver, in contrast to long-acting barbiturates which are excreted mainly unchanged by the kidneys. Patients with renal disease may have prolonged and heightened response to the latter drug.

3 The dentist wants to sedate a very apprehensive child prior to extraction of a fractured mandibular left first permanent molar. The child refuses

pills, lozenges, injections, or syrup. How can sedation be achieved?

Answer: Sedation could be achieved in this situation by giving the drug as a suppository. Barbiturates are not the drugs of choice since they sometimes cause excitation rather than sedation in children. A more predictable sedative in children is chloral hydrate. Children should not receive an adult dose. Instead the dose should be reduced according to the child's weight using Clark's rule: child's dose = adult dose × (child's weight/150).

4 A patient complains of vague facial pain extending from the right temporomandibular joint to the ear and neck. The facial muscles are painful on palpation, indicating a muscle spasm. Occlusal examination reveals prematurities and extensive wear facets in the second premolar–first molar region. The patient is taking a phenothiazine daily as prescribed by his psychiatrist. How should therapy be planned for this patient?

Answer: The muscle spasm may be related to the drug therapy or occlusal trauma from bruxism. Phenothiazine can cause muscle spasms of the head and neck due to extrapyramidal tract stimulation in the central nervous system. The wear facets on the teeth also suggest bruxism. First, a consultation with the patient's psychiatrist is necessary to determine if another drug can be substituted for the phenothiazine. If not, this patient should be provided with an occlusal splint to minimize the occlusal trauma. It is obvious that an occlusal adjustment could not be performed at this time.

5 The dentist would like to prescribe an analgesic for a patient who had a mandibular right second molar extracted. The patient, however, takes an antacid daily to "settle his continually upset stomach." What guidelines should be followed in selecting an analgesic?

Answer: A "continually upset stomach" suggests a gastric ulcer. Therefore, salicylate-containing drugs are contraindicated since they are irritating to the mucosa of the stomach and may produce bleeding, ulcers. Therefore, an acetaminophen-containing drug should be used instead of a salicylate. Because of the minimal postoperative pain expected from this extrac-

tion, it would not be necessary to select a stronger analgesic such as codeine or acetaminophen with codeine.

6 A dentist decides to perform a gingivectomy on an epileptic patient with gingival hyperplasia associated with Dilantin therapy. What can be done to minimize a recurrence of this condition?

Answer: Gingival hyperplasia associated with Dilantin therapy can be minimized if strict plaque control is carried out. This patient should be placed on good plaque control with frequent appointments for recall prophylaxis and reinforcement of plaque control. Plaque control may be more difficult since drowsiness sometimes occurs in patients on anticonvulsants, particularly early in therapy.

The patient's physician should also be consulted about a possible change in medication to a barbiturate, primidone, or other anticonvulsant. These other drugs induce minimal gingival hyperplasia and may be excellent alternatives.

7 Mrs. Smith, a 64-year-old patient, needs a new full denture. She salivates profusely and had sialorrhea (excessive saliva) prior to extraction of her teeth. A reduced salivary flow would enhance the impressions for new dentures. Medically, she is in good health except for tachycardia and low blood pressure. What would be sound management of this case?

Answer: Since the parasympathetic nervous system regulates salivary secretions, one could consider a parasympatholytic drug such as atropine, scopolamine, or propantheline bromide (Pro-Banthine) for reducing salivary flow. Since these drugs may enhance the existing tachycardia, a parasympatholytic drug is not advised.

Alternatively, the patient could rinse with a surface-active mouthrinse (Cēpacol, Scope) which would slightly reduce the distorting effect of secretions, permitting a more accurate impression.

8 Mr. M. Brown, 47, requires dental treatment consisting of:

a Plaque control
b Routine operative dentistry
c Maxillary partial denture

Medically, he is receiving digitalis and has a chronic allergy for which he daily takes an antihistamine. What drug-related problems might be anticipated?

Answer: Chronic administration of some antihistamines can cause a dry and "burning" mouth. In a dry mouth, more plaque may form and more intensive plaque control may be necessary. The dry mouth, however, may be beneficial in maintaining a dry field during operative dentistry and may facilitate the taking of an accurate maxillary impression. It should also be anticipated that digitalis sometimes makes patients more prone to nausea and vomiting when taking the maxillary impression.

9 Many patients take antihypertensive drugs because of elevated blood pressure. What drugs might be prescribed for sedation in such patients that cannot sleep the night before dental appointments?

Answer: As a side effect, many antihypertensive drugs also produce sedation. Therefore, an interaction between these drugs and sedatives would be expected. Because the degree of drug interaction varies with each patient, the sedative dose must be carefully adjusted to prevent oversedation. Initially, the patient should be given half the usual adult dosage 1 h before sleep and 1 h before the appointment. If this does not produce adequate sedation, the dose could be gradually increased. Obviously, the dentist should never alter the dose of the antihypertensive drug in order to administer the usual adult dose of sedative.

10 Mrs. J. Kelly has a hyperthyroid condition. How might this influence her dental treatment?

Answer: Dental treatment may be delayed until the hyperthyroid condition is controlled. In hyperthyroidism, the heart is hyperactive and may possibly be supersensitive to vasoconstrictors. Because the myocardium is overly stressed in hyperthyroidism, the stimulatory effects of exogenous vasoconstrictor could result in a serious cardiac problem. Local anesthetics should therefore be used without vasoconstrictors, providing good anesthesia can be achieved. If good anesthesia is not obtainable, one might use up to 10 mL of a 1/100,000 epinephrine-containing anesthetic solution. In some patients, a local anesthetic with phenylephrine could be used since this vasoconstrictor has minimal effects on the heart.

11 Mr. G. Black has a tooth that must be extracted because of a fracture and decay. However, he has an allergy to all local anesthetics which are benzoic acid esters, and also to lidocaine. Which local anesthetic should be used?

Answer: Obviously, esters of benzoic acid and lidocaine cannot be used because of the allergies. Since the patient is allergic to lidocaine, which is an amide, he may be allergic to other amides, with the possible exception of mepivacaine hydrochloride (Carbocaine Hydrochloride). No cross-allergies have been reported between lidocaine and mepivacaine. As an alternative, an antihistamine could be used as a local anesthetic. Although these drugs are weak local anesthetics, a number of antihistamines have been used with success when large volumes are given (3 to 5 mL): 1% tripelennamine (Pyribenzamine) and 1% diphenhydramine (Benadryl).

12 Mrs. M. Greene has had a history of severe allergies for which she has been receiving corticosteroids for 4 months. She needs periodontal surgery, including three quadrants of osseous recontouring. How should this case be managed?

Answer: Since Mrs. Greene has been taking corticosteroids for a relatively long period of time, the anterior pituitary probably has responded by decreasing its production of ACTH. Therefore, her adrenal cortex is probably not capable of producing adequate amounts of corticosteroid during stress. In view of this, it would be wise to give her extra steroid prior to each surgical procedure. Also, following periodontal surgery, she should be protected from a possible infection by prophylactic antibiotic therapy. This is important because these drugs alter the inflammatory response and decrease the body's defenses against infection.

13 Mr. S. Mack has had arthritis for 6 years and takes 6 g of salicylates per day. He has not had any gastric problems and has tolerated this medication well. He is now scheduled for extraction of the maxillary right second molar.

Would you expect any drug-related problems in Mr. Mack?

Answer: Mr. Mack may have a bleeding problem. Salicylates can alter prothrombin levels in plasma at doses of 6 g or more per day for extended periods of time. It is thought that salicylates influence vitamin K, which is important in prothrombin synthesis. Salicylates at doses as low as 0.3 g can also decrease platelet aggregation, leading to prolonged bleeding time. Therefore, prior to the extraction, a prothrombin time and bleeding time should be determined. If these are abnormal, the patient's physician should be contacted concerning a temporary reduction in salicylate. When the prothrombin and bleeding times are normal, the surgical procedures can be done. For dental emergencies a dose reduction may not be possible, and the dental team should be prepared with measures to control local bleeding after the extraction.

14 A dentist made a well-fitting mandibular partial denture for his patient 8 months ago. Immediately after insertion, the patient had no subjective complaints. Although his mouth was not sore, he then noticed zones of redness under the saddle areas. His medical history showed that 4 months previously he was placed on a tranquilizer. Would you suspect any drug-related problem?

Answer: This patient may have an allergy to the acrylic in the partial saddles, or a monilial infection. Oral, rectal, and vaginal monilial infections have been associated with chronic administration of tranquilizers. It is also possible that during the 8 months since insertion, ridge changes could have occurred which caused denture "sore spots." In this case, an adjustment would be needed.

15 Mrs. C. Kline has a swelling over the maxillary right second premolar and a temperature of 104°F. The tooth is nonvital. The dentist decides to establish drainage through the root canal and place the patient on antibiotics. She has a history of chronic kidney disease and no history of drug allergies. Which antibiotic could be selected?

Answer: Either penicillin or erythromycin are indicated, since these are effective against most microorganisms causing abscesses and do not have adverse renal effects. Although tetracyclines may also be effective for this condition, they are contraindicated in chronic renal disease. A number of studies have established the fact that tetracyclines are nephrotoxic in patients with kidney disease and can aggravate an existing renal problem. Also, they may result in liver damage in these patients.

16 Mrs. J. Wick presents with a similar problem as Mrs. Kline (Case 15). However, she does not have any renal disease but is allergic to penicillin, and has had an adverse drug reaction to erythromycin. She also has a gastric ulcer for which she takes antacids daily. Last, she is leaving for a Caribbean cruise in 2 days. How could she be treated?

Answer: The drug of choice in this case would be a tetracycline. However, since the absorption of a tetracycline is altered by heavy-metal-containing antacids and calcium-containing drugs, the patient should refrain from taking her antacid or dairy products for at least 1.5 h after taking the tetracycline. These instructions should be reinforced by the dental staff as the patient is discharged.

Since Mrs. Wick is about to depart for a Caribbean cruise, she must be warned that tetracycline causes photosensitivity and she should avoid bright sunlight. The dentist should minimize the risk of photosensitivity by not prescribing demeclocyline (Declomycin), which causes more photosensitive reactions than other tetracyclines.

17 A woman who is in her third trimester of pregnancy lives in a nonfluoridated area. What is your recommendation for a fluoride supplement?

Answer: Water used for the infant should be prepared daily by dissolving 2.2 mg of sodium fluoride (1.0 mg fluoride) in 1 qt of water. The value of fluoride tablets for the expectant mother is not clear. It is known that some fluoride passes through the placenta and could deposit in the calcifying teeth. However, because the therapeutic value of prenatal fluoride is not established, postnatal supplementation for the child is necessary.

18 Mr. L. McCarthy has pericoronitis with severe swelling over an unerupted third molar, temperature of 103°F, and a sore throat. His medical history shows that he has been taking oral anticoagulants for 19 months. What antibiotic should be prescribed, and why?

Answer: Antibiotic therapy for patients taking anticoagulants must be carefully considered. Tetracyclines can delay blood clotting by interfering with the absorption of vitamin K from the gastrointestinal tract. This reduced vitamin K, which is required for prothrombin synthesis, leads to lowered prothrombin levels. Oral anticoagulants by themselves can also decrease prothrombin formation. Therefore, synergism between the two drugs may occur, and spontaneous bleeding may result. Sulfonamides are also contraindicated since they can displace anticoagulants from plasma-protein binding sites and result in an increase in available anticoagulant. This anticoagulant interaction is less likely to be clinically significant with erythromycin or penicillin.

Although a minor drug interaction is possible between penicillin and the oral anticoagulants, this interaction is not clinically significant. It should also be noted that elevated temperatures may decrease the effects of anticoagulants on the blood-clotting process. Therefore, both local debridement and systemic antibiotics should be immediately instituted. Prior to the extraction, a prothrombin time should be obtained to determine if there is danger of bleeding. If the prothrombin time is too long, consult with the patient's physician regarding a gradual reduction in anticoagulant therapy before extraction. The reduction in anticoagulant dosage must be gradual since a sudden reduction could result in massive thrombosis.

19 A thorough root planing was scheduled for a patient with a history of rheumatic fever. Would you premedicate this patient and, if so, how?

Answer: If the rheumatic fever caused cardiac valvular damage, then the patient must be premedicated to prevent subacute bacterial endocarditis. If the patient has a history of rheumatic fever with no cardiac valvular damage, no antibiotics are needed. The drug of choice is penicillin, and secondarily, if there are allergies, erythromycin. The dosage regimen for penicillin is 4 tablets of 500 mg each, 1 h before the appointment and 1 tablet thereafter for eight consecutive doses. The dosage regimen for erythromycin is similar, with the exception that the initial dose is 2 tablets of 500 mg each, 1.5 h before the appointment. If the patient is already taking penicillin prophylactically as prescribed by his physician, then erythromycin should be prescribed.

20 A patient was receiving promazine (a phenothiazine-derivative tranquilizer) for a nervous condition. The night before the dental appointment the patient could not sleep and wanted premedication prior to all subsequent appointments. What would you prescribe? Also, if surgery were needed, what factors should be considered?

Answer: Sleep can be facilitated either by increasing the dose of promazine the night before the appointment (in consultation with the patient's physician) or prescribing a sedative. If a sedative is prescribed, less than the usual dosage is necessary since promazine would enhance the sedative's effect.

Regarding surgery, phenothiazines which alter blood cells can result in poor wound healing. Therefore, a complete and differential blood count should be performed in patients on chronic phenothiazine therapy.

21 A patient requiring the extraction of four third molars has a history of rheumatic fever with valvular damage. She is presently taking oxytetracycline for a skin condition and secobarbital for insomnia. After blood tests it was discovered that she has "nutritional megaloblastic anemia" for which she is taking folic acid (quantity unknown). What precautions should be taken?

Answer: The dentist should consult her physician about the severity of the anemia and the possible need to increase the folic acid supplements. Because she has a history of rheumatic heart disease, she must be premedicated with penicillin. She should also be advised to discontinue taking the tetracycline several days prior to administration of penicillin, since it could antagonize the effect of penicillin. Less nitrous oxide should be used on this patient, since nitrous oxide has the same side effects as seco-barbital, i.e., vomiting, nausea, and orthostatic hypotension. These may be additive when administered together. Also, nitrous oxide poses a potential hazard of hypoxia, and unintentional overdosage when used in conjunction with barbiturates could occur, with hypoxia resulting.

22 A 55-year-old male patient is suffering from maturity-onset diabetes which is well controlled with daily dosages of Orinase and diet control. He also had a "heart attack" in April of last year for which he is taking Dicumarol and Valium. The patient's physician indicates his anticoagulant therapy was being monitored monthly, and at the last reading (3 weeks ago) the prothrombin time was within $1\frac{1}{2}$ of normal. The physician recommended that Tylenol could be given in limited dosage and that there was no contraindication to increasing the dosage of Valium. The dental treatment plan called for:

   a Routine operative dentistry
   b Extraction of the mandibular first molar with fabrication of a bridge
   c Periodontal treatment for pocket depths of 4 to 5 mm

Answer: There are no contraindications to the routine operative dentistry; however, there are several precautions that should be observed in the extraction of the tooth and the periodontal treatment.

A complication of diabetes is a compromised blood supply and poor wound healing. This should be a consideration in the extraction and a strong consideration in the definitive periodontal treatment. As long as the diabetes is under control, the extraction could be performed without expected complications. Anticoagulant therapy presents a problem in any surgical procedure, and the prothrombin time should be redone just prior to the extraction. The periodontal conditions should be treated with scaling and root planing to see if there is any resolution of the pockets. Periodontal surgery should be avoided if possible in this situation because the pockets of 4 to 5 mm could possibly be maintained as clean pockets.

Postoperative pain control is another concern in this case because of potential drug interactions. Aspirin potentiates anticoagulants. Also, meperidine (Demerol) and barbiturates are enhanced by diazepam (Valium). Tylenol with codeine (#1 or #2) could be used. A possible adjunct would be to increase the dose of Valium in consultation with his physician to decrease apprehension before and after the surgery.

Dicumarol's anticoagulant activity is rarely enhanced by penicillin, and this interaction, although not usually clinically significant, should be considered when treating any postextraction infection.

Chapter 22

Prescription Writing

"Ms. Jones, what did the doctor mean when he told me to abstain from dairy products while taking this medication? He did explain it to me but I was so confused at the time that I couldn't follow what he said."

Often a patient feels more at ease and less hurried with the dental auxiliary than with the dentist. Therefore, the dental auxiliary must be cognizant of all aspects of prescription writing and be able to discuss the prescription with the patient.

Dental staff should also be aware that drug addicts may complain of severe facial pain hoping to receive a prescription for a narcotic-containing analgesic. Addicts have gone from office to office with these complaints to sustain their addiction. Because of potential drug abuse, blank or pretyped prescriptions should also not be left out in areas accessible to patients. This encourages theft and forgery of these forms.

BASIC PRINCIPLES

In the past, prescriptions were confusing in form and usually written in Latin. Today, prescriptions have been simplified and follow basic guidelines:

1 It should be typed or clearly written in ink. Erasures should not appear on it.

2 The date and name and address of the patient should appear on it. Also, the age may appear as number of years or indicated as child, adult, elderly.

3 The drug name, dosage form, strength, and number of units and number of refills (if any) should appear on the form.

4 The use of Latin abbreviations is discouraged, and carefully worded directions for use should be given.

5 A separate prescription blank should be written for each drug.

6 The dentist must sign the prescription at the time it is given to the patient.

7 If a narcotic is prescribed, the dentist's federal registry number and address must appear on the form.

8 A notation should be made on the patient's chart of the medication dispensed.

THE WRITTEN PRESCRIPTION

The prescription can be thought of as a formal letter to the pharmacist. If it were written as such, it would appear as follows:

John Doe, D.D.S.
3436 Main Street
New Town, N.Y. 14214
Ph. 833-1234

April 4, 1978

Dear Sir:

I would appreciate it if you would place nine (9) 30-mg tablets of codeine sulfate in a container and give the container to Mr. Andrew Young, an adult, who lives at 343 South Street in New Town, New York. Please place the following instructions to Mr. Young on the label: These tablets are to be used to control pain. If pain is experienced, take one tablet every four hours. My narcotic registration number is AC0500101.

Sincerely,

John Doe, D.D.S

When the preceding letter is written as a prescription, it would appear in a simple form as follows:

John Doe, D.D.S   Reg. No. AC0500101
3436 Main Street
New Town, N.Y. 14214

Name: Date: April 4, 1978
   Mr. Andrew Young   Age: Adult
Address: Phone: 833-1234
   343 South Street
   New Town, N.Y.

Rx
   Codeine sulfate tablets, USP   30 mg
   Disp.: Nine (9) tablets
   Sig.: One (1) tablet every four hours if needed
        for pain.

John Doe, D.D.S

The symbol Rx may or may not appear on the prescription. This symbol is an abbreviation for the Latin word recipe, meaning "take thou."

The various parts of a prescription are arranged in a definite sequence and labeled in the following manner.

1 The *superscription*: The patient's name, address, age, the date, and the symbol Rx.

2 The *inscription*: The name of the drug and amount.

3 The *subscription*: Directions to the pharmacist. The dosage form and amount to be given appear in this section of a prescription. The amount to be given may be indicated by the words dispense, number, or the symbol for number, #.

4 The *transcription* or signa: Directions to the patient (Sig.).

5 The *signature*: The signature of the prescribing person must appear on the prescription.

When selecting a drug form, one normally uses standard forms and dosages prepared by the manufacturer. To cite the above example, 30 mg of codeine sulfate was prescribed as a tablet. If another drug form were desirable (capsule or syrup), be certain the desired drug form and quantity are available. In the case of codeine sulfate, tablets containing 8, 15, 30, and 60 mg are available. If the dentist ordered tablets containing 20 mg, the pharmacist would not be able to fill the prescription. The three main information sources about the availability of doses of preparations and dosage form (tablet, capsule, solution, and so on) are the *Physicians' Desk Reference, Accepted Dental Therapeutics,* and the pharmacy.

The first, the *Physicians' Desk Reference,* is an annually revised book in which the pharmaceutical manufacturers pay to list their products. There is a tendency for manufacturers to include only their latest drugs or drugs currently under active promotion.

The second source, *Accepted Dental Therapeutics* (ADT), is revised biannually by the Council on Dental Therapeutics of the American Dental Association. ADT includes drugs of recognized value in dentistry, including their official drug names (those listed in the USP and NF) and generic names. It also contains over-the-counter drugs of recognized safety and efficacy in dentistry which follow the labeling and advertising standards of the Council on Dental Therapeutics.

Prescriptions can either list a brand name of a drug or the generic name. If the generic name is used (as in the above example), the pharmacist can use any brand of drug he or she desires as long as it meets the specifications of the prescription and the USP. This sometimes reduces the cost of the prescription. If a particular brand of codeine sulfate tablet were desired, the prescription should be written with the brand name (see the following example).

Codeine Sulfate Tablets 15 mg
(Vitarine Company)

This prescription is for a substance which is under the Controlled Substances Act and cannot be refilled under any circumstances. If the prescription were not for a narcotic or other controlled substance for which refills are prohibited, and you wanted to have the prescription refilled twice, this can be indicated on the prescription in the lower left corner. The exact number of refills should be specified. The indication p.r.n. (as needed) is not a legal authorization for refills of prescriptions.

Dosage Expressions

Although apples are bought by the pound, gasoline by the gallon, and cloth by the yard, the language of science is the metric system. Because of this, the majority of modern drugs today are prepared in metric units. In the past, however, older drugs were prepared according to the apothecary system, and both physicians and dentists were trained in its use. Gradually the apothecary system is dying out. Tables 22-1 and 22-2 give some approximate relationships between this and the metric system.

Typical metric units are the gram (g), milligram (mg), and microgram (μg) and for volume is the milliliter (mL). A gram is divided into 1000 milligrams (mg), and one milligram is divided into 1000 micrograms (μg). It is generally convenient to note all weights and volumes in terms of the gram, milligram, or milliliter (Table 22-3). If one wants to write a prescription for

Table 22-1 Various Measures of Weight

Metric	Apothecary
1 g (gram)	15 gr (grains)
4 g (grams)	60 gr (grains; 1 dram)
30 g (grams)	1 oz (ounce)
1 kg (kilogram)	2.2 lb (pounds)
60 mg (milligrams)	1 gr (grain)

Table 22-2   Various Measures of Volume

Metric	Apothecary
5 milliliters	1 dram (1 teaspoonful)
30 milliliters	1 fluid ounce
480 milliliters	1 pint
960 milliliters	1 quart

compound X tablets, each containing half a gram, one would write:

Compound X   0.5 g

and the pharmacist would understand that half-gram (500 milligram) compound X tablets are to be dispensed. Similarly, if the prescription reads:

Compound X elixir, USP   120.0 mL

the pharmacist would dispense 120 mL of compound X elixir.

Substances available in *microgram* amounts are written as micrograms rather than grams. For example a substance available in 5 microgram tablets could be written as: 0.000005 g. It

Table 22-3   Commonly Used Metric Equivalents and Their Abbreviations

Abbreviations for the metric system
gram = g
0.000001 gram = 1 microgram (μg or mcg)
0.001 gram = 1 milligram (mg)
1 gram (g) = 1,000 milligrams
= 1,000,000 micrograms
kilogram = kg
1 kilogram (kg) = 1,000 grams (g)
liter = L
microgram = μg or mcg
microliter = μL
milligram = mg
milliliter = mL
0.001 milliliter = 1 microliter (μL)
1 milliliter (mL) = 0.001 liter
1,000 milliliters = 1 liter (L)

is easier and just as correct to write this as: 5 micrograms or 5 μg.

There are exceptions to expressing weights in grams and volumes in milliliters. Sometimes, the quantity of a drug is not expressed as weight or volume, but as units. For instance, a prescription for penicillin might read:

Tabs.: Penicillin G buffered   400,000 units
Disp.: Twenty (20)

This instructs the pharmacist to dispense twenty tablets of buffered penicillin G, each containing 400,000 units. The use of units began in earlier times when drugs were measured by a bioassay system in which their activity was compared to a standard unit. Although this is not usually done today, the doses of some antibiotics such as penicillin are still expressed in units.

Although the use of Latin abbreviations is discouraged, they are still used by some practitioners. Common Latin abbreviations are listed in Table 22-4.

Table 22-4   Commonly Used Latin and Greek Abbreviations

Abbreviations	Latin or Greek	English translation
a.c.	*ante cibos*	Before meals
aq. (or H₂O)	*aqua*	Water
b.i.d.	*bis in die*	2 times a day
c̄, c	*cum*	With
gtt.	*gutta*(e)	Drop(s)
h.s., hor. som., H.S.	*hora somni*	At bedtime
non rep., n.r., N.R.	*non repetatur*	Do not repeat
p.c.	*post cibos*	After eating
p.r.n.	*pro re nata*	As needed
q.h.	*quaque hora*	Each hour, every hour
q.i.d.	*quater in die*	4 times a day
s̄, sine	*sine*	Without
sig.	*signa*	Write on the label
s̄s̄, ss	*semis*	One-half
stat.	*statim*	Immediately
t.i.d.	*ter in die*	3 times a day

Dosage Determination

Most adult doses are recommended by the manufacturer based on a person of average weight. Some manufacturers more accurately recommend doses as *"X"* milligrams of drug per pound or kilogram of body weight. This latter data allows calculation of a dose according to the patient's size. For children, when the dose/weight is not available, the following formulas can be used:

Clark's rule:

$$\frac{\text{Weight of child (lb)}}{150} \times \text{adult dose} = \text{child dose}$$

or

$$\frac{\text{Weight of child (kg)}}{70} \times \text{adult dose} = \text{child dose}$$

The following dosage rules appear in the literature but are used less frequently and are not recommended.

Young's rule:

$$\frac{\text{Age of child}}{\text{Age of child plus 12}} \times \text{adult dose} = \text{child dose}$$

Cowling's rule:

$$\frac{\text{Age at next birthday}}{24} \times \text{adult dose} = \text{child dose}$$

Certain physiologic and metabolic functions as well as many drug effects are known to be proportional to body surface area. The approximate body surface area can be calculated by multiplying weight to the 0.7 power $\times$ 0.055. Updated dosage tables based on body surface area may become available as investigations on this subject continue.

The dosage prescribed must also be modified according to the function of the patient's liver and kidneys. Some drugs are metabolized by the liver and excreted in the metabolized or unmetabolized form by the kidneys. Therefore, if the patient's liver and/or kidneys are not fully functional, the dosage of a drug must be reduced accordingly, or effects of overdosage may be expected.

Laws Affecting Drug Use

There are a number of federal laws which regulate the prescribing of drugs in this country. In addition to the federal laws, a number of states have separate laws affecting the distribution of narcotics, barbiturates, and other drugs. For information on federal, state, or city regulations relative to these laws, a local pharmacist may be the most efficient source of information. A summary of the important federal laws follows:

I Food, Drug and Cosmetic Act of 1938. This law prohibits interstate commerce in drugs that have not been shown to be safe and effective. Regulations are also established for packaging, labeling, strength, and purity of product. These are enforced by the Food and Drug Administration whose offices are in Rockville, Maryland.

II Durham-Humphrey Amendment (part of the Federal Food, Drug and Cosmetic Act) 1952. This important amendment established:
  A Two major drug classifications:
    1 *Drugs sold only on prescription.* These include habit-forming drugs and those not safe for self-medication.
    2 *Drugs sold without prescription.* Over-the-counter (OTC) drugs.
  B The legality of filling an oral order to dispense medication. Oral orders must be promptly written by the prescriber and mailed to the pharmacist.
  C The legality of refilling prescriptions. If authorized by the practitioner, prescriptions may be refilled, except for controlled substances. Prescriptions with p.r.n. or "refill ad lib" (both indicating

refill as necessary or as needed) cannot be refilled. Instead, specific directions for refilling must be given.

D Copies of prescriptions for narcotics, depressants, or stimulants (all controlled substances) cannot be given to the patient. They may only be furnished to any licensed practitioner authorized to write such prescriptions. Copies of other prescriptions may be given to the patient at his or her request. Such prescriptions are for *informational purposes only,* and must be so worded.

E According to this law, there is no ''expiration period'' (controlled substances are exceptions) for a *prescription.* Good judgment is used by the pharmacist.

III Federal Controlled Substance Act of 1970.

The term ''controlled substances'' includes narcotics, stimulants, and depressants. The Federal Controlled Substances Act of 1970 established five ''Schedules'' of these drugs which separate drugs according to potential abuse.

Schedule I drugs are not currently accepted for medical use in treatment in the United States and have a high potential for abuse. The average practitioner, therefore, may not prescribe such drugs. Examples include: heroin, marijuana, LSD, peyote, and so forth.

Schedule II drugs have a high potential for abuse but are currently accepted for medical treatment in the United States, though sometimes with severe restrictions. Examples include: opium, morphine, codeine, meperidine HC1 (Demerol), hydromorphoine (Dilaudid), cocaine, Percodan, amphetamines, methamphetamines, methaqualone, amobarbital (Amytal), pentobarbital (Nembutal), secobarbital (Seconal), and Tuinal (amobarbital and secobarbital combination).

The following drugs, while presently under Schedule III control, have been proposed for Schedule II: butabarbital (Butisol); cyclobar-

bital, heptabarbital, probarbital, and vinbarbital; and talbutal.

Schedule III drugs have less potential for drug abuse than those in Schedules I and II and are currently accepted for medical use in the United States. Examples include: glutethimide (Doriden), methprylon (Noludar), nalorphine, paregoric, APC with codeine (Empirin Compound with codeine except as noted in Schedule V), phenaphen with codeine, Tylenol with codeine (see Schedule V below), some barbiturates (except those in Schedule IV), amphetamine combination products, and some anorexiants (appetite reducers).

Schedule IV drugs have a lower potential for drug abuse than those in Schedule III and are currently accepted for medical use in the United States. Examples include: barbital, phenobarbital, chloral hydrate, etchlorvynol (Placidyl), meprobamate, paraldehyde, chlordiazepoxide (Librium), diazepam (Valium), propoxyphene and salts (Darvon, Darvon Compound, Darvocet), and pentazocine (Talwin).

Schedule V drugs have the lowest potential for drug abuse and are currently accepted for medical use. Examples include: terpin hydrate with codeine, Empirin Compound with codeine, 0.007 g (1/8 gr), Tylenol with codeine, 0.007 g (1/8 gr).

[Note that the following drug is not subject to the Controlled Substances Act, but only the Durham-Humphrey Amendment: ethoheptazate citrate (Zactirin).]

I Prescription requirements under the Controlled Substance Act require that the practitioner must fill in *all* the following information for controlled substances:

A *Full* name and address of the patient.

B Patient's *age.*

C Name (signature), address, registration number (DEA), and telephone number of the practitioner.

D Date (when signed).

E Specific directions for use, including dosage, frequency of dosage, and the maximum daily dosage (MDD).

II The above information *cannot* be added by the pharmacist. "Use as directed" is not acceptable on a controlled substance prescription.

III For Schedule III, IV, and V prescriptions, there is some flexibility. The practitioner may *orally furnish* the pharmacist with *certain* information missing from the prescription, including maximum daily dose and specific directions for use, the patient's age and address, the practitioner's name (not signature) and address, Drug Enforcement Administration or registration number, and telephone number.

IV The following invalidate a prescription:
  A Unsigned prescriptions
  B Undated prescriptions
  C Where the name and quantity of the controlled substance is not specified
  D Where the name of the patient is missing

V A prescription order for drugs in Schedules III, IV, and V may be refilled up to five times within 6 months after the date of issue. After five renewals or after 6 months, a new prescription is required.

VI Pharmacists may not usually dispense more than a 30-day supply of a controlled substance (based on the directions for use). In some cases, prescriptions may be written for longer periods of up to a 3-month supply for:
  A Minimal brain dysfunction (hyperkinesis) in patients not more than 16 years of age (e.g., Ritalin, amphetamines)
  B Convulsive disorders (e.g., phenobarbital)
  C Relief of pain in patients *65 years of age and over* suffering from diseases

VII When a prescription is for more than a 30-day supply of a controlled substance, the diagnosis can be included on the prescription. If this is not done, the pharmacist may telephone to obtain the diagnosis and write it on the back of the prescription. If the prescriber does not wish to divulge the diagnosis, a notation can be made by the pharmacist that the diagnosis is one of the designated exceptions. Whenever the pharmacist adds the diagnosis, he or she must date and sign the back of the prescription.

VIII An application for registration and assignment of a controlled drug registration number can be obtained by writing the United States Department of Justice, Drug Enforcement Administration, P.O. Box 28083, Central Station, Washington, D.C. 20005.

Sample Prescriptions

The following sample prescriptions demonstrate the various aspects presented in this chapter. For the sake of brevity, the superscription and signature are not included.

1 Prescription for an antibiotic to treat an infection of dental origin:

Tetracycline HCl   250 mg
Disp.: 28
Sig.: 1 tablet four times a day with no dairy products within 1½ h of medication.
Refill 1 (one) ×

This same prescription could be written with abbreviations as follows for the directions to the patient:

Sig.: 1 tab q.i.d. s̄ dairy products within 1½ h of medication.

2 Prescription for an antibiotic for a patient with a history of a heart damaged by rheumatic fever in whom a bacteremia is expected from the dental procedure needed by this patient.

Penicillin V tablets   500 mg
#: 12

Sig.: 4 tablets 1 h before appointment and 1 tablet every 6 h thereafter.

The abbreviated directions would be:

Sig.: 4 tab 1 h ā appointment, and 1 tab q6 h thereafter.

3 Prescription for a nonnarcotic analgesic.

Acetaminophen   500 mg
Disp.: 16
Sig.: 1 capsule every 4 h as needed for pain.

The abbreviated directions would be:

Sig.: 1 cap q4 h p.r.n. for pain.

4 Prescription for a narcotic analgesic (requires DEA registration number).

Codeine phosphate tablets   60 mg
Disp.: 6 (six)
Sig.: 1 tablet every 6 h as needed for pain.
Maximum daily dose 6 (six).

The abbreviated directions would be:

Sig.: 1 tab q6 h p.r.n. for pain.
MDD 6 (six)

ANSWER TO CHAPTER CASE

This case demonstrates the fact that a patient sometimes feels more at ease and less hurried with the dental auxiliary than with the dentist and asks numerous questions of the auxiliary personnel.

In this example the dentist probably prescribed a tetracycline antibiotic. Since tetracyclines have an affinity for heavy metal ions such as calcium, they bind with calcium in dairy products and form a compound which cannot be absorbed from the gastrointestinal tract. As a result, therapeutic levels of the antibiotic cannot occur since the drug has not been absorbed into the bloodstream. For this reason the *dentist wanted the patient to abstain from dairy products while taking this antibiotic. Usually, the patient should refrain from dairy products for 1.5 h both before and after taking the medication so that this binding does not occur.*

QUESTIONS

1 What are the basic principles of prescription writing?
2 What are the five parts of a prescription?
3 Compare the metric system to the apothecary system.
4 Name two ways in which drug dosage can be determined for a child.
5 Which laws regulate prescription writing? What are the highlights of each law?
6 What are the requirements for writing a prescription for a controlled substance?
7 Write a prescription for: an antibiotic, an analgesic.

READING REFERENCES

Butler, A. M., and R. H. Richie, "Simplification and Improvement in Estimating Drug Dosage and Fluid and Dietary Allowances for Patients of Varying Sizes," *N. Eng. J. Med.,* **262:**903–908, 1960.

Drug Enforcement Administration, U.S. Department of Justice, *A Manual for the Medical Practitioner—An Informational Outline of the Controlled Substances Act of 1970,* Washington, 1977.

Friend, D. G., "Principles and Practices of Prescription Writing," *Clin. Pharmacol. Ther.,* **6:**411–416, 1965.

Stewart, R. B., and L. E. Cluff, "A Review of Medication Errors and Compliance in Ambulatory Patients," *Clin. Pharmacol Ther.,* **13:**463–468, 1972.

Wynn, R. L., *Fundamentals of Drug Prescribing in Dentistry—An Independent Student Learning Program,* University of Maryland, School of Dentistry Publication, Baltimore, 1972.

Part Six

Appendixes

Tables of Nonprescription Drugs

The tables in Appendix A are from the *Handbook on Non-Prescription Drugs,* American Pharmaceutical Association, Washington, D.C., 1977, pp. 259–263. Copyright 1977, all rights reserved, reproduced with permission of the American Pharmaceutical Association.

Toothpaste

Product (manufacturer)	Ingredients
Aim (Lever Bros)	Stannous fluoride, 0.4%; alcohol; sorbitol; glycerin; hydrated silica; polethylene glycol 32; sodium lauryl sulfate; sodium and potassium carrageenans; saccharin sodium; sodium benzoate; flavor
Amosan (Cooper)	Sodium peroxyborate monohydrate, sodium bitartrate
Caroid Tooth Powder (Breon)	Papain
Chloresium (Rystan)	Chlorophyll
Close-up (Lever Bros)	Sorbitol, hydrated silica, glycerin, polyethylene glycol 32, sodium lauryl sulfate, alcohol, saccharin sodium, cellulose gum, sodium benzoate, sodium phosphate, disodium phosphate, flavor
Colgate with MFP (Colgate-Palmolive)	Sarcosinate, sodium monofluorophosphate

Toothpaste (*Continued*)

Product (manufacturer)	Ingredients
Crest (Procter & Gamble)	Stannous fluoride, 0.40%; calcium pyrophosphate; cellulose gum; glycerin; sorbitol; stannous pyrophosphate; flavor
Depend (Warner-Lambert)	Alcohol, 23.8%; sorbitol; glycerin; polysorbate 80; saccharin sodium phosphate; caramel; disodium phosphate; flavor
Extar (Extar)	Sodium polymetaphosphate, extra heavy mineral oil, magnesium oxide, tragacanth, sodium lauryl sulfate, saccharin sodium, spralene mint, silica gel, calcium carbonate, mint oil flavor
Gleem II (Procter & Gamble)	Sodium fluoride, 0.22%; calcium pyrophosphate; glycerin; sorbitol; blend of anionic surfactants; cellulose gum; flavor
Ipana (La Maur)	Stannous fluoride
Listerine (Warner-Lambert)	Dicalcium phosphate
Listermint (Warner-Lambert)	Alcohol, 12.8%; glycerin; poloxamer 407; polysorbate 80; saccharin sodium; zinc chloride; saccharin; flavoring
Macleans (Beecham Products)	Dicalcium phosphate dihydrate, glycerin, calcium carbonate
Macleans Fluoride Toothpaste (Beecham Products)	Sodium monofluorophosphate, 0.76%; calcium carbonate, 38%; glycerin, 26%; sodium lauryl sulfate, 1.15%
NDK Liquid (NDK Co.)	Fluorophosphate, benzethonium chloride
Pearl Drops Liquid (Carter)	Dicalcium phosphate, aluminum hydroxide, sorbitol, carboxymethylcellulose
Pepsodent (Lever Bros)	Sorbitol, alumina, hydrated silica, glycerin, polyethylene glycol 32, sodium lauryl sulfate, dicalcium phosphate, cellulose gum, titanium dioxide, saccharin sodium, sodium benzoate, flavor
Pepsodent Ammoniated Tooth Powder (Lever Bros)	Sodium metaphosphate, tricalcium phosphate, diammonium phosphate, urea, sodium lauryl sulfate, polyethylene glycol, carrageenan, saccharin, flavor
Pepsodent Tooth Powder (Lever Bros)	Sodium metaphosphate, dicalcium phosphate, magnesium trisilicate, sodium lauryl sulfate, polyethylene glycol, carrageenan, saccharin, flavor
Pycopay Tooth Powder (Block)	Sodium chloride, sodium bicarbonate, calcium carbonate, magnesium carbonate, tricalcium phosphate, flavor
Revelation Tooth Powder (Alvin Last)	Calcium carbonate, soap, sodium bicarbonate, sodium chloride, menthol, methyl salicylate
Sensodyne (Block)	Strontium chloride
Thermodent (Leeming)	Magnesium carbonate, calcium carbonate, sodium chloride, potassium sulfate, formaldehyde

Denture Cleaner

Product (manufacturer)	Ingredients
Denalan (Whitehall)	Sodium peroxide, 9.5%; sodium chloride, 90%
Efferdent Tablets (Warner-Lambert)	Potassium monopersulfate, 960 mg; sodium borate perhydrate, 480 mg; sodium carbonate; sodium lauryl sulfoacetate; sodium bicarbonate, 1.116 g; citric acid, 362 mg; magnesium stearate; simethicone
Effervescent Denture Tablets (Rexall)	Sodium bicarbonate, citric acid, sodium perborate, sodium acid pyrophosphate, sodium benzoate, trisodium phosphate, sodium lauryl sulfate, poloxamer 188, sorbitol, silica, peppermint oil, povidone
K.I.K. (K.I.K. Co.)	Sodium perborate, 25%; trisodium phosphate, 75%
Mersene Dental Cleaner (Hoyt)	Troclosene potassium, sodium perborate, trisodium phosphate

Denture Cleaner (*Continued*)

Product (manufacturer)	Ingredients
Polident Denture Cleanser Powder (Block)	Sodium perborate, potassium monopersulfate, sodium carbonate, sodium tripolyphosphate, surfactant, sodium bicarbonate, flavor
Polident Tablets (Block)	Potassium monopersulfate, sodium perborate, sodium carbonate, surfactant, sodium bicarbonate, citric acid, flavor

Toothache/Cold Sore/Canker Sore

Product (manufacturer)	Ingredients
Baby Orajel (Commerce)	Benzocaine, viscous water-soluble base
Benzodent (Vick)	Benzocaine, 20%; eugenol, 0.4%; 8-hydroxyquinoline sulfate, 0.1%; denture adhesive-like base
Betadine Mouthwash/Gargle (Purdue Frederick)	Povidone-iodine, 0.5%; alcohol, 8.8%
Blistex Ointment (Blistex)	Phenol, 0.4%; camphor, 1%; ammonia; mineral oil; lanolin; petrolatum; paraffin; alcohol; sorbitan sesquioleate; peppermint oil; lanolin alcohol; soya sterol; ammonium carbonate; fragrance
Cold Sore Lotion (DeWitt)	Camphor, 3.6%; tincture of benzoin, 4.2%; phenol, 0.3%; menthol, 0.3%; alcohol, 90%
Dalidyne (Dalin)	Methylbenzethonium chloride; benzocaine; tannic acid; camphor; chlorothymol; menthol; benzyl alcohol; alcohol, 61%; aromatic base
Dr. Hands Teething Gel (Roberts)	Tincture of pellitory; menthol; clove oil; hamamelis water; alcohol, 10%
Dr. Hands Teething Lotion (Roberts)	Tincture of pellitory; menthol; clove oil; hamamelis water; alcohol, 10%
Jiffy (Block)	Benzocaine; eugenol; alcohol, 56.5%
Numzident (PurePac)	Benzocaine, eugenol, peppermint oil, polyethylene glycol-like base
Numzit (PurePac)	Glycerin; alcohol, 10%; gel vehicle
Orabase (Hoyt)	Benzocaine
Orajel (Commerce)	Benzocaine, polyethylene glycol-like base
Ora-Jel-d (Commerce)	Benzocaine, clove oil, benzyl alcohol, adhesive base
Pain-A-Lay (Roberts)	Boric acid, cresol
Proxigel (Reed & Carnrick)	Urea carbamide, gel vehicle
Rexall Cold Sore Lotion (Rexall)	Phenol; benzoin; camphor; menthol; alcohol, 90%
Rexall Cold Sore Ointment (Rexall)	Phenol; benzoin; camphor; menthol; alcohol, 30%; viscous base
Tanac (Commerce)	Benzalkonium chloride, tannic acid
Teething Lotion (DeWitt)	Propylene glycol, 44%; glycerin, 29%; benzocaine, 5.6%; benzyl alcohol, 2.5%; tincture of myrrh, 4.5%; alcohol
Toothache Drops (DeWitt)	Clove oil, 9.98%; benzocaine, 5.01%; creosote beechwood, 4.83%; flexible collodion (base); alcohol, 20%

Denture Adhesive

Product (manufacturer)	Ingredients
Brace (Norcliff-Thayer)	Cellulose gum, 2.5%; methyl vinyl ether–maleic anhydride and/or acid copolymer, 1.5%; povidone, 1%; petrolatum, 3.5%; mineral oil, 1.5%; flavor, 0.02%
Confident (Block)	Carboxymethylcellulose gum, 32%; ethylene oxide polymer, 13%; petrolatum, 42%; liquid petrolatum, 12%; propylparaben, 0.05%

Denture Adhesive (*Continued*)

Product (manufacturer)	Ingredients
Corega Powder (Block)	Karaya gum, 94.6%; water-soluble ethylene oxide polymer, 4.76%; calcium silicate, 0.07%; flavor, 0.4%
Effergrip Denture Adhesive Cream (Warner-Lambert)	Carboxymethylcellulose sodium, 39%; cationic polyacrylamide polymer, 10%
Effergrip Denture Adhesive Powder (Warner-Lambert)	Carboxymethylcellulose sodium, 40%; cationic polyacrylamide polymer, 10%
Fasteeth (Vick)	Karaya gum, sodium borate
Firmdent (Moyco)	Karaya gum, 90.91%; sodium tetraborate, 9.05%; powdered flavor essence of peppermint, 0.04%
Fixodent (Vick)	Calcium, sodium, polyvinyl methyl ether maleate, petrolatum base
Orafix (Norcliff-Thayer)	Karaya gum, 51%; petrolatum, 30%; mineral oil, 13%; peppermint oil, 0.08%
Orafix M (Norcliff-Thayer)	Karaya gum, 51%; benzocaine, 2%; allantoin, 0.2%; petrolatum, 28%; mineral oil, 13%; peppermint oil, 0.08%
Orahesive Powder (Hoyt)	Gelatin, 33.3%; pectin, 33.3%; carboxymethylcellulose sodium, 33.3%
Perma-Grip Powder (Lactona)	Polyethylene wax, 50.9%; carboxymethylcellulose sodium, 39.0%; cationic acrylic polymer, 10.0%; flavor
Polident Dentu-Grip (Block)	Carboxymethylcellulose gum, 49%; ethylene oxide polymer, 21%; flavor, 0.4%
Poli-Grip (Block)	Karaya gum, 51%; petrolatum, 36.7%; liquid petrolatum, 9.4%; magnesium oxide, 2.7%; propylparaben; flavor
Wernet's Cream (Block)	Carboxymethylcellulose gum, 32%; petrolatum, 42%; liquid petrolatum, 12%; ethylene oxide polymer, 13%; propylparaben, 0.05%; flavor, 0.5%
Wernet's Powder (Block)	Karaya gum, 94.6%; water-soluble ethylene oxide polymer, 4.76%; calcium silicate, 0.07%; flavor, 0.4%

Mouthwash

Product (manufacturer)	Ingredients
Astring-O-Sol (Breon)	Tincture of myrrh; methyl salicylate; alcohol, 70%; zinc chloride
Cherry Chloraseptic Mouthwash and Gargle (Eaton)	Phenol, sodium phenolate
Chloraseptic (liquid) (Eaton)	Phenol, sodium phenolate
Chlorazene Aromatic Powder (for solution) (Wisconsin Pharmacal)	Chloramine-T, 5%; sodium chloride, 88%; sodium bicarbonate, 5%; eucalyptol; saccharin sodium
Cēpacol (Merrell National)	Cetylpyridinum chloride, 0.05%; alcohol, 14%; aromatics
Forma-Zincol Concentrate (Ingram)	Formaldehyde, zinc chloride, anise oil, menthol
Gly-Oxide (International Pharmaceutical)	Carbamide peroxide, 10%; anhydrous glycerin; flavor
Greenmint Mouthwash (Block)	Chlorophyll, alcohol; urea; glycine; flavor
Isodine Mouthwash/Gargle Concentrate (Blair)	Povidone-iodine, 7.5%; alcohol, 35%
Kasdenol Powder (Kasdenol)	Available chlorine 5–6% (as oxychlorosene)
Lavoris (Vick)	Zinc chloride, 0.22%; alcohol, 5%; cinnamaldehyde and clove oil, 0.06%
Listerine (Warner-Lambert)	Menthol; boric acid; thymol; eucalyptol; methyl salicylate; benzoic acid; alcohol, 25%

Mouthwash (*Continued*)

Product (manufacturer)	Ingredients
Micrin Plus Gargle & Rinse (Johnson & Johnson)	Alcohol, glycerin, poloxamer 407, flavor, saccharin sodium, monosodium glutamate–glutamic acid buffer, cetylpyridinium chloride
Mouthwash and Gargle (McKesson)	Cetylpyridinium chloride; alcohol, 14%
Odara (Lorvic)	Phenol (less than 2%); zinc chloride; glycerin; potassium iodide; methyl salicylate; eucalyptus oil; myrrh tincture; alcohol, 48%
Oral Pentacresol (Upjohn)	Secondary amyltricresols, 100 mg/100 ml; alcohol, 30%; sodium chloride, 861 mg/100 ml; calcium chloride, 33 mg/100 ml; potassium chloride, 29.9 mg/100 ml
Proxigel (Block)	Carbamide peroxide; 11%; anhydrous glycerin; thickeners; flavor
Scope (Procter & Gamble)	Cetylpyridinium chloride; domiphen bromide, 0.005%; alcohol, 18.5%; glycerin; saccharin; polisorbate 80; flavor
S.T. 37 (Calgon)	Hexylresorcinol, 0.1%; glycerin

Categories of commonly used Drugs— Brand Names

Based on *Physician's Desk Reference*, 32d ed., Medical Economics, Oradell, N.J., pp. 201–222, 1978.

Anorexics—Appetite Curbers

Amphetamines: Benzedrine Sulfate; Biphetamine; Delcobese; Desoxyn; Dexamyl; Dexedrine; Didrex; Eskatrol; Fetamin; Obetrol; Obotan;

Nonamphetamines: Bontril PDM; Fastin; Ionamin; Melfiat; Metamucil; Obe-Nil TR; Pondimin; Preludin; Pre-Sate; Sanorex; Tenuate; Tepanil; Voranil;

Other: Bacarate; Plegine; Pretts; Statobex

Antacids Alka-Seltzer Effervescent Antacid; Alks-2 Chewable Antacid; Aludrox; Alurex; Amphojel; Camalox; Delcid; Dicarbosil; Ducon; Equilet; Escot; Gaviscon; Gelusil; Kolantyl; Kudrox; Maalox; Magnatril; Marblen; Neutralox; Oxabid; Riopan; Robalate; Romach; Titralac; Trisogel; WinGel

Antianxiety and Antipsychotic Agents

Butyrophenones and combination: Haldol; Inapsine; Innovar

Chlordiazepoxide: Libritabs; Menrium

Chlordiazepoxide hydrochloride: Librax; Librium

Diazepam: Valium

Hydroxyzines: Atarax; Vistaril

Lithium carbonate: Eskalith; Lithane; Lithium; Lithonate; Lithotabs; Pfi-Lithium

Meprobamate and combination: Deprol; Equanil; Meprospan; Meprotabs; Milpath; Milprem; Miltown; Miltrate; PMB-200, PMB-400; Pathibamate; SK-Bamate

Other: Hydromox R; Kutrase; Loxitane; Moban; Raudixin; Rau-Sed; Serax; Serpasil; Sinequan; Trancopal; Tranxene; Tybatran

Phenothiazines and combination: Chlor-PZ; Compazine; Etrafon; Mellaril; Permitil; Prolixin; Quide; Repoise; Serentil; Stelazine; Thorazine; Tindal; Triavil; Trilafon; Vesprin

Reserpine: Sandril

Thioxanthenes: Navane; Taractan

Antiarthritics

Antiarthritics: Arthropan; Ascodeen; Ascriptin; Azolid; Butazolidin; Cama; Celestone; Cirin;

Clinoril; Decadron; Delta-Dome; Deronil; Duragesic; Ecotrin; Empirin Compound; Gaysal; Ger-O-Foam; Hyalex; Indocin; Kenacort; Kenalog; Meticortelone; Meticorten; Mobidin; Motrin; Os-Cal-Gesic; Oxalid; Pabalate; Pabirin; Plaquenil Sulfate; Solganal; Sterazolidin; Tandearil

Antigout: Anturane; Azolid; Benemid; Butazolidin; ColBenemid; Colchicine; Hyalex; Indocin; Oxalid; Tandearil; Zyloprim

Antiasthma Aarane; Brethine; Bronchobid; Elixophyllin; Intal; Lixaminol; microNefrin; Norisodrine; Slo-phyllin; Synophylate; Theobid; Theolair

Antibacterials and Antiseptics

Antibacterial with analgesics (urinary): Azo-Gantrisin; Azo-Mandelamine; Azotrex; Cyantin; Hiprex; Mandelamine; Suladyne; Thiosulfil; Trac; Urised; Urobiotic-250; Urolene Blue

Antibacterial (urinary): Furadantin; Hexalet; Macrodantin; NegGram; Neosporin; Septra; Thiosulfil; Urex; Uristat; Uro-Phosphate; Uroquid-Acid

Anticoagulants Coumadin; Dicumarol; Heparin Sodium; Lipo-Hepin; Miradon; Panheprin; Panwarfin; Phenindione; Protamine Sulfate; Sintrom

Anticonvulsants Amytal Sodium; Celontin; Clonopin; Dilantin; Diphenyl; Ekko; Gemonil; Luminal; Mebaral; Mebroin; Mesantoin; Milontin; Mysoline; Paradione; Peganone; Phelantin; Phenurone; Tegretol; Tridione; Zarontin

Antidepressants Adapin; Aventyl; Deprol; Elavil; Etrafon; Imavate; Imipramine; Janimine; Marplan; Nardil; Norpramin; Parnate; Pertofrane; Presamine; Sinequan; SK-Pramine; Tofranil; Trivil; Vivactil

Antidiabetic Agents DBI; Diabinese; Dymelor; Illetin; Insulin; Meltrol; NPH Illetin; Orinase; Protamine; Tolinase

Antihistamines Actidil; Actifed; Allerest; Ambenyl; Antagonate; Benadryl; Chlor-Trimeton; Citra; Codimal; Co-Pyronil; Coricidin; Coriforte; Deconamine; Dehist; Demazin; Dimetane; Dimetapp; Disomer; Disophrol; Dramamine; Drinus;

Drixoral; Duadacin; Emesert; Extendryl; Fedahist; Fedrazil; Fiogesic; Forhistal maleate; Hispril; Histabid; Hista-Clopane; Histadyl; Histaspan; Historal; Isoclor; Marhist; Matropinal Forte; Napril Plateau; Narine; Narspan; Neotep; Nolamine; Oraminic; Phenergan; Polaramine; Pyribenzamine; Quelidrine; Rondec DSC & T; Rynatan; Rynatuss; Sinovan; Sinulin; Tacaryl; Teldrin; Triaminic; Triaminicin; Triten; Tussagesic; Ursinus; Vistaril; Zipan

Antiinflammatory Agents Ananase; Avazyme; Chymoral; Orensyme; Papase; Varidase; Acthar; Allersone; Aristocort; Arthropan; Azolid; Azulfidine; Betapar; Butazolidin; Celestone; Chloresium; Cortef Acetate; Cortenema; Cortifoam; Cortisporin; Decaderm in Estergel; Decadron; Delta-Dome; Derma Medicone-HC; Deronil; Dexone; Diprosone; Fluonid; Flurobate; Halog; Herpecin-L; Hysone; Kenacort; Kenalog; Medrol; Meticortelone Acetate; Metreton; Mobidin; Motrin; Myoflex; Orabase HCA; Orasone; Oxalid; Plaquenil Sulfate; Proctocort; Protofoam-HC; Sterazolidin; Synalar; Synemol; Tandearil; Valisone; Vioform-Hydrocortisone

Antiparkinsonism Drugs Akineton; Antitrem; Artane; Artane Sequels; Bendopa; Cogentin; Disipal; Dopar; Kemadrin; Larodopa; Levsin; Levsinex; Pagitana Hydrochloride; Pipanol Hydrochloride; Sinemet; Symmetrel; Tremin

Antispasmodics and Anticholinergics Anaspaz; Antrenyl bromide; Antrocol; Arco-Lase Plus; Atropine Sulfate; Barbidonna; Bar-Tropin; Belap; Belladenal; Bentyl; Butibel; Cantil; Chardonna; Combid; Darbid; Daricon; Donnatal; Donphen; Dyspas; Eldonal; Enarax; Eta-Lent; Festalan; Gustase-Plus; Homapin; Hybephen; Kinesed; Kutrase; Levsin; Levsinex; Librax; Matropinal; Milpath; Octin; Pamine Bromide; Papaverine Hydrochloride; Pathibamate; Pathilon; Prantal; Pro-Banthine; Probital; Prydon; Robinul; Robinul w/Phenobarbital; Sedadrops; Sidonna; Tral; Trasentine; Trest; Trocinate; Valpin; Vistrax

Cancer Chemotherapy Adriamycin; Alkeran; Amnestrogen; Blenoxane; Cytoxan; Delalutin; Delestrogen; Drolban; Efudex; Estinyl; Fluoroplex;

Fluorouracil; FUDR; Hydrea; Imuran; Imuran Injection; Kenacort; Leukeran; Lysodren; Matulane; Megace; Methosarb; Methotrexate; Meticorten; Methracin; Mutamycin; Myleran; Oncovin; Oreton; Purinethol; TACE; Tesiac; Thioguanine; Thiotepa; Velban; Vercyte

Cardiovascular Preparations

Antianginal preparations: Amyl Nitrite; Antora; Duotrate; Inderal; Iso-Bid; Isordil Oral; Miltrate; Nitro-Bid; Nitroglyn; Nitrong; Nitrostat; Papaverine Hydrochloride; Paveril Phosphate; Peritrate; Persantine; SK-Petn; Sorbide; Sorbitrate

Antiarrhythmics: Cardioquin; Inderal; Isuprel; Oaubain; Pronestyl

Digitalis: Acylanid; Cedilanid; Crystodigin; Digoxin; Gitaligin; Lanoxin

Hypotensives: Aldactazide; Aldactone; Aldomet; Apresoline hydrochloride; Arfonad; Catapres; Diucardin; Diuril; Dralserp; Dralzine; Enduron; Esidrix; Eutonyl; Exna; Harmonyl; Hydro-DIURIL; Hydro-Z-50; Hygroton; Ismelin; Lasix; Lexxor; Moderil; Naqua; Naturetin; Nipride; Oretic; Raudixin; Rau-Sed; Renese; Saluron; Sandril; Serpasil; Unitensen; Aldactazide; Aldoclor; Aldoril; Apresoline-Esidrix; Butiserpazide; Butizide; Combipres; Diupres; Diutensen; Dyazide; Enduronyl; Esimil; Eutron; Exna-R; Hydromox; Hydropres; Hydrotensin-50; Metahydrin; Metatensin; Naquival; Oreticyl; Rauzide; Regroton; Renese-R; Salutensin; Ser-Ap-Es; Serpasil-Esidrix; Singoserp-Esidrix; Theocalcin

Other cardiovasculars: Dilor; Miradon; Ouabain; Paredrine; Proternol; Quinaglute; Thiomerin

Quinidine: Quinaglute; Quinidex; Quinidine; Quinora

Vasodilator, cerebral: Cebral; Cerespan; Circubid; Cyclospasmol; Ethaquin; Ethatab; Isovex-100; Kavrin; Menic; Pavabid; Pavacen; Pavased; Pavaspan; Pavatran; Pava-Wol; Sustaverine; Vasodilan; Vasospan

Vasodilator and combination: Cardilate; Duotrate; Isordil; Isuprel; Menic; Sorbitrate

Vasodilator, coronary: Aerolate; Amyl Nitrite; Antora; Cardilate; Cardilate-P; Cartrax; Corovas; Duotrate; Eta-Lent; Iso-Bid; Isordil; Kavrin; Nitro-Bid; Nitroglyn; Nitrol; Nitrong; Nitrospan; Papavatral; Pavacen; Pavadel; Pavased; Pavatran; Pava-Wol; Pentritol; Peritrate; Persantine; Sorbide;

Sorbitrate; Sustaverine; Tensodin; Theocalcin; Vasal; Vasospan

Vasodilator, general: Arlidin; Athemol; Cebral; Cerebid; Cerespan; Circubid; Ethatab; Isovex-100; Kavrin; Pava-Wol; Sustaverine

Vasodilator, peripheral: Arlidin; Athemol; Athemol-N; Cebral; Circubid; Cyclospasmol; Dibensyline; Eta-Lent; Ethaquin; Ethatab; Isovex-100; Kavrin; Menic; Niac; Nico-400; Pavabid Plateau; Pavadel; Pavased; Pavatran TD; Pava-Wol; Priscoline; Roniacol; Sustaverine; Tensodin; Vasodilan; Vasospan

Vasopressor: Aramine; Intropin; Levophed Bitartrate; Vasoxyl

Contraceptives, Oral
Brevicon; Demulen; Demulen-28; Enovid; Loestrin; Lo/Ovral; Micronor; Norinyl; Norlestrin; Nor-Q.D.; Norquen; Oracon, Oracon-28; Ortho-Novum; Ovral; Ovrette; Ovulen; Zorane

Diuretics

Mercurial: Dicurin Procaine; Thiomerin Injection

Other: Aldactone; Diamox; Diamox, Sequels; Dyrenium; Edecrin; Hydromox; Hydromox R; Hygroton; Lasix; Mannitol; Theocalcin; Ureaphil; Zaroxolyn

Thiazide and combination: Aldactazide; Anhydron; Aquatag; Aquatensen; Diupres; Diuril Intravenous Sodium; Diutensen; Diutensen-R; Dyazide; Enduron; Enduronly; Esidrix; Exna; Exna-R; Hydrochlorothiazide; HydroDIURIL; Hydropres; Hydrotensin-50; Hydrotensin-Plus; Hydro-Z-50; Lexxor; Metahydrin; Metatensin; Naqua; Naquival; Naturetin; Oretic; Renese; Renese-R; Saluron

Hemostatics
Amicar; Gelfoam; Konakion; Oxycel; Surgicel Absorbable Hemostat; Thrombin

Hormones
ACTH: Acthar

Anabolic: Deca-Durabolin; Dianabol; Durabolin; Os-Cal Mone; Winstrol

Androgens: Anadrol-50; Android-5; Delatestryl; Depo-Testosterone Cypionate; Halotestin; Metandren; Methosarb; Oreton; Testred; Virilon

Estrogens: Amnestrogen; Delestrogen; Depo-Estradiol; Diethylstilbestrol; Estinyl; Estradurin;

Evex; Feminone; Femogen; Hormonin; Menagen; Menest; Menrium; Milprem; Ogen; Premarin; SK-Estrogens; TACE

Androgen and estrogen, combination: Android-G; Deladumone; Depo-Testadiol; Ditate-DS; Estratest; Formatrix; Gevrine; Gynetone; Halodrin; Mediatric; Os-Cal Mone; Testand-B; Test-Estrin; Tylosterone

Glucocorticoid: Aristocort; Aristospan; Ataraxoid; Benisone; Celestone; Cortef; Cortenema; Cortifoam; Cortisone; Decaderm; Decadron-La; Delta-Cortef; Delta-Dome; Deltasone; Depo-Medrol; Deronil; Dexamethasone; Dexone; Florinef; Gammacorten; Haldrone; Hexadrol; Kenacort; Medrol; Meticorten; Orasone; Oxylone; Prednisone; Solu-Medrol; Sterane; Sterapred; Triamcinolone

Gonadotropin: A.P.L.; Follutein

Mineralocorticoid: Florinef Acetate; Percorten

Progestogens: Amen; Delalutin; Depo-Provera; Gynorest; Micronor; Norlutate; Norlutin; Nor-Q.D.; Prolutin; Provera

Progestogens and estrogens, combination: Brevicon; Demulen; Duphaston; Enovid; Norinyl; Norquen; Ortho-Novum; Ovral; Ovulen; Zorane

Immunosuppressive Imuran

Laxatives Bu-Lax; Colace; Comfolax; Dialose; DILAX-100; DioMedicone; Di-Sosul Forte; Doctate-P; Dorbantyl; Doxinate; Effersyllium; Geriplex-FS; Konsyl; L.A. Formula; Maltsupex; Metamucil; Milkinol; Movicol; Neolax; Sarolax; Sof-Cil; Stimulax; Surfak; Syllact; Syllamalt; Trilax; Turicum

Mineral oil: Fleet Mineral Oil

Muscle Relaxants, Skeletal Muscle Anectine; Dantrium; Metubine; Norflex; Paraflex; Quelicin; Quinamm; Robaxin; Robaxin Injectable; Robaxin-750; Skelaxin; Soma; Sucrostrin; Tubocurarine Chloride; Valium

Nutritional Aids (*see also* **Vitamins**) A/G-PRO; Android-G; Beelith; Ca-PLUS; Chlorophyll Complex; Citrotein; Compleat-B; Controlyte; Dietene; Flexical Elemental Diet; Gevral Protein; Hycal; Incremin w/Iron; Isocal Complete Liquid Diet; K-Phos Neutral; Lolactene; Lysmins; Magnesium

Gluconate; Magora-Forte; Mediatric; Meritene; Mevanin-C; Neutra-Phos; Niarb; Niferex w/Vitamin C; Norlac; Nuclomin; Nutri-1000; P.D.P. Liquid Protein; Precision Moderate Nitrogen Diet; Support; Vivonex; Zinc-220; Zn-PLUS

Parasympathetic Agents and Parasympathomimetics Andro Medicone; Mestinon; Myotonachol; Prostigmin; Urecholine

Parasympatholytic Agents Akineton; Antrenyl bromide; Antrocol; Bellergal; Bentyl; Cantil; Combid; Darbid; Homapin; Kinesed; Levsin; Levsinex; Matropinal; Oxoids; Trac; Tral; Trasentine; Trest

Sedatives

Barbiturates: Alurate; Amytal; Belap; Butisol Sodium; Carbrital; Corovas; Dialog; Donphen; Duotrate; Eskabarb; Luminal; Matropinal; Mebaral; Nebralin; Nembutal; Oxoids; Pamine PB; Pento-Del; Plexonal; Qui-A-Zone III; Repan; S.B.P.; Seconal; Sedadrops; Sedapap; Sed-Tens; Solfoton; Tuinal

Nonbarbiturates: Aquachloral; Beta-Chlor; Bromural; Dalmane; Equanil; Felsules; Levoprome; Noctec; Noludar, Noludar 300; Parest; Phenergan; Placidyl; QIDbamate; Quaalude; Quadnite; Sopor; Tranxene; ZIPAN

Sympatholytics Bellergal; Regitine

Sympathomimetics and Combination Aerolate; Aerolone; Amesec; Arlidin; Benzedrine Sulfate; Biphetamine; Brethine; Bronkometer; Bronkosol; Delcobese; Demazin; Desoxyn; Dexamyl; Dexedrine; D-Feda; Didrex; Drinus; Extasule; Entex; Extendryl; Fedrazil; Histabid; Hista-Clopane; Intropin; Isuprel; Levophed Bitartrate; Metaprel; microNEFRIN; Napril Plateau; Neo-Synephrine; Nolamine; Obetrol; Otrivin; Oxoids; Rondec; Sinacet; Slo-Fedrin; Sudafed; Sus-Phrine; Triaminic; Trimtabs; Tussagesic; Tussaminic; Ursinus; Vasoxyl; Ventaire

Thyroid Preparations

Antithyroid: Propylthiouracil; Tapazole

Synthetic thyroid hormone: Choloxin; Letter; Synthroid; Thyrolar

Thyroid: Armour Thyroid; Cytomel; Euthroid;

Letter; Proloid; S-P-T; Synthroid; Thyroid Strong; Thyrolar

Thyrotropic hormone: Thytropar

Thyroxine sodium: Choloxin; Cytolen; Levoid; Synthroid

Tonics Betacrest; Bironate-B; C-B Time; Hep-Forte; Hytinic; I.L.X.; Nicotinex; Niferex; Nutricol; Panafort

Vitamins

B Complex with C: B-C-Bid; Becotin with Vitamin C; Thex Forte

Multivitamins: A.C.N.; Adabee; Al Vite; Allbee w/C; B-C-Bid; Becotin; Beminal; Berocca; Betalin Complex; Bironate-B; C-B Time; Cefol; Clusivol; Dayalets; Feosol Plus; Folbesyn; Fortespan; Gerilets; Larobec; Lederplex; Mega-B; Monster; Multicebrin; Mulvidren; M.V.I.; Peridin-C; Probec-T; RoeriBeC; Sigtab; Solu-B; Stresscaps; Stuart Therapeutic; Surbex; Therabid; Theracebrin; Thera-Combex II-P; Theragran; Thex Forte; Trophite; Vi-Aqua; Vicon Forte; Vi-Daylin; Vigran; Vi-Magna; Vio-Bec; Vi-Zac

Multivitamins with minerals: Adabee w/Minerals; Cardenz; Clusivol; Dayalets plus Iron; En-Cebrin; Engran-HP; Feminins; Foralicon Plus; Fosfree; Gevrabon; Gevrite; Hemo-Vite; Iromin-G; Livitamin; Lysmins; Mega-Vita; Mevanin-C; Mg-+C; Mi-Cebrin; Myadec; Niarb; Nuclomin; Optilets; Poly-Vi-Sol; Pramocon; Probec; Sclerex; Tagus; Testand-B; Thera-Delmal; Theragran; Theron; Troph-Iron; Ulvical; Vi-Aquamin; Vi-Daylin; Vigran plus Iron; Vi-Sorbin; Vitacrest; Viterra; Vi-Zac

Parenteral: AquaMephyton; Berocca-C; Hexa-Betalin; Illopan; M.V.I.; Rubramin PC; Vicam

Pediatrics: AquaMephyton; C-B Time; Cari-Tab; Hepp-Iron; Monster; Monster with Iron; Mulvidren; PALS; PALS plus Iron; Poly-Vi-Sol; Tri-Vi-Sol; Vi-Daylin; Vi-Daylin ADC; Vi-Daylin Plus Iron ADC; Vi-Daylin Plus Iron; Vi-Penta

Pediatrics with fluoride: Adeflor B; Adeflor; Mulvidren-F; Novacebrin; Poly-V-Flor; Tri-Vi-Flor; Vi-Daylin/F ADC; Vi-Daylin with Fluoride; Vi-Penta; Vi-Penta F Multivitamin

Therapeutic: Al Vite; B-C-Bid; Becotin-T; Betazyme; Cetane; Cevi-Bid; Folic Acid; Gevral T; Hep-Forte; Hexa-Betalin; Mega-B; Mi-Cebrin T; Niac; Nico-400; Nicobid; Nicolar; Stresstabs 600; Therabid; Theron; Thex Forte; Tokols; Vicon Forte; Vicon-Plus; Vio-Bec; Vi-Zac

Recognition of Medical Problems from a Patient's Medication

This table is designed to facilitate identification of a patient's medical problem on the basis of the patient's medication. Often patients will be taking medications without full knowledge of their medical problems. Also, some patients will tell you the medications they are taking but will fail to give the reason for this medication. The table is designed so that the generic or group name is written in parentheses after the trade name.

Medical problem	Trade and Group or generic names of common medications
Addison's disease	Cortisone (corticosteroids)
Allergy	Benadryl, Chlortrimeton, Dimetane (antihistamines)
Angina pectoris	Amylnitrate (amylnitrate), Nitro-Bid, Nitrostat (nitro-glycerin), Inderal (propranolol)
Birth control	Enovid, Ovulen (estrogen-progestogen combination)
Cancer	Mustargen, Alkeran (alkylating agents); methotrexate, fluorouracil (antimetabolites); Velban (alkaloid); doxorubicin, dactinomycin (antibiotics)
Convulsions, epilepsy	Dilantin (diphenylhydantoin or phentyoin), Mysoline (primidone), Luminal (barbiturate)
Diabetes	Iletin (insulin), Orinase (tolbutamide), Diabinese (chlorpropamide), Dymelor (acetohexamide), DBI (phenformin hydrochloride)

Medical problem	Trade and Group or generic names of common medications
Heart failure	Digoxin, Lanoxin (digitalis), Quindex (quinidine), Inderal (propranolol), Pronestyl (procainamide), Diamox (acetazolamide and other diuretics)
Heart murmur related to rheumatic fever history	Various forms of penicillin or erythromycin (see Chap. 4 and App. F).
Hypertension	Reserpine (Rauwolfia alkaloids), Thiazide (diuretics), Apresoline (hydralazine), Ismelin (guanethidine), Aldomet (methyldopa).
Hyperthyroidism	Propylthiouracil (thiouracils)
Hypothyroidism	Cytomel, Proloid (thyroid extract), Choloxin, Synthroid (thyroxine)
Mental problems	Chlorpromazine, Compazine, Sparine (phenothiazines); Miltown, Equanil (meprobamates); Parnate (monamine oxidase inhibitor); Tofranil, Elavil (tricyclic antidepressants); Benzadrine, Dexedrine (amphetamines); Desoxyn, Norodin, Fetamin, Phelantin (methamphetamines)
Myasthenia gravis	Prostigmin (neostigmine, a cholinesterase inhibitor)
Parkinson's disease	Cogentin (benzotropine); Artane (trihexyphenidyl); Larodopa, Bendopa (levodopas)
Pemphigus	Cortisone (corticosteroids)
Peptic or duodenal ulcer	Banthine (methantheline); Probanthine (propantheline); Digel, Gelusol, Maalox (antacids); Prydon, Chardonna (atropine); Butibel (belladonna)
Predisposed to blood clots	Dicumarol, Coumadin (bishydroxycoumarin), Panwarfin (warfarin sodium), Hedulin (phenindione)
Rheumatoid arthritis, allergies	Cortisone (corticosteroids)

Toxicity Reports*

ASBESTOS[1]

Asbestos is chiefly used in dentistry as a binder in periodontal dressings and as a lining material for casting rings and crucibles. Asbestos is a generic term for a number of hydrated silicate minerals which, under crushing or other processing procedures, separate into flexible fibers. There are many such minerals, including chrysotile, asmosite, crocidolite, anthophyllite, tremolite, and actinolite. Most asbestos is classified as chrysotile and it appears to be the most hazardous fiber in the group.

It has been documented that airborne asbestos is related causally to the development of pulmonary asbestosis and fibrosis,[2-4] lung cancer,[5-7] and pleural and peritoneal mesotheliomas.[8-10] Recent epidemiologic studies also have indicated that the chance of lung cancer developing in smokers ex-posed to airborne asbestos is greater than it is in nonsmokers.[11-13]

The potential danger to dental personnel in preparation of asbestos-containing periodontal packs is of sufficient concern that the Council on Dental Therapeutics will no longer consider such products as eligible for its Acceptance Program. Airborne asbestos may become hazardous during the mixing of these asbestos-containing periodontal dressings, particularly when large amounts are being prepared in poorly ventilated areas and when the powder is shaken prior to mixing.[14,15] Also, exposure to airborne fibers may occur in dental laboratories where asbestos is used to line casting rings or crucibles for casting machines and in general is kept in the laboratory in large rolls. Here, the danger lies in the tendency for personnel to carelessly cut sections off these rolls and thus release asbestos into the ambient air. The maximum permissible exposure of an employee to airborne concentrations of asbestos fibers over an eight-hour, time-weighted average has been established as five fibers (longer than 5 μm) per cubic centimeter of air.[16] On July 1, 1976, the maximum was reduced to two such fibers per cubic centimeter of air. This is of importance to the dentist operating his own laboratory as well as to the employees in commercial dental laboratories. To prevent release of fibers into the air, asbestos should be handled, applied, removed, cut, or otherwise worked in a wet state to reduce the emission of airborne asbestos. Personnel should be aware that soaking of asbestos liners in water releases fibers into the community sewage line and, therefore, suitable trapping of such wastes is recommended.

There is no apparent health danger from inhalation to patients for whom asbestos-containing periodontal dressings are used, since the fibers cannot be appreciably released from the dressings once they are mixed and applied. In addition, present information indicates that there is little danger to patients should the dressings be accidentally swallowed. According to the Food and Drug Administration, "evidence concerning the possible hazard from ingestion of asbestos particles is contradicting and inconclusive."[17]

There is, however, evidence that parenteral administration of asbestos in animals can result in local malignancies, malignant mesothelioma, and dissemination of fibers in lymph nodes, spleen, kidneys, and brain.[18-20] Therefore, the Council on Dental Therapeutics is concerned about the asbestos concentration of filters used for preparing drugs that may be injected parenterally by dentists. Such filters may release asbestos particles into the solution and thus be injected into the patient. The Food and Drug Administration is surveying the industry for information concerning the use of such filters.

MERCURY[21]

Specific comments on hair analyses as a means to assess mercury exposure by the dentist and his staff are appropriate. There is no danger of a chronic low-level exposure to mercury for the patient who may have amalgam restorations,[22,23] but there is concern for the dentist and his staff.[24,25]

Current Status

Current data suggest that absorption of atmospheric mercury through the lungs is the primary route of absorption by the dental team. Vaporization of mercury results from the various mercury spills. Another potential source of mercury exposure is the routine use of hand expression of mercury from a wet trituration mix. Although mercury is not absorbed to any appreciable extent through intact skin, the combination of frequent contact with mercury and minor skin abrasions could result in significant mercury absorption via this route. Still another source is the inhalation of amalgam particulates during removal of old restorations. A study with animals[26] has shown that the animals breathing the total atmosphere during air-cooled high-speed grinding of fresh amalgam absorbed significant quantities of mercury. In the study no attempt was made to differentiate the amount of mercury absorbed from the mercury vapor and that absorbed from the amalgam particulate. There are no data to substantiate the significance of absorption from amalgam particulates.

Hair is an attractive substrate for mercury analysis.[27-30] It is easy to sample and is stable. Since the hair surface reacts with atmospheric mercury, data from hair analysis for mercury could be a composite of the mercury absorbed systemically and incorporated into the hair during formation and the mercury adsorbed on the hair from the atmosphere. A fourfold to sevenfold higher level of mercury has been reported for the mercury content of exposed hair and nails of dental personnel than for the clothing-covered tissues of these same personnel; this indicates that atmospheric, direct contact and systemic sources of mercury contribute to the total mercury levels.[31]

The amount of mercury adsorbed onto the hair surface depends on vapor concentration, duration of exposure, and the individual characteristics of the hair. In general the tip of a long hair will have more mercury per unit of length than the tip of a short hair. The surface mercury can be removed by appropriate sample preparation, but the mercury incorporated during hair formation is not readily removed, according to Giovanoli-Jakubczak and co-workers[32] and unpublished data by Hefferren. A recent study[33] has attempted to use a mathematic model to account for the mercury content from systemic and topical sources. This study was based on mercury analyses of sequential head hair segments from the tip to the root. Analytical, unpublished data by Hefferren accumulated to date on total mercury levels of hair have not shown good general correlation with mercury exposure and absorption as measured by atmospheric monitoring and assay of biologic fluids—blood, urine, and saliva.

Recommendation: Until this situation is resolved by further studies, it is well to consider conservatively mercury levels in hair as indicative and not a definitive measure of mercury absorption by dental personnel.

RECOMMENDATIONS IN MERCURY HYGIENE

Council on Dental Materials and Devices

The Council on Dental Materials and Devices is preparing, as directed by the 1975 House of Delegates, standards for mechanical amalgamators, capsules, and proportioners to minimize spillage of mercury. The following recommendations for mercury hygiene are being republished for the information of our readers.

1 Store mercury in unbreakable, tightly sealed containers.

2 Perform all operations involving mercury over areas that have impervious and suitably lipped surfaces so as to confine and facilitate recovery of spilled mercury or amalgam.

3 Clean up any spilled mercury immediately. Droplets may be picked up with narrow bore tubing connected (via a wash-bottle trap) to the low-volume aspirator of the dental unit.

4 Use tightly closed capsules during amalgamation.

5 Use a no-touch technique for handling the amalgam.

6 Salvage all amalgam scrap and store it under water.

7 Work in well-ventilated spaces.

8 Avoid carpeting dental operatories as decontamination is not possible.

9 Eliminate the use of mercury-containing solutions.

10 Avoid heating mercury or amalgam.

11 Use water spray and suction when grinding dental amalgam.

12 Use conventional dental amalgam compacting procedures, manual and mechanical, but do not use ultrasonic amalgam condensors.

13 Perform yearly mercury determinations on all personnel regularly employed in dental offices.

14 Have periodic mercury vapor level determinations made in operatories.

15 Alert all personnel involved in handling of mercury, especially during training or indoctrination periods, of the potential hazard of mercury vapor and the necessity for observing good mercury hygiene practices.

REFERENCES

[1] From: *Journal of the American Dental Association,* April 1976, V. 92, pp. 777–778.

[2] Cooke, W. E. Fibrosis of lungs due to the inhalation of asbestos dust. Br Med J 2:147 July 26, 1924.

[3] Cooke, W. E. Pulmonary asbestosis. Br Med J 2:1024 Dec 3, 1927.

[4] McDonald, S. Histology of pulmonary asbestosis. Br Med J 2:1025 Dec 3, 1927.

[5] Doll, R. Mortality from lung cancer in asbestos workers. Br J Industr Med 12:81 April 1955.

[6] Cordova, J. F.; Tesluk, H.; and Knudtson, K. P. As-

[7] Selikoff, I. J.; Churg, J.; and Hammond, E. C. Asbestos exposure and neoplasia. JAMA 188:22 April 6, 1964.

[8] Hammond, E. C.; Selikoff, I. J.; and Churg, J. Neoplasia among insulation workers in the United States with special reference to intraabdominal neoplasia. Ann NY Acad Sci 132:519 Dec 31, 1965.

[9] Lieben, J., and Pistawka, H. Mesothelioma and asbestos exposure. Arch Environ Health 14:559 April 1967.

[10] Owen, W. G. Mesothelial tumors and exposure to asbestos dust. Ann NY Acad Sci 132:674 Dec 31, 1965.

[11] Warnock, M. L., and Churg, A. M. Association of asbestos and bronchogenic carcinoma in a population with low asbestos exposure. Cancer 35:1236 April 1975.

[12] Berry, G.; Newhouse, M. L.; and Turok, M. Combined effect of asbestos exposure and smoking on mortality from lung cancer in factory workers. Lancet 2:476 Sept 2, 1972.

[13] Selikoff, I. J.; Hammond, E. C.; and Churg, J. Asbestos exposure, smoking and neoplasia. JAMA 204:106 April 1968.

[14] Otterson, E. J., and Arra, M. C. Potential hazards of asbestos in periodontal pact. J Wis Dent Assoc 50:435 Nov 1974.

[15] Dyer, M. R. The possible adverse effects of asbestos in gingivectomy packs. Br Dent J 122:507 June 6, 1967.

[16] Federal Register 39:23543 June 27, 1974.

[17] Federal Register 38:27076 Sept 28, 1973.

[18] Harington, J. S., and Roe, F. J. Studies of carcinogenesis of asbestos fibers and their natural fibers. Ann NY Acad Sci 132:439, 1965.

[19] Roe, F. J., and others. The pathological effects of subcutaneous injections of asbestos fibres in mice: migration of fibres to submesothelial tissues and induction of mesotheliomata. Int J Cancer 2:628 Nov 15, 1967.

[20] Kanazawa, K., and others. Migration of asbestos fibres from subcutaneous injection sites in mice. Br J Cancer 24:96 March 1970.

[21] From: J Am Dent Assoc, June 1976, V. 92, pp. 1213–1217.

[22] Frykholm, K. O. On mercury from dental amalgam. Its toxic and allergic effects and some comments on occupational hygiene. Acta Odontol Scand 15:7 (Suppl 22) 1957.

[23] Frykholm, K. O., and Odeblad, E. Studies on the penetration of mercury through the dental hard tissue, using ^{203} Hg in silver amalgam fillings. Acta Odontol Scand 13:157 Nov 1955.

[24] Criteria for a recommended standard . . . Occupational exposure to inorganic mercury. Department of Health, Education, and Welfare, Public Health Service, National Institute for Occupation Safety and Health, 1973.

[25] Council on Dental Materials and Devices, Council on Dental Research. Rupp, N. W., and Paffenbarger, G. C. Significance to health of mercury used in dental practice: a review. JADA 82:1401 June 1971.

[26] Cutright, D. E., and others. Systemic mercury levels caused by inhaling mist during high-speed amalgam grinding. J Oral Med 28:100 1973.

[27] Lenihan, J. M. A.; Leslie, A. C. D.; and Smith, H. Mercury in the hair of Robert Burns. Lancet 2:1030 Nov 6, 1971.

[28] Perkons, A. K., and Jervis, R. E. Hair individual studies. Trans 2nd Int Conf Modern Trends in Activation Analysis, 1965, p 295.

[29] Yamaguchi, S., and others. Relationship between mercury content of hair and amount of fish consumed. HSMHA Health Rep 86:904 Oct 1971.

[30] Nord, P. J.; Kadaba, M. P.; and Sorenson, J. R. J. Mercury in human hair. Arch Environ Health 27:40 July 1973.

[31] Nixon, G. S., and Smith, H. Hazard of mercury poisoning in dental surgery. J. Oral Ther 1:512 March 1965.

[32] Giovanoli-Jakubczak, T., and others. Determination of total and inorganic mercury in hair by flameless atomic absorption and of methylmercury by gas chromatography. Clin Chem 20:222, 1974.

[33] Giovanoli-Jakubczak, T., and Berg, G. G. Measurement of mercury in human hair. Arch Environ Health 28:139 March 1974.

Hepatitis and Dental Practice[1]*

Recent publications in the medical literature[2,3] indicate that an increased risk of viral hepatitis infections exists not only for physicians, as has been documented in the past, but also for dentists, and particularly for some dental specialists. An increased hazard in dentistry had not previously been clearly recognized. The specialty groups in dentistry at greatest risk of contracting viral hepatitis are those whose work includes surgery with frequent exposure to blood. Oral surgeons are known to be at greater risk,[4] and periodontists also may be a high risk group because of their exposure to blood.

Since 1968, when the "Australia" antigen, now known as the hepatitis B surface antigen (HBsAg), was recognized as a serologic marker of hepatitis B virus (HBV) infection, it has been possible to differentiate type B from non-B hepatitis and to identify carriers of the type B virus.[5] As more and more carriers are identified through serologic testing, epidemiologic evidence tends to indicate that the traditional concept that HBV is transmitted only by obvious percutaneous introduction is no longer valid. In addition to transfer of serum as the means of transmission, it now appears that saliva can be a primary vehicle in oral-oral or even repiratory transmission of type B hepatitis.[6] Air-borne droplets from sneezing or coughing are a possible means of transmitting the disease, and saliva-contaminated objects such as dental instruments could conceivably be responsible for transmitting type B hepatitis.

It now appears that carriers of type B hepatitis do not present as great a risk to casual contacts as was thought in the late 1960s,[7] but contact with a person with acute hepatitis or contact with a carrier does pose the risk of acquiring this serious and debilitating disease. If contact is made with a person with an acute case or with a carrier and the disease is transmitted, the incubation period for type B hepatitis ranges from 28 to 180 days, with most cases occurring 65 to 95 days after exposure.

In the typical case, HBsAg develops 20 to 100 days after exposure, is detectable in the serum for 1 to 120 days, and then disappears. The serum becomes negative for surface antigen and in most instances antibody to HBsAg (anti-HBs) develops and is detectable in the serum for many years thereafter.[8] Immunity is evidenced by the presence of anti-HBs, and the antibody is a serum marker for previous HBV infection.

Approximately 5% to 10% of persons infected with the disease will circulate HBsAg for up to 2 years or for as long as 25 years. This situation is referred to as the chronic carrier state, and all present data indicate that blood and possibly other body fluids from the chronic HBsAg carrier are infectious for type B hepatitis. The serum of some persons who have been carriers for several years has converted from being positive for HBsAg to being negative for the antigen.[9]

The course of the acute illness is usually divided into two symptomatic phases: a prejaundiced and a jaundiced phase. The prejaundiced (anicteric) phase is characterized by loss of appetite, nausea, vomiting, abdominal discomfort, general weakness, and in some patients headache, fever, and muscle soreness. This phase may last from several days to more than a week. In the jaundiced (icteric) phase, the eyes become yellow, stools are white or gray in color, and the urine is brownish. Within two to six weeks, jaundice and other symptoms gradually subside.[8] In many instances, the patients do not become jaundiced but have most of the other symptoms, as well as serologic and biochemical evidence of the disease; this immunity or the carrier state may develop without prior knowlege of infection.

It is very important to examine the issue of whether health care personnel who become chronic antigen carriers should continue to have contact with patients.[10] Some dentists are reported to have been restricted from having direct contact with patients when there was definite evidence that they were chronic antigen carriers and were transmitting the disease to their patients. They have been forced to give up their practices until their serum no longer is positive for HBsAg or until antibody to HBsAg develops. The economic impact for a dentist, un-

able to continue practice, is much more overwhelming than the possible loss of two to six weeks from the practice during an acute episode of the disease. The carrier state, the prevalence of the disease in dentists, and its transmission and possible prevention are discussed in this paper in a question-and-answer format.

PREVALENCE AMONG DENTAL PERSONNEL

Question *What proportion of viral hepatitis in dental personnel is serologically identifiable as type B?*

Answer Among 1,245 general dentists participating in the Health Screening Program at the 1972 annual session of the American Dental Association in San Francisco, there was a 13.6% frequency of serologic evidence for prior infection by HBV.[11] There are no data available to indicate the incidence among dental personnel of other serologic types of hepatitis (that is, type A hepatitis and "non-A, non-B" hepatitis), but type B hepatitis probably accounts for at least a half of those cases that occur during professionally active life.[11,12] Measures that will prevent the occurrence of type B hepatitis, therefore, should reduce by a substantial proportion the rate of viral hepatitis among dental personnel.

Question *Are members of the dental profession (dentists, dental hygienists, and dental assistants) at greater risk in contracting type B hepatitis than the general population?*

Answer Yes. Several studies[2,3,11–13] indicate that dentists are at higher risk than the general population and that the incidence of type B hepatitis antigen and antibody in dentists is similar to that in physicians.[14] Epidemiologic data indicate that approximately 0.5% of the general population may be carriers of HBsAg, whereas the percentage of carriers among health care workers is estimated to be 1% to 2%.[15] It is estimated that dentists in general practice have two to four times the risk of acquiring type B hepatitis than do persons not in health care professions. The risk for other dental personnel, including dental hygienists and dental assistants, appears to be lower and may not be different than for a comparable socioeconomic group in the general population according to J. L. Smith of the Phoenix

Laboratories Division, Bureau of Epidemiology, Center for Disease Control.

Question *Are certain dental specialty groups at higher risk than dentists in general practice?*

Answer Yes. Those who have greater exposure to blood in their practices show a higher incidence of serologic evidence of type B hepatitis. In unpublished data by Mosley and coworkers from a recent survey conducted at the 1974 national meeting of the American Society of Oral Surgeons, these rates were found among 650 participants:

—prevalence of presumed carriers (serum positive on a single occasion for HBsAg), 2.3%;

—prevalence of humoral immunity (serum positive for type B hepatitis antibodies, 27%; and

—incidence of overt hepatitis during active professional life, 13%.

At the present time, published reports[2-4] and unpublished data by Mosley and co-workers indicate that oral surgeons are at greater risk than any other professional group. Orthodontists have been surveyed, but the results are not yet available. There is insufficient data on other specialty groups to make a valid statement at this time. The prevalence of probable carriers of HBsAg among oral surgeons of approximately 2% to 3% justifies intensive examination of means to prevent further transmission of the disease.

Question *Are additional surveys required to identify specialists at risk?*

Answer Yes. Surveys are just now beginning to identify groups at greatest risk, and additional groups must be examined. This is especially true if passive (hepatitis B immune globulin) or active immunization is to be most effectively used.

SERUM TESTING

Question *When serum is tested and found to be positive for HBsAg, is this equivalent to the presence of virus in the blood?*

Answer Yes. The assumption should be made that antigenemia is synonymous with viremia. Most, but not all, of the evidence favors this view. It is possible, however, for individuals to be viremic (capable of transmitting the virus itself) even though the HBsAg level is too low to be detected by present serologic techniques. In most posttransfusion studies, the majority of persons who have received HBsAg-positive units of blood have subsequently had serologic evidence of infection—either subsequent positivity for HBsAg, a late antibody response, clinical evidence of the disease, or a combination of these.

Question *Should serologic testing of dental personnel be done routinely?*

Answer Routine serologic testing of dental personnel is not recommended at this time, and anyone who is asked to be tested should be permitted to decline without any adverse action or censure. However, it is extremely important to assess fully the risk in various groups and, therefore, testing in an investigative situation, such as a survey, in which anonymity can be maintained, is encouraged.

Question *Is there a time or circumstance when a person with hepatitis or a carrier is most likely to transmit the disease?*

Answer Individuals with either acute or chronic type B hepatitis infection can transmit the disease. At the present time it is assumed that the disease is infectious and, therefore, potentially contagious in any person whose serum is HBsAg positive. Whether variations occur in the ease with which the person can transmit the infection is not known.

IMMUNOLOGICAL PROTECTION AGAINST HEPATITIS B

Question *Are there effective agents for preexposure and postexposure prophylaxis against type A and type B hepatitis?*

Answer Normal immune serum globulin preparations have been effective against type A hepatitis from the very first experiments and continue to be effective. The risk of type A hepatitis in routine dental practice, however, is too low to make routine preexposure prophylaxis worthwhile, with the possible exception of dental personnel working in institutions in which type A hepatitis is endemic or epidemic. There are no situations in the United States in which immune serum globulin is used routinely except for postexposure prophylaxis.

There is no ready answer to the question of using normal immune serum globulin preparations for preexposure or postexposure prophylaxis against hepatitis B virus. Until hyperimmune serum globulin (containing high levels of anti-HBs) has been established as useful, it is probably worthwhile to use normal globulin only if there is serum-to-serum or serum-to-saliva contact with an infected person.

Question *If an oral surgeon found it absolutely necessary to perform surgery on a known carrier of HBsAg, should he receive normal immune serum globulin prophylactically?*

Answer No.

Question *If an oral surgeon performs surgery on a known carrier of HBsAg and receives a needle prick or cuts his hand, should he receive normal immune serum globulin?*

Answer Each situation must be evaluated individually on the basis of the extent of the exposure and the immune status of the surgeon with respect to HBV. If the patient's blood is positive for HBsAg, the surgeon has had definite exposure. If the surgeon's serum is negative for anti-HBs or cannot be promptly tested for antibody, a 5-ml injection from a recently prepared lot of normal immune serum globulin is recommended.

Question *Are special immune serum globulin preparations for prevention of type B hepatitis available and if so, are they effective?*

Answer Hepatitis B immune globulin preparations are not yet licensed for clinical use, although the material is sometimes obtainable through institutions approved to use it as an Investigational New Drug. Availability, however, is limited to situations in which there is definite percutaneous exposure to known type B hepatitis. Uncontrolled studies already published[16] and controlled investigations for which reports are now in press show modest to good levels of effectiveness for preexposure and postexposure prophylaxis in various situations. The only apparent disadvantage to its use is that it suppresses not only clinical disease, but also subclinical infection, thereby preventing active immunity from developing as passive immunity wanes.

For at least dentists and dental specialists with a sufficiently high risk of type B hepatitis (for example, oral surgeons), routine preexposure prophylaxis may be advised when recommendations are formulated. The dose and frequency of injection will have to be determined.

Question *What is the status of the specific vaccines that have been discussed in the recent medical literature?*

Answer Research groups that have developed type B hepatitis vaccines are now in the process of testing their safety, immunogenicity, and effectiveness in chimpanzees. The vaccines thus far do appear to be safe, and it is estimated that the data from the animal model will be evaluated within the next six months. These vaccines can then be tested for safety and effectiveness in humans. The vaccine may be available in five to ten years if the safety and efficacy studies are successful.

THE HIGH-RISK PATIENT

Question *In an effort to prevent the transmission of type B hepatitis to the dentist or dental personnel, is there information from a patient's medical history or clinical signs on physical examination that can be helpful in identifying those individuals likely to have HBV infection?*

Answer Seldom can a patient's history be relied on to yield information that would indicate whether the person is likely to be a carrier. Even if the history reveals that a patient has had hepatitis, this does not necessarily mean that he had type B hepatitis or that the disease is still infectious. In fact, the disease would be infectious in no more than 5% to 10% of patients with a history of icteric type B hepatitis six months or more in the past. There is nothing that can be determined from a physical examination that would alert the dentist to a possible hepatitis carrier unless the patient is jaundiced or has needle marks characteristic of illicit self-injection.

Question *What are the groups that pose the highest risk of HBV infection in the dental office?*

Answer Patients undergoing chronic hemodialysis for renal disease; patients institutionalized for mental retardation, especially Down's syndrome; patients with malignancy treated with frequent transfusions and immunosuppressive drugs; patients who receive blood and blood derivatives in large volumes, such as hemophiliacs; percutaneous drug abusers; and male homosexuals.[17]

Question *Should patients known to be in a high-risk group be asked to have serum tested for HBsAg before treatment?*

Answer No. For patients in a high-risk group, their personal physician should perhaps be contacted before a treatment program is begun, but testing should not be required before they are treated.

Question *Should dentists and dental personnel who treat patients in high-risk groups be advised to wear gloves in treating these patients?*

Answer Yes. The protection that gloves may provide should outweigh the inconvenience or cost of wearing them. The gloves should be disposable, and discarded immediately after treatment is concluded.

Question *Should oral surgeons be advised to wear gloves while treating all patients?*

Answer Yes. Bleeding often occurs with procedures used by oral surgeons, and there is the possibility of infection through minor inflammations or abrasions of the fingers.

Question *Should all dental care personnel be advised to wear gloves in treating all patients?*

Answer There does not seem to be enough evidence that gloves will provide sufficient protection to justify a universal recommendation of this type at the present time.

Question *Should all dental schools be urged to train their dental students to wear gloves?*

Answer Yes. Although very little evidence exists to support the use of gloves in preventing the spread of hepatitis, the use of gloves certainly should be encouraged in operative procedures that may result in bleeding. Gloves may be of particular value in protecting the dentist from viremic patients.

Question *Can a dentist refuse treatment to a known carrier of HBsAg?*

Answer A dentist can legally deny treatment to any patient, particularly one who is not a regular patient. The patient with unusual problems, such as a carrier of HBsAg, may be referred to a medical center or a hospital with clinics that are well equipped for handling these problems, provided that such a facility is available to the patient. The patient who is a carrier should receive a careful and considerate explanation of the problem, so that he is not made to feel that he is a social outcast because of his medical problem.

THE DENTIST WITH HEPATITIS

Question *Should a dentist with acute viral hepatitis practice?*

Answer No. A dentist who is acutely ill with the disease should not practice. In addition to his possible infectivity, it is very likely that the dentist will not be physically able to practice effectively, and resolution of his illness may be delayed. When the dentist's physician believes he is physically able to return to work, he can do so.

Question *Should a dentist whose serum is positive for HBsAg—the acute or chronic antigen carrier—discontinue his practice?*

Answer At the present time information is insufficient to permit a satisfactory answer to this question. There are reports in the literature of cases of hepatitis arising in patients treated by dentists whose serum was positive for HBsAg.[18,19] In contrast, another report shows no transmission to patients who were treated by two dentists in the late incubation period and early phase of illness; the serum of both these dentists was positive for HBsAg.[20] Another study reported two acute antigen carriers and two chronic antigen carriers who were nondental health care workers. Patient contacts of these four carriers did not contract the illness as a result of their exposure to the carriers.[21]

The factors that determine the infectivity of a carrier of type B hepatitis are unknown at the present time, but it appears that communicability from chronically infected dentists is negligible. A dentist who has HBsAg-positive serum should not be restricted from practice unless there is evidence that he is transmitting the disease to his patients. The dentist with HBsAg-positive serum, however, should make every effort to prevent transmission by good hygienic and sterilization practices. There is not enough evidence at the present time to indicate that all carrier dentists must be prevented from practicing.

Question *Can a dentist with serum positive for antibody to HBsAg safely practice?*

Answer Yes, definitely. The presence of anti-HBs indicates that a prior infection has resolved, and that immunity is present. The dentist whose serum is positive for anti-HBs is least likely to transmit the disease.

Question *When can a dentist return to his practice after an infection of hepatitis?*

Answer When the dentist's physician agrees that his health has returned to normal and he is able to practice effectively, he could return to his practice. If he had type B hepatitis but HBsAg is no longer detectable, then there is no known danger of person-to-person communicability.

PREVENTING TRANSMISSION

Question *What aspects of dental practice are particularly likely to result in transmission of HBV?*

Answer Certainly those procedures in which blood may be transferred from patient to dentist, patient to patient, and dentist to patient are likely to result in transmission of HBV. Blood on the hands and instruments and blood that gets into the eyes or oral or nasal cavities of dentists and dental personnel has the potential to transmit the virus. HBsAg has been detected in whole saliva of humans, but it is not known whether this is attributable to blood in whole saliva or is derived from gingival crevicular fluid. Studies have been done with pure parotid saliva and whole saliva in known carriers. HBsAg has not been detected in pure saliva but has been detected in whole saliva.[6,22] There is one instance of reported transmission by a human bite.[23]

While there are no specific data on perspiration as a possible means of transmission, it is possible that this may be a real problem for oral surgeons who perspire under surgical gloves while they operate. Nicks in a glove during surgery could theoretically permit the spread of virus from dentist to patient by way of perspiration or small amounts of blood.

Blood and whole saliva are possible means of type B hepatitis transmission in dental practice and these body fluids may be carried from patient to patient by contamination of the dentist's hand, gloves, or instruments. Another possible route may be the accidental transfer of blood during surgery into the eyes or onto mucosal surfaces. There is no direct evidence that the virus is aerosolized with saliva during use of the high-speed dental handpiece, but there is the possibility that the virus may be transmitted by this route.

Question *Can dentists who are carriers take satisfactory precautions to prevent transmission to their patients? If so, what precautions can they take?*

Answer Dentists and dental care personnel who know that they are carriers should be encouraged to wear gloves and face masks. This should be considered as a preventive measure, because there is no direct evidence that gloves and masks will significantly reduce the chances of transmission. There is evidence that the virus may be spread by transfer of saliva; therefore, any effort to reduce extrusion of droplets is encouraged. Studies should be done to determine if these measures are effective in reducing the spread of infection.

Question *Can all dental instruments be effectively sterilized to prevent the transmission of the hepatitis virus?*

Answer No. The manufacture of some dental handpieces is such that they cannot be sterilized. However, some handpieces now on the market can be sterilized by autoclaving or exposure to ethylene oxide gas.

Question *What agents and methods of sterilization are virucidal for HBV?*

Answer Several agents and methods are known to be effective sterilization procedures for HBV. Their efficacy has been confirmed by epidemiologic data from clinics and hospitals in which there was known evidence of type B hepatitis infection or the potential for its transmission. These methods include immersion in 100°C (boiling) water for 30 minutes, or exposure to saturated steam at 121°C and 15 psi pressure for 30 minutes, or dry heat at 160°C for one hour, or ethylene oxide gas at 10% concentration in carbon dioxide at 55 to 69°C for eight to ten hours.[24]

At the present time, it is not possible to culture HBV in tissue culture. The chimpanzee can be infected with HBV and is an excellent laboratory model of the disease. The chimpanzee with HBV can be tested for residual infectivity after treatment for the disease, but the limited availability of animals and the expense of using this model make it impractical for testing disinfecting agents.

The Center for Disease Control in Phoenix, Ariz, has developed an effective in vitro testing method that measures quantitatively, using a radioimmunoassay technique, the residual concentration of HBsAg after application of a disinfecting agent. The rationale for this approach is that any procedure or agent that can destroy the surface coat of the virus (the source of the HBsAg) will probably cause loss of viral viability. This is reasoned because some procedures known to inactivate the virus itself do not reduce the level of HBsAg. Therefore, it seems likely that any procedure effective enough to destroy the surface coat of the virus, which is more resistant to destruction than the intact virus, is also inactivating the virus. It is believed that by the time the antigen is destroyed, the virus has long since disappeared.

These methods or agents have been shown by the Center for Disease Control to be effective in significantly inactivating HBsAg: immersion in 100°C (boiling) water for ten minutes, or immersion in a 1% solution of sodium hypochlorite (10,000 ppm free chlorine) for ten minutes. In addition, it is likely that sporicidal disinfectants will destroy HBV. These include tincture of iodine, formaldehyde, alkaline glutaraldehyde, and ethylene oxide. At the present time, their effectiveness against HBV is speculative since actual tests of these agents and the determination of exposure times for significant inactivation of HBsAg have not been made.

The effectiveness of the chemical agents is assumed if the surfaces being disinfected are clean, if the solutions are freshly prepared in the proper use dilution, and if the recommended temperature and length of exposure are followed.

Question *What agents and methods of disinfection are known to be ineffective in preventing the spread of HBV?*

Answer Solutions of ethyl or isopropyl alcohol, 70% to 90%, and quaternary ammonium compounds are not considered to be effective in inactivating HBV.

RECOMMENDATIONS

The risk of acquisition of type B hapatitis and the carrier state should be examined very carefully for all dental care personnel as soon as possible, using questionnaire surveys and blood tests. Testing for type B hepatitis antigenemia should be done anonymously so that no person—other than the one being tested for HBsAg—should be given the opportunity to know if the serum is positive. The individual should be told before the testing that he should consult an appropriate physician if the test result is positive. In this way, anonymity can be maintained.

State and local dental societies should be encouraged to set up and help staff special clinics in medical schools or hospitals that are equipped for handling patients with infectious diseases. Dentists in the area should be informed that these special clinics are available and able to handle such patients.

A special effort should be made within the dental profession to encourage all personnel to follow time-proven methods of sterilization, disinfection, and good hygiene with every patient contact to reduce the incidence of infectious disease, particularly type B hepatitis. In addition, the use of gloves in a practice should be encouraged through dental school training for those procedures in which there is bleeding.

REFERENCES

[1] From: *Journal of the American Dental Association,* Jan. 1976, V. 92, pp. 153–159.

Participants in a workshop on viral hepatitis and dental practice, held June 5, 1975 in the ADA Headquarters Building, were James W. Mosley, MD, workshop chairman, (hepatology), University of Southern California, George G. Blozis, DDS, (oral diagnosis), Ohio State University; Alan J. Drinnan, MD, DDS, (oral medicine), State University of New York at Buffalo; Martin S. Favero, PhD, (epidemiology), Center for Disease Control; John Gillis, PhD, (microbiology), American Sterilizer Co.; Lionel Id, DDS, MS, (oral surgery), Cherry Hill, NJ; Jay H. Hoofnagle, D, (blood and blood products), National

Institutes of Health; Stuart N. Kline, DDS, (oral surgery), University of Miami; Charles P. Pattison, MD, (epidemiology), Center for Disease Control; David Rimland, MD, (epidemiology), Grady Memorial Hospital, Atlanta; Charles B. Sabiston, Jr., DDS, PhD, (microbiology), University of Iowa; Eugene R. Schiff, MD, (hepatology), University of Miami, Joseph L. Smith, MD, (epidemiology). Center for Disease Control; Wolf Szmuness, MD, (epidemiology), New York Blood Center, and David S. Topazian, DDS, MS, (oral surgery), member, ADA Council on Dental Therapeutics.

[2] Feldman, R. E., and Schiff, E. R. Hepatitis in dental professionals JAMA 232:1228 June 23, 1975.

[3] Mosley, J. W. and White, E. Viral hepatitis as an occupational hazard of dentists JADA 90:992 May 1975.

[4] Glazer, R. I.; Spatz, S. S.; and Catone, G. A. Viral hepatitis: a hazard to oral surgeons. J Oral Surg 31:504 July 1973

[5] Prince, A. M., and others. The serum hepatitis virus specific antigen (SH): a status report. In Pollard, M., ed. Perspectives in virology. From molecules to man. New York, Academic Press, 1971, vol 7, p 241.

[6] Villarejos, V. M., and others. Role of saliva, urine and feces in the transmission of type B hepatitis. N Engl J Med 291:1375 Dec 26, 1974.

[7] Mosley, J. W. Epidemiology of viral hepatitis: an overview. Am J Med Sci 270:253 Sept-Oct 1975.

[8] Maynard, J. E. Viral hepatitis. In Brenneman's practice of pediatrics. Scranton, Pa, Harper and Row, 1972, vol 11.

[9] Redeker, A. G. Viral hepatitis: clinical aspects. Am J Med Sci 270:9 July-Aug 1975.

[10] Mosley, J. W. The HBV carrier—a new kind of leper? Editorials N Engl J Med 292:477 Feb 27, 1975.

[11] Mosley, J. W., and others. Hepatitis B virus infection in dentists N Engl J Med 293:729 Oct 9, 1975.

[12] Hepatitis B said occupational hazard. News. J Can Dent Assoc 5:348, 1974.

[13] Berris, B., and others. Frequency of hepatitis in dentists in Ontario. Letters. Ann Int Med 81:699 Nov 1974.

[14] Lewis, T. L., and others. A comparison of the frequency of hepatitis-B antigen and antibody in hospital and nonhospital personnel. N Engl J Med 289:647 Sept 27, 1973.

[15] Chalmers, T. C., and Alter, H. J. Management of the asymptomatic carrier of the hepatitis-associated (Australia) antigen. Tentative considerations of the clinical and public-health aspects. N Engl J Med 285:613 Sept 9, 1971.

[16] Desmyter, J., and others. Hepatitis B immunoglobulin in prevention of HBs antigenemia in hemodialysis patients. Lancet 2:377 Aug 30, 1975.

[17] Szmuness, W., and other. On the role of sexual behavior in the spread of hepatitis B infection. Ann Intern Med 83:489 Oct 1975

[18] Levin, M. L., and others. Hepatitis B transmission by dentists. JAMA 228:1139 May 27, 1974.

[19] Rimland, D., and Parkin, W. E. An outbreak of hepatitis B traced to an oral surgeon. J Gastroenterology (Abst) 67:822 Oct 1974.

[20] Williams, S. V., Pattison, C. P.; and Berquist, K. R. Dental infection with hepatitis B. JAMA 232:1231 June 23, 1975.

[21] Alter, J. J., and others. Health-care workers positive for hepatitis B surface antigen: are their contacts at risk? N Engl J Med 292:454 Feb 27, 1975.

[22] Ward, R., and others. Hepatitis B antigen in saliva and mouth washings. Lancet 2:726 Oct 7, 1972.

[23] MacQuarrie, M. B.; Forghani, B.; and Wolochow, D. A. Hepatitis B transmitted by a human bite. JAMA 230:723 Nov 4, 1974.

[24] Miller, W. V.; Walsh, J. H.; and Paskin, S. Ethylene oxide sterilization to prevent post-transfusion hepatitis. N Engl J Med 280:386 Feb 13, 1969.

Prevention of Bacterial Endocarditis: A Committee Report of the American Heart Association*

Periodically, the American Heart Association through its councils and committees reviews its recommendations for the prevention of bacterial endocarditis. The ADA Council on Dental Therapeutics has representation on the Committee on Prevention of Rheumatic Fever and Bacterial Endocarditis of the American Heart Association and, thereby, the Council members are able to review the recommendations being proposed. The statement that follows, directed to physicians and dentists, has been prepared by that committee. It has been approved by the Council on Dental Therapeutics as it relates to dentistry. This 1977 revision is reproduced here with the permission of the American Heart Association. The section of the committee report on genitourinary tract and gastrointestinal tract surgery or instrumentation has been omitted. The complete report appears in Circulation 65:139A July 1977.

Bacterial endocarditis remains one of the most serious complications of cardiac disease. The morbidity and mortality remain significant despite advances in antimicrobial therapy and cardiovascular surgery. This infection occurs most often in patients with structural abnormalities of the heart or great

---

* From: *Journal of the American Dental Association*, Sept. 1977, V. 95, pp. 601–605. Members of the Committee on Prevention of Rheumatic Fever and Bacterial Endocarditis of the American Heart Association are Edward L. Kaplan, MD, chairman; Bascom F. Anthony, MD; Alan Bisno, MD; David Durack, MB, D Phil; Harold Houser, MD; H. Dean Millard, DDS; Jay Sanford, MD; Stanford T. Shulman, MD; Max Stillerman, MD; Angelo Taranta, MD; and Nanette Wenger, MD. The address of the American Heart Association is 7320 Greenville Ave, Dallas, 75231. Copyright by the American Dental Association. Reprinted by permission.

vessels. Effective measures for prevention of this infection by physicians and dentists are highly desirable.

Dental treatment, or surgical procedures or instrumentation involving the upper respiratory tract, genitourinary tract, or lower gastrointestinal tract, may be associated with transitory bacteremia. Bacteria in the bloodstream may lodge on damaged or abnormal valves such as are found in rheumatic or congenital heart disease or on endocardium near congenital anatomic defects, causing bacterial endocarditis or endarteritis. However, it is not possible to predict specific patients with structural heart disease in whom this infection will occur, nor the specific causal event.

Prophylaxis is recommended in those situations most likely to be associated with bacteremia since bacterial endocarditis cannot occur without a preceding bacteremia. Certain patients (e.g., those with prosthetic heart valves) appear to be at higher risk to develop endocarditis than are others (eg, those with mitral valve prolapse syndrome). Likewise, certain dental (e.g., extractions) and surgical (e.g., genitourinary tract surgery) procedures appear to be much more likely to initiate significant bacteremia than are others. These factors, although difficult to quantitate, have been considered in developing these recommendations.

Since there have been no controlled clinical trials, adequate data for comparing various methods for prevention of endocarditis in man are not available. However, an experimental animal model permitting consistent induction of bacterial endocarditis with microorganisms which often cause the infection in man has allowed experimental evaluation of both prophylaxis and treatment. Data from these studies, although derived from animal rather than clinical investigations, represent the only direct information on the efficacy of prophylaxis that is presently available. This information has influenced formulation of the current recommendations. The significant morbidity and mortality associated with infective endocarditis and the paucity of conclusive clinical studies emphasize the need for continuing research into the epidemiology, pathogenesis, prevention, and therapy of infective endocarditis.

When selecting antibiotics for bacterial endocarditis prophylaxis, one should consider both the variety of bacteria that is likely to enter the blood stream from any given site and those organisms most likely to cause this infection. Certain species of microorganisms cause the majority of cases of infective endocarditis, and their antimicrobial sensitivity patterns have been defined. The present recommendations are based on a review of available information about the organisms responsible for endocarditis including their in vivo and in vitro sensitivity to specific antibiotics and the pharmacokinetics of these drugs.

In general, parenteral administration of antibiotics provides more predictable blood levels and is preferred when practical, especially for patients thought to be at high risk. Optimal prophylaxis requires close cooperation between physicians, and between physicians and dentists.

DENTAL PROCEDURES AND UPPER RESPIRATORY TRACT SURGICAL PROCEDURES

Patients at risk to develop infective endocarditis should maintain the highest level of oral health to reduce potential sources of bacterial seeding. Even in the absence of dental procedures, poor dental hygiene or other dental disease such as periodontal or periapical infections may induce bacteremia. Patients without natural teeth are not free from the risk of bacterial endocarditis. Ulcers caused by ill-fitting dentures should be promptly cared for since they may be a source of bacteremia.

Antibiotic prophylaxis is recommended with *all* dental procedures (including routine professional cleaning) that are likely to cause gingival bleeding. Chemoprophylaxis for dental procedures in children should be managed in a similar manner to the way in which it is handled in adults. Although not a procedure, one exception to this is the spontaneous shedding of deciduous teeth; there are no data to suggest a significant risk of bacteremia accompanying this common event.

Devices which utilize water under pressure to clean between teeth and dental flossing may improve dental hygiene, but they also have been shown to cause bacteremia. However, bacterial endocarditis associated with the use of these devices has not been reported. Present data are insufficient to make firm recommendations with regard to their use in patients susceptible to endocarditis. How-

Table 1 Prophylaxis for Dental Procedures and Surgical Procedures of the Upper Respiratory Tract*

Procedures	Most congenital heart disease;† rheumatic or other acquired valvular heart disease; idiopathic hypertrophic subaortic stenosis; mitral valve‡ prolapse syndrome with mitral insufficiency.	Prosthetic heart valves§
All dental procedures that are likely to result in gingival bleeding.¶	Regimen A or B	Regimen B
Surgery or instrumentation of the respiratory tract.**	Regimen A or B	Regimen B

* Please see Table 2 for explanation of regimens.

† For example, ventricular septal defect, tetralogy of Fallot, aortic stenosis, pulmonic stenosis, complex cyanotic heart disease, patent ductus arteriosus or systemic to pulmonary artery shunts. Does *not* include uncomplicated secundum atrial septal defect.

‡ Although cases of infective endocarditis in patients with mitral valve prolapse syndrome have been documented, the incidence appears to be relatively low and the necessity for prophylaxis in all of these patients has not yet been established.

§ Some patients with a prosthetic heart valve in whom a high level of oral health is being maintained may be offered oral antibiotic prophylaxis for routine dental procedures except the following: parenteral antibiotics are recommended for patients with prosthetic valves who require extensive dental procedures, especially extractions, or oral or gingival surgical procedures.

¶ Does not include shedding of deciduous teeth or simple adjustment of orthodontic appliances.

** For example, tonsillectomy, adenoidectomy, bronchoscopy, and other surgical procedures of the upper respiratory tract involving disruption of the respiratory mucosa (see text).

ever caution is advised in their use by patients with cardiac defects, especially when oral hygiene is poor.

Several studies suggest that local gingival degerming immediately preceding a dental procedure provides some degree of protection against bacteremia. However, use of this technique is controversial, since gingival sulcus irrigation itself could theoretically induce bacteremia. If local degerming is employed, it should be used only as an adjunct to antibiotic prophylaxis.

Since alpha hemolytic streptococci (e.g., viridans streptococci) are the organisms most commonly implicated in bacterial endocarditis following dental procedures, antibiotic prophylaxis should be specifically directed toward them. Certain procedures on the upper respiratory tract (e.g., tonsillectomy or adenoidectomy, bronchoscopy—especially with a rigid bronchoscope—and surgical procedures involving respiratory mucosa) also may cause bacteremia. Since bacteria entering the blood stream after these procedures usually have similar antibiotic sensitivities to those recovered following dental procedures, the same regimens are recommended.

Table 1 contains suggested regimens for chemo-prophylaxis for dental procedures, or surgical procedures and instrumentation of the upper respiratory tract. The order of listing does not imply superiority of one regimen over another although parenteral administration is favored when practical (see Table 2). The committee also favors the combined use of penicillin and streptomycin or the use of vancomycin in the penicillin-allergic patient (regimen B) in those patients felt to be at high risk (e.g., prosthetic valves).

Table 2 For Dental Procedures and Surgery of the Upper Respiratory Tract

Regimen A—penicillin

1 Parenteral-oral combined:

  a *Adults:* Aqueous crystalline penicillin G (1,000,000 units intramuscularly) mixed with procaine penicillin G (600,000 units intramuscularly). Give 30 min to 1 h prior to procedure and then give penicillin V (formerly called phenoxymethyl penicillin) 500 mg orally every 6 h for 8 doses.†

  b *Children:** Aqueous crystalline penicillin G (30,000 units/kg intramuscularly) mixed with procaine penicillin G (600,000 units

Table 2   For Dental Procedures and Surgery of the Upper Respiratory Tract (*Continued*)

intramuscularly). Timing of doses for children is the same as for adults. For children less than 60 lb, the dose of penicillin V is 250 mg orally every 6 h for 8 doses.†

2 Oral:‡

  a *Adults:* Penicillin V (2.0 g orally 30 min to 1 h prior to the procedure and then 500 mg orally every 6 h for 8 doses.)†

  b *Children:** Penicillin V (2.0 g orally 30 min to 1 h prior to procedure and then 500 mg orally every 6 h for 8 doses.† For children less than 60 lb, use 1.0 g orally 30 min to 1 h prior to the procedure and then 250 mg orally every 6 h for 8 doses.)†

3 *For patients allergic to penicillin:* Use either vancomycin (see Regimen B) *or* use:

  a *Adults:* Erythromycin (1.0 g orally 1½–2 h prior to the procedure and then 500 mg orally every 6 h for 8 doses.)†

  b *Children:* Erythromycin, (20 mg/kg orally 1½–2 h prior to the procedure and then 10 mg/kg every 6 h for 8 doses.)†

Regimen B—penicillin plus streptomycin

1 *Adults:* Aqueous crystalline penicillin G (1,000,000 units intramuscularly) mixed with procaine penicillin G (600,000 units intramuscularly) plus streptomycin (1 g intramuscularly). Give 30 min to 1 h prior to the procedure; then penicillin V 500 mg orally every 6 h for 8 doses.†

2 *Children:** Aqueous crystalline penicillin G (30,000 units/kg intramuscularly) mixed with procaine penicillin G (600,000 units intramuscularly) plus streptomycin (20 mg/kg intramuscularly). Timing of doses for children is the same as for adults. For children less than 60 lb the recommended oral dose of penicillin V is 250 mg every 6 h for 8 doses.†

3 *For patients allergic to penicillin:*

  a *Adults:* Vancomycin (1 gm intravenously over 30 min to 1 h). Start initial vancomycin infusion ½ to 1 h prior to procedure; then erythromycin 500 mg orally every 6 h for 8 doses.†

  b *Children:** Vancomycin (20 mg/kg intravenously over 30 min to 1 h).** Timing of doses for children is the same as for adults. Erythromycin dose is 10 mg/kg every 6 h for 8 doses.†

Footnotes to Regimens:

  † In unusual circumstances or in the case of delayed healing, it may be prudent to provide additional doses of antibiotics even though available data suggest that bacteremia rarely persists longer than 15 min after the procedure. The physician or dentist may also choose to use the parenteral route of administration for all of the doses in selected situations.

CARDIAC SURGERY

Patients undergoing cardiac surgery utilizing extracorporeal circulation—especially those requiring placement of prosthetic heart valves or needing prosthetic intravascular or intracardiac materials—are at risk to develop infective endocarditis in the preoperative and postoperative periods. Because the morbidity and mortality of infective endocarditis in such patients are high, maximal preventive efforts are indicated, including the use of prophylactic antibiotics.

Early postoperative infective endocarditis following these surgical procedures is most often due to *Staphylococcus aureus* (coagulase positive) or *Staphylococcus epidermidis* (coagulase negative). Streptococci, gram negative bacteria, and fungi are less frequently responsible. No single antibiotic regimen is effective against all these organisms. Furthermore, the prolonged use of broad spectrum antibiotics may itself predispose to superinfection with unusual or highly resistant microorganisms. Therefore, antibiotic prophylaxis at the time of open heart surgery should be directed primarily against staphylococci and should be of short duration. The choice of antibiotic should be influenced by each individual hospital's antibiotic sensitivity data, but penicillinase resistant penicillins or cephalosporin antibiotics are most often selected. Antibiotic prophylaxis should be started shortly before the operative procedure and usually is continued for no more than three to five days postoperatively to reduce the likelihood of emergence of resistant microorganisms. The physician or surgeon should consider the effects of cardiopulmonary bypass on serum antibiotic levels and time the doses accordingly.

Careful preoperative dental evaluation is recommended so that any required dental treatment can be carried out several weeks prior to cardiac surgery

  * Doses for children should not exceed recommendations for adults for a single dose or for a 24-h period.

  ** For vancomycin the total dose for children should not exceed 44 mg/kg per 24 h.

  ‡ For those patients receiving continuous oral penicillin for secondary prevention of rheumatic fever, alpha hemolytic streptococci which are relatively resistant to penicillin are occasionally found in the oral cavity. While it is likely that the doses of penicillin recommended in regimen A are sufficient to control these organisms, the physician or dentist may choose one of the suggestions in Regimen B or may choose oral erythromycin.

whenever possible. Such measures may decrease the incidence of late postoperative endocarditis (occuring later than six to eight weeks following surgery) which is often due to the same organisms which are responsible for causing infective endocarditis in the unoperated patient.

STATUS FOLLOWING CARDIAC SURGERY

Following cardiovascular surgery, the same precautions should be observed that have been outlined for the unoperated patient undergoing dental, gastrointestinal, genitourinary, and other procedures. As far as is known, the risk of endocarditis probably continues indefinitely; it appears particularly significant in patients with prosthetic heart valves. Exceptions are patients with an uncomplicated secundum atrial septal defect repaired by direct suture without a prosthetic patch, and patients who have had ligation and division of a patent ductus arteriosus; these patients do not appear to be at increased risk of developing endocarditis. For these two defects, prophylaxis for prevention of infective endocarditis is not necessary following a healing period of six months after surgery. Although prophylactic antibiotics are often given intraoperatively, there is no evidence to suggest that patients who have undergone coronary artery operations are at risk to develop endocarditis in the months and years following surgery unless there is another cardiac defect present; prophylactic antibiotics to protect against endocarditis are not needed in these postoperative patients.

OTHER INDICATIONS FOR ANTIBIOTIC PROPHYLAXIS TO PREVENT ENDOCARDITIS

In susceptible patients chemoprophylaxis to prevent endocarditis is also indicated for surgical procedures on any infected or contaminated tissues, including incision and drainage of abscesses. Antibiotic prophylaxis for the indicated dental and surgical procedures should also be given to those patients who have had a documented previous episode of infective endocarditis, even in the absence of clinically detectable heart disease.

Indwelling vascular catheters, especially those which reside in one of the cardiac chambers, present a continual danger. Particular care should be given to maintaining the sterility of these catheters and to avoiding unnecessarily prolonged use.

Indwelling transvenous cardiac pacemakers appear to present a low risk of endocarditis; however dentists and physicians may choose to employ prophylactic antibiotics to cover dental and surgical procedures in these patients. The same recommendations apply to renal dialysis patients with implanted arteriovenous shunt appliances. Although no firm recommendation can be made on the basis of current information, antibiotic prophylaxis for prevention of endocarditis provoked by dental and surgical procedures also deserves consideration in patients with ventriculoatrial shunts placed to relieve hydrocephalus since there are documented cases of infective endocarditis in these patients.

Prophylactic antibiotics are not required in diagnostic cardiac catheterization and angiography since, with standard techniques, the occurrence of endocarditis following these procedures has proven to be extremely uncommon.

It is important to recognize that antibiotic doses used to prevent recurrences of acute rheumatic fever (''secondary'' rheumatic fever prophylaxis) are inadequate for the prevention of bacterial endocarditis (see reference). Special attention should be paid to these patients and appropriate antibiotics should be prescribed in addition to the antibiotic they are receiving for prevention of group A beta hemolytic streptococcal infections (the addition of an aminoglycoside to appropriate doses of penicillin, or the use of erythromycin or vancomycin).

WARNING

The committee recognizes that it is not possible to make recommendations for all possible clinical situations. Practitioners should exercise their clinical judgment in determining the duration and choice of antibiotic(s) when special circumstances apply. Furthermore, since endocarditis may occur despite antibiotic prophylaxis, physicians and dentists should maintain a high index of suspicion in the interpretation of any unusual clinical events following the above procedures. Early diagnosis is important to reduce complications, sequelae, and mortality.

Additional Book References

A number of excellent reference books are available and are listed below with a brief description.

I In-depth coverage of general and specific topics in pharmacology

  A *Drill's Pharmacology,* 4th ed., J. DiPalma (ed.), McGraw-Hill, New York, 1971.

  B L. S. Goodman and A. Gilman (eds.), *Pharmacological Basis of Therapeutics,* 5th ed., Macmillan, New York, 1975.

II Information on drugs according to generic and trade names

  A *Physician's Desk Reference,* 33d ed., Medical Economics Company, Oradell, N.J., 1979. One should note that the information presented is prepared by the manufacturer of the drug described and is the same as that found in the "package insert" of the drug.

  B *AMA Drug Evaluations,* 3d ed., American Medical Association, Department of Drugs, Publishing Sciences Group, Inc., Littleton, Mass., 1977. This book describes all scientific, recognized uses of drugs, irrespective of the statements in the manufacturer-prepared package insert.

III Specific information on pharmacology and therapeutics in dentistry: *Accepted Dental Therapeutics,* 38th ed., Council on Dental Therapeutics, American Dental Association, Chicago, 1979.

Part Seven

Glossary

Terms are included here which are not defined in all chapters but which may be of value in improving the reader's understanding of a topic.

Acidogenic That which is capable of producing acids; plaque is sometimes called acidogenic.

Anaphylaxis A severe, exaggerated response of an organism to a foreign substance; such a reaction often results in death.

Aromatic A medicinal substance with a spicy odor and sometimes stimulant properties.

Arrhythmia A variation from a normal rhythm; usually refers to abnormal heart activity.

Arthralgia Pain in a joint.

Bradycardia A slow heart rate.

Bulla A large blister or vesicle filled with serous fluid.

Capsule A soluble container in which a drug, in powdered form, is placed.

Cardiac infarct An area of necrosis in cardiac tissue due to obstruction of circulation to that area; the lay term for this is "heart attack."

Cariogenic That which promotes caries.

Covalent bonds A chemical bond of atoms formed by the sharing of an electron and found in most organic compounds.

Diplopia Double vision.

Dyscrasia (blood) An abnormal or pathological condition of blood.

Ectopic A location or occurrence away from that which is normal. For example, an ectopic pacemaker is one which produces a heart beat from a site other than that of the normal pacemaker.

Elixir   A sweetened liquid containing a chemical in solution and appropriate flavoring agents.

Endogenous   Developing or originating within the organism.

Enzyme   An organic compound, composed of protein, capable of accelerating or producing a change in a substrate for which it is usually specific.

Extravascular   Occurring outside a blood or lymphatic vessel.

Feces   Solid wastes from the body. Unabsorbed drugs can usually be detected in it.

Fibrillation   An irregular contraction of muscles.

Gestation   The period of development of a child from the time of fertilization of the ovum to birth.

Glossitis   Inflammation of the tongue.

Glycosemia   The presence of sugar in the blood.

Hemolysis   The separation of hemoglobin from a red blood cell and its appearance in the fluid containing the red blood cells.

Hemostasis   A stoppage in the flow of blood.

Henderson-Hasselback equation   An equation used to determine the pH of a mixture of an acid and a base in terms of the pK_a of the acid and the concentration of the acid and base.

Hirsutism   Abnormal hairiness.

Hydrogen bond   A chemical bond occurring when a hydrogen atom joins two other atoms.

Hyperglycemia   An increase in the amount of sugar in the blood.

Hyperplasia   An increase in size due to an increase in the number of cells making up a tissue or organ.

Hyperpnea   Abnormally rapid and deep breathing.

Hypoglycemia   A decrease in the amount of sugar in the blood.

Ionic bond   A bond formed by atoms of opposite charge; each atom contributes an electron to the bond formed. Common in inorganic compounds.

Lymphadenopathy   A disease of the lymph nodes in which they usually enlarge.

Lymphoma   A general term applied to a tumorlike growth of lymphatic tissue.

Metabolism   The sum of all the physical and chemical processes by which living, organized substance is produced and maintained.

Metastasis   The spread of disease from one organ or part to another not directly connected with it.

Myalgia   Pain in a muscle.

Neutropenia   A disorder in which the number of white blood cells in the body is decreased.

Nonmyelinated nerves   Nerves which are not surrounded by myelin, which is a fatlike substance forming a sheath around some nerve fibers.

Nystagmus   An involuntary, rapid movement of the eyeball.

Ointment   A semisolid preparation which usually contains a medication.

Osteolysis   A term referring to the dissolution of bone.

Osteoporosis   A decrease in bone density.

Osteosclerosis   An increase in bone density.

Pacemaker   That which influences the rate at which something occurs. In the heart, the sinoatrial node establishes heart rate and is the cardiac pacemaker.

Palliative   That which brings relief, usually of pain.

Paresthesia   A feeling of numbness.

Paroxysmal   Occurring at varying intervals.

Perfusion   The passage of a fluid through cells or vessels of a specific body part.

Photosensitivity   A response to light in which the patient cannot tolerate light, and harmful effects can result to the patient. Tetracyclines produce a photosensitivity to sunlight whereby the patient will burn when exposed.

pK_a   The dissociation of a substance in solution into its constituent parts so that 50 percent is in the ionized form and 50 percent is in the un-ionized form.

Puberty   The period between the initial appearance of secondary sex characterics and the completion of their development.

Purkinje fibers   Specialized cardiac fibers which carry nerve conduction from the atria to the ventricles.

Quaternary ammonium compound   A compound with surface-active properties which contains the chemical radical $(CR)_4N^+$.

Solution   A liquid preparation in which a chemical has been dissolved.

Stomatitis   Inflammation of the oral mucosa which may involve the buccal and labial mucosa, palate, tongue, floor of the mouth, and gingivae.

Suspension   A liquid preparation containing fine particles.

Synapse   The region of contact between processes of two adjacent nerves.

Syrup A concentrated solution of a sweetening agent, usually a sugar, which is combined with medicinal agents.

Systole The contraction or period of contraction of the heart.

Tachycardia A rapid heart rate.

Thromboembolus Obstruction of a blood vessel with a clot which has broken loose from its site of formation.

Thrombophlebitis An inflammation in the blood vessel wall, usually of the legs, with the concomitant development of a risk of the formation of blood clots.

Urticaria A skin rash which is often associated with severe itching.

van der Waals forces Weak intermolecular forces which hold molecules together.

Index

Page numbers in *italic* indicate tables and illustrations.